TILTED

*A Medical Memoir of Dysautonomia
and Other Horizontal Pursuits*

By: **Dr. Khalid Saeed, D.O.**

Legal Stuff (Because Lawyers Get Lightheaded Without This)

Medical Disclaimer
This book is intended for educational, informational, and sharply sarcastic purposes only. It is not medical advice. It is not a substitute for professional diagnosis, treatment, or care. And it will not refill your fludrocortisone or teach your cardiologist how baroreceptors work.

Although the author is a licensed physician who personally has dysautonomia, unless you've met him face-to-face, completed an exhausting amount of paperwork, and tried not to pass out while explaining your tilt table results, he is not your doctor.

Always consult your own licensed healthcare provider before making any changes to your medications, fluids, salt intake, exercise regimen, vagal nerve stimulation practices, or tendency to faint near household appliances. Especially if you are pregnant, nursing, taking medications, or are currently horizontal and wondering if it's normal to sweat through your socks.

Reading this book does not create a doctor–patient relationship. Educational sarcasm is not a clinical service. Autonomic dysfunction is real, and this book helps you laugh through the wreckage — but do not confuse insight with prescriptive advice.

Copyright Notice
© 2025 Khalid Saeed, D.O. / *TILTED: A Medical Memoir of Dysautonomia and Other Horizontal Pursuits*™ / ISBN 979-8-218-72456-6

All rights reserved. No part of this book may be copied, reprinted, scanned, screenshot, transcribed, memed, repurposed, translated, turned into a slideshow, or dramatized in a social media video without prior written permission from the author — except for brief excerpts used in reviews, research, commentary, or dark humor tweets that properly cite the source.

This work is protected under the Copyright Act of 1976 (Title 17, United States Code) and international copyright agreements. Unauthorized reproduction may result in legal action, bad karma triggering a dysautonomia flare, and a prescription for unflavored electrolyte powder.

Trademarks, Satire, and Nominative Fair Use

This book contains satire, parody, commentary, and criticism on topics including but not limited to: food marketing, wellness industry nonsense, ableist healthcare bias, diagnostic gaslighting, and public health slogans that pretend posture and hydration can cure everything.

All brand names, product references, diagnostic labels, public health jargon, wearable medical devices, and institutional names remain the property of their respective trademark holders. Use of these terms is strictly nominative, educational, or satirical, and does not imply endorsement, sponsorship, affiliation, or mutual respect.

References to "the cardio bros," "electrolyte capitalism," or "your nervous system's passive-aggressive tantrum" are metaphors, not diagnoses. If you feel personally attacked by a metaphor, consider whether your product or professional conduct deserves a closer look.

Use of trademarks and brand names in this book is protected under nominative fair use, as recognized by *New Kids on the Block v. News America Publishing, Inc.*, 971 F.2d 302 (9th Cir. 1992), and under the Lanham Act, 15 U.S.C. § 1115(b)(4). The content of this book also qualifies as fair use under 17 U.S.C. § 107, as reinforced by the U.S. Supreme Court in *Campbell v. Acuff-Rose Music*, 510 U.S. 569 (1994).

In plain English: it's legal to mention brands or terms for the purpose of critique, education, and commentary — especially when no other clear way exists to talk about them without confusing the reader. Which, given the autonomic chaos we're covering, is already challenging enough.

Liability Disclaimer

The author and publisher disclaim all liability, loss, injury, or damage — real, imagined, or existential — that may arise from reading this book, attempting to self-diagnose, confronting your doctor with a symptom log color-coded by salt cravings, or attempting to microwave soup while pre-syncopal.

You are responsible for your own health decisions. Use caution, use science, and if you're using this book as a substitute for a treatment plan, please lie down immediately and rethink your life choices. Snark ≠ scope of practice.

ACKNOWLEDGMENTS

First, to the patients living in the Tilt Zone™ — the ones who fainted in bathrooms, got dismissed in exam rooms, and still showed up with symptom logs, compression gear, and sheer defiance: This book is for you. You made dysautonomia visible when medicine tried to ignore it. You turned salt into strategy and survival into science. You are not "just tired." You are walking, sitting, and reclining proof of human resilience.

To the clinicians who believed us before the tilt table did — thank you for listening, learning, and not blaming anxiety when our baroreceptors rage-quit. You made this a safer world for all of us with dysautonomia, and frankly, you deserve salted caramel medals and better reimbursement codes.

To my friends and family who tolerated years of half-finished sentences, heat-induced flares, and sudden horizontal lifestyle shifts — thank you for adapting, adjusting, and only occasionally asking, "Are you sure it's not stress?"

To my colleagues and fellow chronic illness rebels — thank you for your late-night messages, snarky memes, research rabbit holes, symptom charts, and dark humor. If community is a form of medicine, you are high-dose IV therapy.

To the grammar overlords — thank you for helping turn a pile of autonomic chaos, diagnostic rage, and neuro-cardiovascular despair into a book that's actually readable — and sometimes funny on purpose.

To my nervous system — I don't forgive you, but I accept that we are in this together.

And finally, to every reader who's been gaslit by a normal lab result or told to "drink more water" after collapsing in a grocery store — thank you for picking up this book. Thank you for choosing laughter alongside science, strategy alongside struggle, and rebellion over resignation.

You're not alone. You're adaptive. You're Tilted™. And you're proof that resistance is not only possible — it's personal.

DEDICATION

For everyone who's ever passed out in public and was told it was probably just anxiety.

For the ones who live in the in-between — upright, but only barely.

For the salt-shakers, the spreadsheet trackers, the quiet warriors managing an autonomic rebellion with compression gear and relentless determination.

This is for you.

Not because you need fixing.

But because you deserve to be seen.

Stay salty. Stay standing (or sitting, or lying down — whatever works).

You are the revolution in motion.

TABLE OF CONTENTS

Acknowledgments i
Dedication iii

Introduction: You're the Rebel Pulse Beating Beneath the Status Quo. 7

Part I: Acute Tilt Syndrome 11
Chapter 1: Tilt Happens... 13
Chapter 2: Symptoms, Science, and Shenanigans....................... 23
Chapter 3: Diagnostics, Data, and "It's Just Anxiety"................. 31

Part II: Chronic Tilt Management 45
Chapter 4: Management, Meds, and Maneuvering Your Way
    Through This Circus.. 47
Chapter 5: Triggers, Flares, and the Plot Twists That Take You
    Down Without Warning 59
Chapter 6: Daily Tilt Survival Guide 67

Part III: Functional Tilt Living... 73
Chapter 7: Feeding Yourself Without Passing Out 75
Chapter 8: Exercising While Tilted 81
Chapter 9: Managing Your Environment................................... 91
Chapter 10: Parenting While Chronically Exhausted 99
Chapter 11: Traveling While Tilted... 107
Chapter 12: Romance, Dating, and Other Forms of Cardiovascular
    Exercise 115
Chapter 13: Relationships, Boundaries, and the People Who Love
    You (Even When You're Horizontal) 121

Part IV: Systemic Tilt Disruption **131**
Chapter 14: Chronic Illness in the Age of Algorithms 133
Chapter 15: Insurance, Paperwork, and Bureaucratic Gaslighting........141
Chapter 16: How to Talk to Doctors Without Losing Your Mind........149
Chapter 17: Living with Chronic Uncertainty..157
Chapter 18: What I Wish I Knew Sooner..165

Final Tilted Thoughts — Looking Back, Tilting Forward **171**
About the Author **175**
References **177**
Suggested Reading & Tools **181**
Glossary of Terms **187**
Credits **195**

INTRODUCTION:
YOU'RE THE REBEL PULSE BEATING BENEATH THE STATUS QUO.

If you're reading this, chances are your nervous system is doing something weird. Not cute-weird. Not quirky-weird. I'm talking full-blown, physiology-defying, how-do-I-explain-this-to-my-boss weird. Maybe you've passed out in the shower. Maybe you've had a heart rate of 150 while sitting still. Maybe you've been told, in no uncertain terms, that it's "just anxiety" while watching your vision tunnel and your limbs turn into sweat-soaked spaghetti.

Welcome. You've found your people.

This book isn't a gentle exploration of symptoms through rose-colored compression stockings. It's a field guide for the medically gaslit, a tactical playbook for the functionally horizontal, and a survival manual for anyone whose baroreceptors rage-quit sometime around their third specialist visit. If you're tired of being "interesting" to doctors but invisible to protocols, this one's for you.

Who Am I to Write This?

I'm a physician. And I'm a patient. I have dysautonomia, which means I've diagnosed the chaos and been flattened by it. I've worn the white coat, and I've also worn the compression gear under it. I've read the studies and lived the flares. I've held the stethoscope, managed the meds, and still carry electrolyte packets and sarcasm everywhere I go.

This dual identity gives me a particular vantage point. I understand the science — and I understand the challenges that comes from having to explain your own condition to the person allegedly treating it.

Nothing I found did justice to the absurdity, the complexity, and the daily negotiations required to live with dysautonomia. I needed something that could hold both the science and the sarcasm. The facts and the fury. The treatment plans and the tantrums. And I needed to say all of it in a voice that didn't condescend, minimize, or try to "fix" the reader. So I wrote it myself.

What You'll Find in These Pages

This is not a linear story, because dysautonomia doesn't behave in straight lines. It's a rollercoaster, a plot twist, a non-Euclidean maze with symptoms that rotate like playlists on shuffle. So this book mirrors that structure: part science, part satire, part strategy manual.

You'll find:

- Clear, referenced explanations of how the autonomic nervous system breaks down — and what that looks like in real life.
- Diagnostic guides that cut through the gaslighting fog and help you collect data like a clinical investigator maverick.
- Management plans built on salt, spreadsheets, compression garments, and defiant hope.
- Chapters that break down everything from feeding yourself, to traveling, to managing relationships while Tilted.
- Sharp commentary on the systemic failures of medicine, insurance, social media, and self-care culture.
- Survival hacks, symptom lists, nerdy sidebars, and enough sarcasm to qualify as emotional ballast.

You'll also find validation. A lot of it. Because if you've been living with this condition without a clear diagnosis, treatment, or support, you're not weak. You're elite-level adaptive. This book won't ask you to "stay positive." It will ask you to stay resourced, informed, and unapologetically Tilted.

What This Book Won't Do

It won't cure you. That's not the goal. It won't promise easy answers, miracle protocols, or five-step plans to perfect health — because chronic illness doesn't care about your vision board.

What it *will* do is help you understand what's happening, figure out what to track, advocate for what you need, and laugh just enough to stay dangerous.

This isn't about passive acceptance. This is about strategic defiance. It's about learning to navigate a system that often fails to see you — and refusing to disappear anyway.

Who This Book Is For

- People with POTS, OH, NCS, or other forms of dysautonomia who are tired of explaining that "no, really, it's not anxiety."
- Undiagnosed patients whose bodies are misfiring and whose labs are "normal."
- Caregivers, spouses, and friends trying to understand why the person they love lives in compression gear and carries salt packets like holy relics.
- Clinicians who want to stop dismissing patients and start listening like lives depend on it. (Spoiler: they do.)

- Rebels, misfits, and medically mysterious types who have figured out how to function in a world that wasn't built for them — and who want a book that meets them at their level.

Final Word Before the First Chapter

You didn't ask for this condition. But you get to decide how you navigate it. This book won't make the dysautonomia disappear, but it might help you feel less alone, less confused, and way more equipped to call out bad advice and half-baked protocols.

So grab your compression socks, your hydration bottle, and your emotional support sarcasm.

Let's get Tilted™.

PART I:
ACUTE TILT SYNDROME

Initial Collapse, Unwanted Opinions, and Too Many Normal Labs

CHAPTER 1:
TILT HAPPENS

When Your Autonomic Nervous System Declares Mutiny

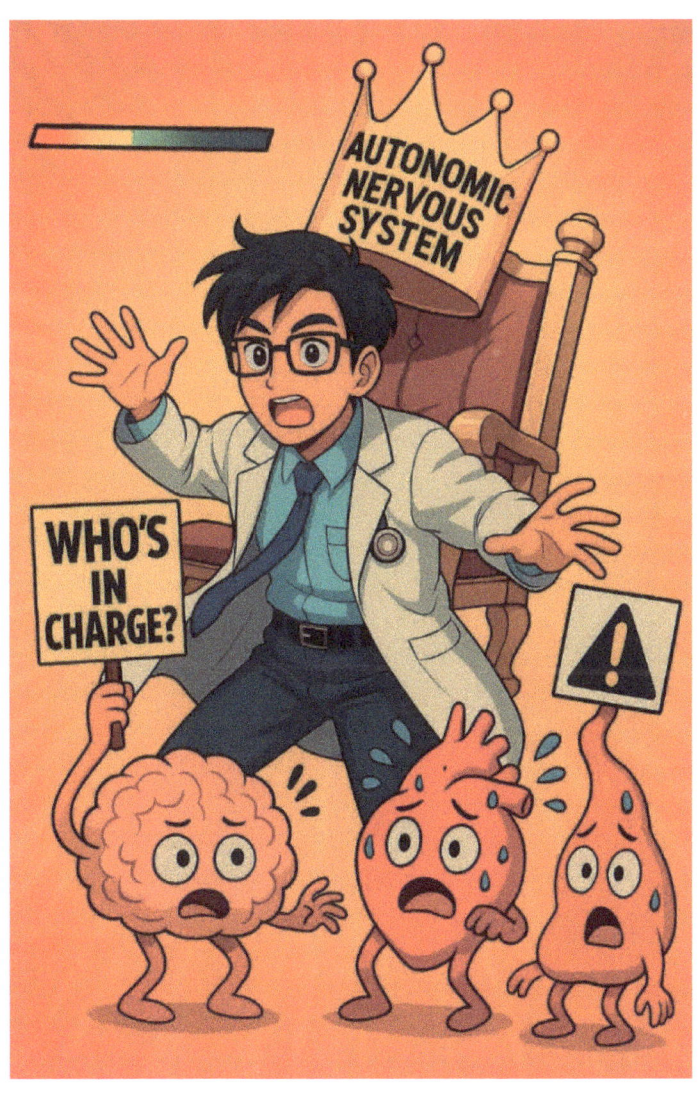

A Nervous System Walks Into a Bar (And Promptly Faints)

An Unexpected Plot Twist, Sponsored by Physics and Biology.

So, you've stumbled in here wondering why your body feels like it's buffering in real life. Maybe you've fainted in the shower. Maybe your heart rate does parkour when you brush your teeth. Maybe some earnest healthcare provider looked deep into your soul, nodded sagely, and whispered: "It's probably anxiety."

Let's get one thing straight — you are not imagining it. Your body is throwing a full-scale autonomic rebellion, and the only thing you're guilty of is trying to function in a system designed for bodies that don't issue cardiovascular alerts every time they assume standing won't trigger a system reboot.

Welcome to dysautonomia, where homeostasis is a myth and gravity is your final boss.

This Isn't "Just Anxiety" — It's Systemic Betrayal with a Pulse

If you've ever been told to "just breathe" while your heart rate hit 160 from standing still, you're in the right place.

You're not exaggerating. You're not slacking. And no, you're not "just tired." You are reverse-engineering a malfunctioning command center with nothing but salt and sarcasm.

The part of your body that's supposed to regulate blood pressure, heart rate, digestion, temperature, and everything else you never asked to think about... has quit mid-sentence.

Meet your autonomic nervous system (ANS): the backstage crew of your internal Broadway production. Its job is to run the show quietly so the stars — your organs — can shine without stage direction. But in dysautonomia? That crew locked itself in the bathroom and lit the script on fire.

The Dysfunctional Cast of Characters: Your ANS in Crisis

Division	Job Description	Personality Quirk
Sympathetic (SNS)	Fight or flight	A chaos goblin on six espresso shots
Parasympathetic (PNS)	Rest and digest	A burnout intern microdosing melatonin

These two systems normally perform a beautifully choreographed physiological waltz — smooth, synchronized, and impressively unconscious. The sympathetic and parasympathetic branches take turns like a well-rehearsed duo: one revs you up, the other calms you down.

- The **sympathetic nervous system (SNS)** is your gas pedal. It's responsible for the "fight, flight, or faint" response. It raises heart rate, constricts blood vessels, opens airways, and dumps adrenaline like your life depends on it — because sometimes, it does. It's the reason you can run from a bear or stand up quickly without passing out. (Usually.)
- The **parasympathetic nervous system (PNS)** is your brake. It promotes "rest and digest" mode — slowing the heart rate, aiding digestion, and sending the body into repair mode. It's what

helps you chill, recover, and not live in a constant state of hormonal arson.

When these two branches work in harmony, your body adjusts fluidly to daily stressors: standing up, digesting food, surviving group texts. But when dysautonomia shows up, the ballroom turns into a slam-dancing mosh pit and your organs start improvising choreography like a drunk bar band that lost the sheet music.

Science Snapshot

The autonomic nervous system is a complex, integrated web of central, peripheral, and neuroendocrine components that controls involuntary functions like cardiovascular regulation, thermoregulation, GI motility, and respiratory rhythm. Dysautonomia represents the failure of this system to maintain homeostasis under physiologic or environmental stress.

— *Freeman et al., 2011; Goldstein, 2013*

Translation: Your body's autopilot spilled coffee on the controls and is now flying blind while using a banana as a joystick and vibes for navigation.

This Isn't a Diagnosis — It's a Dysfunctional Cinematic Universe

Dysautonomia isn't a disease. It's a genre. Think of it as an entire ecosystem of nervous system errors, multiple overlapping spin-offs and plot twists — with fewer capes and more electrolyte powders.

Subtype	Core Failure	Symptoms Include
POTS (Postural Orthostatic Tachycardia Syndrome)	HR spikes ≥30 bpm on standing	Dizziness, fatigue, palpitations, brain fog
OH (Orthostatic Hypotension)	BP drops ≥20/10 mmHg within 3 minutes	Lightheadedness, fainting, blurry vision
NCS (Neurocardiogenic Syncope)	Reflex crash of BP + HR	Fainting with stress or heat
PPS (Paradoxical Parasympathetic Syndrome)	Vagus nerve panic attacks	Post-meal collapses, bradycardia, nausea
PAF (Pure Autonomic Failure)	Nerve degeneration	Severe instability, urinary dysfunction
Secondary Dysautonomia	Linked to other illness (e.g., Ehlers-Danlos, lupus)	Symptom chaos in stereo

Autonomic Breakdown: What is Actually Falling Apart?

This isn't one system breaking down. It's a total-body group project where nobody did the required reading and your circulatory system is using crayons on the budget spreadsheet.

- **Baroreceptor Failure:** Your pressure sensors used to know how to stabilize BP. Now they're either asleep (OH), hyper-dramatic (POTS), or just bored and destructive (NCS).

- **Sympathetic Overflow:** Your fight-or-flight system now thinks brushing your hair requires full tactical alert.
- **Parasympathetic Malfunction:** The vagus nerve swings between underachiever and control freak. Either way, you're nauseated and horizontal.
- **Small Fiber Neuropathy:** Your tiny nerves freelanced into chaos — random sweating, cold extremities, heat intolerance, and sudden episodes of "why does my skin feel like microwaved TV static?"
- **RAAS Dysfunction (Renin-Angiotensin-Aldosterone System):** This hormone system manages salt, fluid, and BP. Yours? On a gap year in Ibiza.
- **Brainstem Confusion:** The CPU of your bodily operations is interpreting "stand up" as DEFCON-1.

Science Snapshot

Up to 70% of POTS patients show hypovolemia, impaired norepinephrine clearance, low aldosterone, and autonomic neuropathy.

— Raj et al., 2005; Thieben et al., 2007

Translation: You're under-filled, over-alert, and led by nerves in full panic delegation mode.

The Great Multi-System Dumpster Fire

System	What's Going Wrong
Cardiovascular	HR spikes, BP drops, syncope
Neurologic	Brain fog, migraines, dizziness
Gastrointestinal	Bloating, nausea, constipation, food sit-ins
Thermoregulatory	Sweating roulette, heat/cold intolerance
Respiratory	Air hunger, shallow breathing, tight chest
Urogenital	Problems peeing, sexual dysfunction, menstrual cycle chaos
Musculoskeletal	Fatigue, weakness, post-exertional flares

Science Snapshot

Autonomic disorders often mimic psychiatric disease due to their multi-system nature and inconsistent presentation.

— Benarroch, 2008; Stewart et al., 2012

Translation: You're not overreacting — your body is just throwing full-cast tantrums over minor plot points like "standing up" or "digesting lunch."

Why You? (Besides the Universe Being Fickle)

Trigger	Mechanism of Mayhem
Viral Infections	Post-viral glitch (e.g., COVID, EBV)
Autoimmune Illnesses	Friendly fire on your own nerve fibers
Genetic Conditions	Ehlers-Danlos, defiant nerves
Trauma or Surgery	Vagus nerve insult, brainstem damage
Idiopathic	Latin for: "We have no idea"

Tilt Tip: Signs You're in the Tilt Zone

- You faint in the shower, but your doctor says you're "fine."
- Salt makes you feel invincible.
- You consider brushing your teeth cardio.
- You've been misdiagnosed with anxiety more times than you've flossed this year.

Horizontal Summary –- Tilt Breakdown at a Glance

Concept	Reality Check
Dysautonomia = Autonomic Failure	Your autopilot crashed and burned
Multi-system Mayhem	It's not "just stress"
Subtype Differences Matter	Not all fainting is created equal
RAAS + Small Fiber Damage	The unsung villains of your daily disaster reel
Normal Labs ≠ Normal Life	"We didn't find anything" ≠ "There's nothing wrong"

Final Thought

This isn't in your head. It's in your baroreceptors, your blood volume, your vagus nerve, and your neurotransmitters playing tug-of-war in the hypothalamus.

You're not malfunctioning. You're operating under a radically altered user manual. You're a circulatory strategist executing high-stakes survival inside a nervous system that forgot the script.

And no, you're not just a patient. You're a full-blown neurovascular revolutionary — armed with salt, science, and the audacity to rise while tilted.

CHAPTER 2:
SYMPTOMS, SCIENCE, AND SHENANIGANS

A Guided Tour Through the Daily Chaos

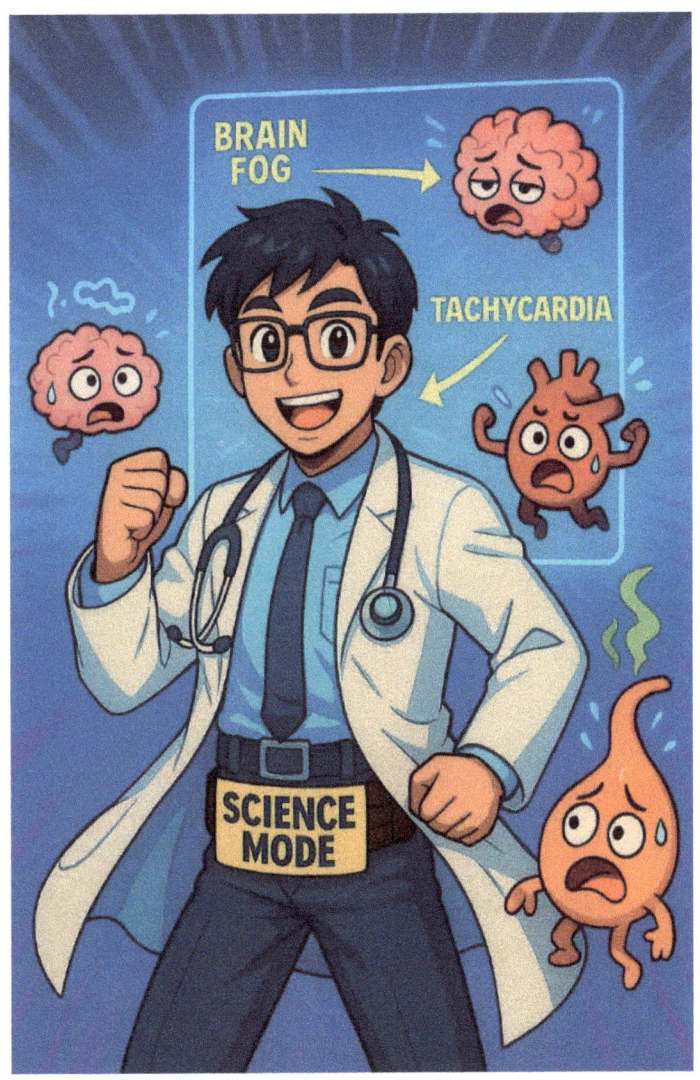

The Dysfunctional Variety Hour — Now Featuring Gastrointestinal Betrayal and Existential Sweats

Your nervous system checked out, and your body is throwing symptoms like it's trying to win a raffle. Dizziness, nausea, fatigue, sweats — it's a multi-system variety show with no intermission. Let's start decoding the signal in all that static.

Now that we've established your autonomic nervous system is the least reliable teammate since the group project days of high school, it's time to dive into its greatest hits. And by "hits," we mean symptoms. Dozens of them. Often in sequence. Occasionally in harmony. Sometimes all at once.

If your medical history reads like a malfunctioning slot machine — tachycardia, dizziness, nausea, bloating, chest tightness, brain fog, back to tachycardia — you're not inconsistent. You're starring in a one-person bodily improv show that never rehearses and loses the script mid-performance.

Let's break this circus down system-by-system before your brain fog files for early retirement.

1. Cardiovascular Chaos: When Gravity Is a Personal Insult

Symptoms:
- Heart rate spikes when standing (tachycardia)
- Palpitations during laundry
- Dizziness, tunnel vision, "I need to sit down right now"
- Chest pressure, especially when doing nothing heroic

- Blood pressure swings that make roller coasters look stable

What's Happening: Your internal pressure sensors — baroreceptors — are misfiring. In a healthy body, standing up triggers a smooth cardiovascular adjustment. In dysautonomia, your heart rate leaps 30+ beats per minute as if you're fleeing a predator — while folding socks.

Science Snapshot

POTS is defined by a heart rate increase of ≥30 bpm in adults or ≥40 bpm in adolescents within 10 minutes of standing, in the absence of orthostatic hypotension.

— *Raj et al., 2013*

Translation: You're not nervous — you're biologically over-stimulated by posture.

2. Neurologic Dysfunction: Your Brain Is Buffering

Symptoms:
- Brain fog (also known as "where did I put my vocabulary")
- Dizziness, lightheadedness, vertigo
- Sensory overload (light, sound, crowds)
- Twitching, tremors, zaps
- Orthostatic migraines

What's Happening: Reduced blood flow to your brain = neurons running on low battery mode. This turns your mind into a lagging browser with 32 tabs open and one rogue window playing music that you can't seem to find.

Science Snapshot

Cerebral blood flow reductions in POTS patients are linked with impaired attention, memory, and executive function.

— Stewart et al., 2012

Translation: You're not flaky — your brain is operating on a dimmer switch.

3. Gastrointestinal Treason: When Your Stomach Stages a Sit-In

Symptoms:

- Nausea (from merely thinking about food)
- Bloating (after three bites)
- Constipation, diarrhea, or both — nature's sadistic roulette wheel
- Cramping and digestive mutiny
- Food just... sits there

What's Happening: The vagus nerve, which oversees digestion, is either underperforming or catastrophizing. Add in small fiber neuropathy and you get a gastrointestinal tract that thinks sequencing is optional and timing is a personal decision.

Science Snapshot

Over 70% of patients with autonomic dysfunction report symptoms of GI dysmotility, including delayed gastric emptying.

— Camilleri et al., 2011

Translation: Your stomach isn't broken. It's just on strike.

4. Thermoregulatory Mayhem: A Malfunctioning Human Thermostat

Symptoms:

- Sweating inappropriately — or not at all
- One cold foot, one sweaty armpit: the asymmetry special. Neat.

- Flushing, chills, skin changing colors like mood lighting

What's Happening: Small fiber neuropathy disrupts your thermoregulatory system. Your sweat glands and blood vessels are getting mixed signals — and reacting with the enthusiasm of toddlers at a sleepover.

Science Snapshot
Abnormal sweating patterns due to small fiber neuropathy and central dysfunction are common in dysautonomia.

— Low et al., 2003

Translation: Your internal thermostat has joined the rebellion.

5. Respiratory Confusion: Your Lungs Are Fine — Your Brain Isn't Convinced

Symptoms:
- Air hunger ("I can't get a full breath")
- Shallow breathing
- Excessive yawning or sighing
- Sensation of suffocating, despite normal oxygen levels

What's Happening: Chemoreceptors and brainstem signaling misfire, triggering false alarms. Your lungs work fine — but your brain insists you're drowning on dry land.

Science Snapshot
Respiratory symptoms in dysautonomia stem from altered autonomic control and chemoreflex sensitivity, not pulmonary pathology.

— Garland et al., 2015

Translation: Your oxygen levels are normal. Your nervous system just wants attention.

6. Urogenital Shenanigans: The Systems Nobody Talks About (But We Will)

Symptoms:
- Urinary urgency, frequency, or hesitancy
- Incontinence or retention
- Sexual dysfunction
- Menstrual irregularities

What's Happening: Autonomic nerves regulate bladder and reproductive functions. When they go rogue, you get contradictory messages — like needing to pee constantly but not being able to, or menstrual cycles that treat calendars as a loose suggestion.

7. Musculoskeletal & Energy Deficits: Fatigue That Redefines the Word

Symptoms:
- Crushing, non-restorative fatigue
- Muscle weakness and heaviness
- Exercise intolerance
- Post-exertional malaise (aka post-activity crash)

What's Happening: Low blood volume, poor perfusion, and mitochondrial dysfunction form an unholy alliance. Even basic movement becomes high-stakes negotiation with your cellular energy reserves.

Science Snapshot

Dysautonomia is associated with low stroke volume, poor muscle perfusion, and prolonged post-exertional recovery.

— *Shibata et al., 2012*

Translation: You're not lazy. You're rationing energy like it's currency in a blackout.

Tilt Break: Symptom Rotation Is a Feature, Not a Bug

If your day starts with palpitations, peaks with bloating, detours into brain fog, and ends with shivering in a cold sweat — you're not inconsistent. You're living in the Tilt Zone, where symptom roulette is the house game and the odds are always weird.

In the Tilt Zone, the laws of physiology take a personal day and your nervous system spins the symptom wheel every morning like it's auditioning for a game show you never signed up for. Will it be dizziness? GI rebellion? That weird buzzing in your limbs again? All of the above? Who knows! Even your body doesn't check the schedule.

Here's the secret — rotating symptoms aren't a sign of failure — they're proof that your autonomic nervous system is still wildly creative. It's not a glitch. It's a high-maintenance feature with zero documentation and patchy tech support.

Consistency is for home thermostats and basic cable. You, my friend, are running an autonomic improv show where no two performances are ever the same — and that's just how it works here.

Horizontal Summary –- Tilted System Status Report

System	Dysfunction Highlights
Cardiovascular	Tachycardia, hypotension, fainting
Neurologic	Brain fog, dizziness, cognitive lapses
Gastrointestinal	Delayed emptying, nausea, bloating, constipation
Thermoregulatory	Heat/cold intolerance, unpredictable sweating
Respiratory	Air hunger, sighing, shallow breathing
Urogenital	Incontinence, urgency, dysfunction, irregularity
Musculoskeletal	Fatigue, crashes, weakness

Final Thought

Dysautonomia doesn't show up with one tidy symptom. It floods every system with chaotic signals and wildly inconsistent behavior. And still — somehow — you brush your teeth, send emails, answer texts, and maybe even make dinner.

That's not just coping. That's elite-level adaptation. You're doing multi-system crisis management in real-time — and you're doing it while vertical, conscious, and possibly salt-covered. That's Tilt brilliance in motion.

CHAPTER 3:
DIAGNOSTICS, DATA, AND "IT'S JUST ANXIETY"

How to Survive the Gaslighting Gauntlet With Your Sanity

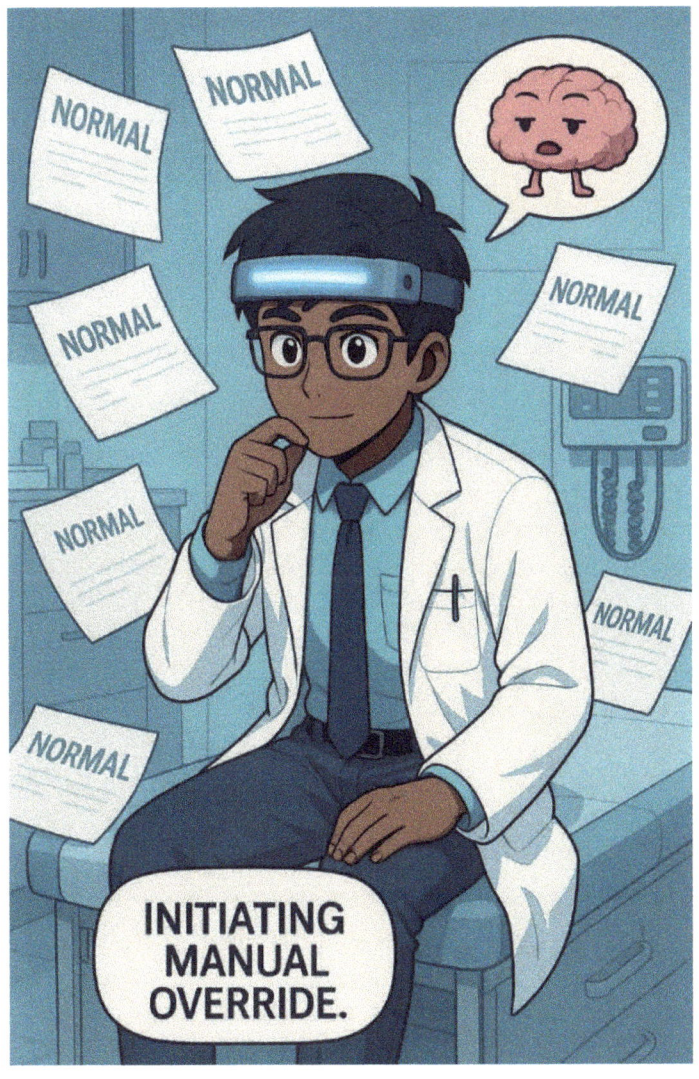

You walked in with a multi-system meltdown and walked out with a suggestion to "relax more." Apparently, when tests are normal, reality becomes optional. Time to explore what actually gets tested — and what gets missed entirely.

You've passed out in the shower. Your heart races while brushing your hair. You ate half a sandwich and your body staged a coup. And after enduring a parade of specialists, labs, and expressions of vague concern, you've been handed a diagnosis of… dehydration. Or hormones. Or — you guessed it — "just anxiety."

Let's clarify something — anxiety does not explain why your heart rate spikes to 150 every time you load the dishwasher. It doesn't explain the crash after lunch, the sweat-storm in air conditioning, or the fact that standing still now feels like an Olympic sport.

It's time to ditch vague reassurances and get diagnostic. Not with vibes — with verifiable, trackable, reproducible data. Because when your nervous system is conducting its own rogue symphony, you don't need a pep talk. You need a playbook.

Why Getting Diagnosed Can Feel Like a Side Quest With No Map

Roadblock	Reality Check
"You don't look sick"	Ableism in a lab coat
Symptoms fluctuate	"You looked fine last time" doesn't mean anything

Roadblock	Reality Check
No autonomic testing	Normal labs ≠ functional nervous system
Medical curriculum fails	Most physicians get <30 minutes on dysautonomia in training
Anxiety gets blamed	HR spikes cause anxiety — not the other way around
You look "well"	Your appearance is not a diagnostic tool

Step 1: Know the Real Diagnostic Criteria

This is where you stop explaining how you feel and start explaining how you qualify. Peer-reviewed criteria are your shield.

A. Postural Orthostatic Tachycardia Syndrome (POTS)

Your nervous system doesn't adjust correctly when you go from lying down to standing. Instead of smoothly keeping your blood moving, your heart rate jumps dramatically. That fast heartbeat is your body's attempt to keep blood flowing to your brain — but it doesn't always work.

Metric	Threshold
HR Increase	≥30 bpm (≥40 in adolescents) within 10 mins of standing
Blood Pressure	No significant drop
Duration	Symptoms present ≥6 months
Exclusions	Rule out anemia, thyroid issues, dehydration

B. Orthostatic Hypotension (OH)

Your blood pressure drops too much when you stand up. Unlike POTS — where the heart speeds up — OH is about your blood pressure not rising fast enough to keep blood flowing to your brain. It's often worse in the morning, after meals, or during hot weather, and it can make getting through daily life feel like walking uphill through molasses.

Metric	Threshold
Systolic Drop	≥20 mmHg within 3 minutes standing
Diastolic Drop	≥10 mmHg within 3 minutes standing

C. Neurocardiogenic Syncope (NCS)

Also known as vasovagal syncope. Drop in heart rate and blood pressure triggered by heat, stress, fear, pain, dehydration, or prolonged standing. Diagnosis often involves a tilt table test or ambulatory heart rhythm monitors (like Holter or event monitors) to capture changes in heart rate and blood pressure during a symptomatic episode.

Key signs:

- Nausea or abdominal discomfort before fainting
- Sweating (often cold or clammy)
- Visual changes — tunnel vision or spots before the eyes
- Brief loss of consciousness (typically less than a minute)

D. Paradoxical Parasympathetic Syndrome (PPS)

Not officially listed in most textbooks — but unmistakably familiar to people living in Tilt Town. PPS describes a backwards over-activation of the parasympathetic nervous system, which shows up not to calm things down, but to aggressively misfire at exactly the wrong time.

Key signs:
- Sudden bradycardia
- Post-meal collapses
- Heat-induced blackouts
- A vagus nerve that treats upright posture like a personal threat

Step 2: Get the Right Tests (Not Just — "Do a Medical Party Trick While We Judge You")

A quick heart listen does not count. Real evaluation involves tools, numbers, and strategy. You deserve more than a stethoscope shrug and an "everything looks normal." Here's what real autonomic testing actually involves — and why it matters.

1. Active Stand Test

- **What it does:** Measures heart rate (HR) and blood pressure (BP) after moving from lying to standing.
- **How it works:** Lie down for 10 minutes. Then stand. Take vitals at 1, 3, 5, and 10 minutes.
- **What it shows:** A ≥30 bpm HR increase (≥40 bpm in teens) within 10 minutes = POTS. A ≥20/10 mmHg BP drop = orthostatic hypotension.
- **Where to do it:** At home with a BP cuff, a stopwatch, and a chaperone (you know, just in case you pass out). Bonus if you color-code the flares.
- **Why it matters:** It's free, effective, and doesn't require being restrained on a table like a medieval torture subject.

2. Tilt Table Test (TTT)

- **What it does:** Recreates orthostatic stress in a controlled setting while tracking vitals.
- **How it works:** You're strapped to a table, tilted to 60–70 degrees upright, and monitored for 10–45 minutes. Sometimes they give you medication to trigger the symptoms. Fun.
- **What it shows:** Diagnostic criteria for POTS, OH, or neurocardiogenic syncope (NCS).
- **Why it matters:** It's the gold standard for confirming positional chaos.
- **Reality tip:** Cancel all plans for the rest of the day. You'll be a human puddle.

3. QSART (Quantitative Sudomotor Axon Reflex Test)

- **What it does:** Measures sweat response to stimulation.
- **How it works:** Acetylcholine is coaxed via electrodes to provoke sweat.
- **What it shows:** Small fiber autonomic nerve function.
- **Why it matters:** If your sweat glands ignore the command, it points to autonomic neuropathy.
- **The catch:** Only a few centers offer this test.

4. Thermoregulatory Sweat Test (TST)

- **What it does:** Evaluates head-to-toe sweating response in a heated chamber.
- **How it works:** You're dusted with indicator powder and gently baked. Sweat patterns show up as color changes.
- **What it shows:** Whether your body can regulate temperature — or not.

- **Bonus:** You'll look like a purple neon zebra. Cool.
- **Why it matters:** Dysfunction here supports a diagnosis of generalized autonomic failure.

5. Valsalva Maneuver (Hold Your Breath, Bear Down, Confuse Your Heart)

- **What it does:** Measures baroreflex (BP and HR recovery) during pressure strain.
- **How it works:** You bear down like you're trying to win a staring contest with gravity while monitors watch your vitals.
- **What it shows:** Your ability to recover from sudden internal pressure changes.
- **Why it matters:** It directly assesses autonomic tone — especially vagus nerve function.

6. Deep Breathing Test

- **What it does:** Measures HR variability during controlled breathing.
- **How it works:** You breathe slowly (approximately 6 breaths/min) while an ECG tracks beat-to-beat changes.
- **What it shows:** Parasympathetic nervous system function.
- **Why it matters:** Blunted response = impaired vagal tone = parasympathetic crash.

7. Skin Biopsy

- **What it does:** Tests small nerve fiber density in the skin.
- **How it works:** A tiny punch biopsy is taken from the leg or thigh and analyzed.

- **What it shows:** Nerve fiber loss = small fiber neuropathy, a common POTS co-pilot.
- **Why it matters:** Validates symptoms when other tests are "normal" such as electromyography (EMG) and nerve conduction studies.

8. Autonomic Reflex Screen (ARS)
- **What it does:** Rolls multiple tests into one.
- **How it works:** Combines TTT, deep breathing, Valsalva, QSART, and BP/HR monitoring.
- **What it shows:** A full snapshot of sympathetic and parasympathetic function.
- **Why it matters:** This is the autonomic grand slam. It's definitive. It's data-rich. It's usually only found at top-tier centers (insert shameless plug for our clinic here).

Step 3: Order Labs That Actually Tell You Something

No, there's no single "dysautonomia blood test." You can't just stick a needle in your arm and get a printout that says "Congratulations, you're Tilted." But the right labs can help rule out mimics, uncover root causes, and give your diagnosis some biochemical street cred. You're not chasing unicorns — you're collecting data. Here's how to do it smarter.

Lab Test	Why It Matters
CBC (Complete Blood Count)	Screens for anemia, infection, or chronic inflammation — all of which can mimic fatigue and tachycardia. Low hemoglobin? That's not dysautonomia, that's a red blood cell shortage.

Lab Test	Why It Matters
CMP (Comprehensive Metabolic Panel)	Checks sodium, potassium, glucose, liver, and kidney function. Electrolyte imbalance = crash fuel. Hypoglycemia = false alarm with real consequences.
TSH, Free T3, Free T4	Because your thyroid can go rogue and pretend to be your autonomic nervous system. Hypo or hyperthyroidism both play dirty.
Cortisol, ACTH	Rules out adrenal insufficiency. If your body can't mount a stress response, orthostatic symptoms are just the tip of the dysfunction iceberg.
Plasma Norepinephrine (supine and upright)	Upright levels >600 pg/mL suggest hyperadrenergic POTS. Translation: adrenaline is your new baseline.
Renin & Aldosterone	Low levels = RAAS dysfunction. That means salt wasting, volume depletion, and an internal plumbing system that leaks like a bad faucet.
24-Hour Urine Sodium	<100 mEq/day? You're not just salt deficient — you're practically a salt vampire. Helps confirm volume depletion even if labs look "normal."

Lab Test	Why It Matters
ANA, ESR, CRP	Screens for autoimmune or inflammatory processes. Could point to lupus, Sjögren's, or something else with alphabet-soup potential.
Anti-ganglionic AChR Antibodies	Rare, but worth checking if symptoms are severe and unexplained. Associated with autoimmune autonomic ganglionopathy.
Vitamin B12 & Methylmalonic Acid (MMA)	Low B12 = nerve dysfunction. If MMA is elevated, your nerves are starving. And no, subclinical deficiency isn't harmless.
Vitamin D	Because being deficient in this common vitamin makes everything worse. Bone pain, fatigue, immune dysfunction — pick your poison.
Ferritin & Iron Panel	Low ferritin = poor oxygen delivery = brain fog + fatigue + POTS-y symptoms. Especially in menstruating humans.
Hemoglobin A1c + Fasting Insulin	Screens for blood sugar issues. Dysautonomia doesn't cause insulin resistance — but it definitely doesn't get along with it.

Lab Test	Why It Matters
Catecholamines (plasma or 24-hr urine)	Helps evaluate adrenal overdrive. If you're marinating in epinephrine, we should know.
Urinary Metanephrines	Rules out pheochromocytoma — rare, but real. If your BP spikes like a rollercoaster, don't skip this one.
Celiac Panel	Because gluten sensitivity isn't just a social media trend — celiac disease can cause autonomic symptoms, and untreated cases are sneakier than you think.
MCAS Markers (Tryptase, Histamine, Chromogranin A)	If your symptoms scream histamine overload — flushing, tachycardia, wheezing — you might be dealing with mast cell shenanigans too.

Tilt Tip: Testing Goes Smoother When You're Not Guessing the Dress Code and Drug List

Many of these need to be drawn under specific conditions — supine (ie. lying down), upright, fasting, no meds — so check protocols before showing up in a tangled mess of compression gear and beta-blocker withdrawal.

Science Snapshot

Elevated standing norepinephrine (>600 pg/mL) indicates hyperadrenergic POTS. Low renin and aldosterone levels suggest RAAS dysfunction and volume dysregulation.

— Raj et al., 2005; Stewart et al., 2009

Translation: Your labs might look "normal" to someone skimming. But to someone trained? They're screaming "Autonomic Dysfunction Ahoy!"

The Gaslighting Gauntlet: What They Say vs. What You Can Say

They Say…	You Say…
"Your labs are normal."	"So's my BP when lying down. Want to see my HR log?"
"It's just anxiety."	"Anxiety doesn't cause post-meal syncope. This does."
"Everyone gets tired."	"Not everyone crashes after microwaving soup."
"You need to exercise more."	"When I try, I collapse. Got another suggestion?"
"You should push through it."	"That's how I ended up horizontal in a grocery store."

Tilt Tip: Bring Your Medical Binder To Every Appointment
Pack a dossier of:

- HR/BP logs
- Symptom timelines
- Menstrual tracking (if applicable)
- Highlighted test results
- Peer-reviewed studies (printed, tabbed, fabulous)
- Photos or video clips (if safe and appropriate)

You're not over-explaining. You're leading the investigation. This isn't overkill — it's survival with footnotes. Bonus if your binder is digital. Hand your doctor that flash drive with a side of sass.

Horizontal Summary -- Diagnostic Recon Toolkit

Step	Action
1	Know the criteria for POTS, OH, NCS
2	Log your vitals and symptoms
3	Ask for real autonomic testing
4	Use labs to clarify the bigger picture
5	Show up prepared. Lead with data, not description

Final Thought

You don't need to convince anyone that you're suffering to deserve care. But in a system that runs on checkboxes and printouts, learning to speak the language of data protects your time, energy, and sanity.

Every log you track, every test you request, every binder you build — it's armor. You're not just trying to get answers. You're reclaiming control — one chart, one result, one salty spreadsheet at a time.

PART II:
CHRONIC TILT MANAGEMENT

Treatment Plans, Trial-and-Error, and Tactical Salt Usage

CHAPTER 4:
MANAGEMENT, MEDS, AND MANEUVERING YOUR WAY THROUGH THIS CIRCUS

Salt, Compression, and the Unshakable Will to Stay Upright

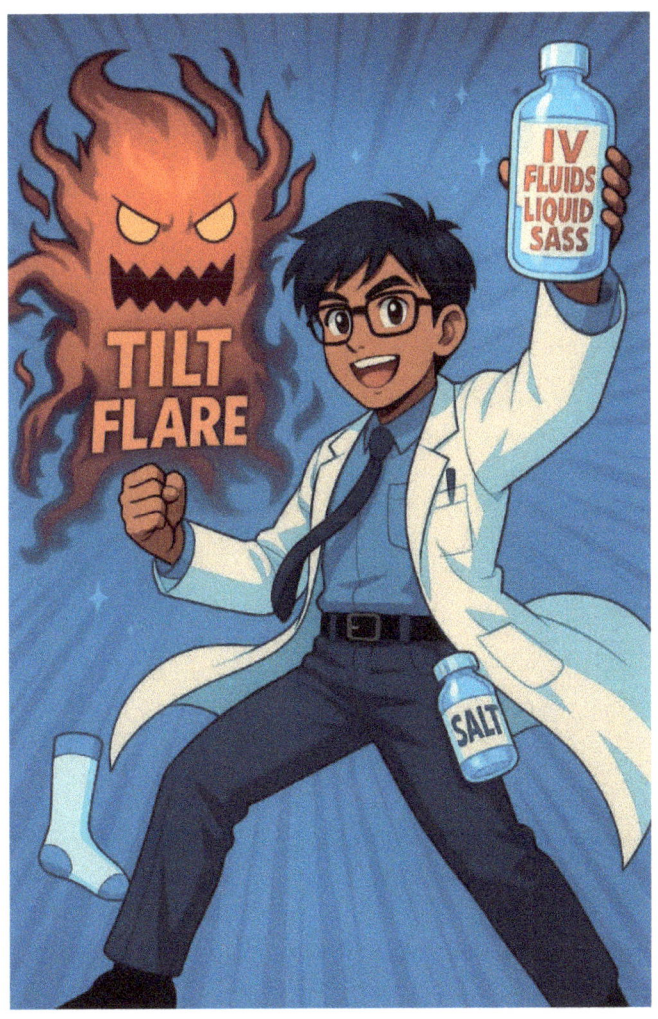

If no one's coming to rescue you, you build your own rescue plan. You've got salt, a spreadsheet, and just enough spite to make it work. Let's turn half-baked guidance into something usable.

Getting a name for your autonomic chaos is only half the battle. The next part? Building a treatment plan that makes your body less of a biohazard and more of a semi-reliable partner in daily life.

Here's the kicker — there is no single pill, protocol, or magic fix. No reset button. No miracle juice cleanse. What you do have is strategy. Options. Tactical awareness forged in the fires of super-market collapses and shower fainting incidents.

This isn't about finding a cure. It's about assembling a personalized operating system — a toolkit you tweak, test, and finesse until you can function on your own terms. Sometimes upright.

The Five Pillars of Dysautonomia Management

Every autonomic warrior builds their plan from five foundational goals. Not everyone needs all five, but most pull from several to create a cocktail of functionality:

1. Volume Expansion
2. Vasoconstriction
3. Heart Rate Control
4. Neuromodulation
5. Symptom-Specific Tools

This isn't linear. It's "choose-your-own-treatment-path" — complete with detours, trial periods, and occasional dramatic side effects.

1. Volume Expansion: Because You're Basically a Dehydrated Houseplant

Goal: Increase blood volume → stabilize blood pressure → reduce heart rate spikes → extend time upright.

A. Salt Loading
- Target: 3–10 grams sodium/day (medically supervised)
- Sources: Salt tablets, electrolyte powders, bouillon cubes, salted nuts, ramen packets, pickle juice (aka briny goodness)
- Caution: Monitor for high blood pressure, swelling, or headaches

B. Fluid Intake
- Target: 2–3 liters/day
- Key Rule: Electrolyte fluids > plain water. Too much water without salt = dilution disaster
- Tactic: Front-load fluids early in the day before gravity starts winning

C. Compression Gear
- Tools: Compression stockings (30–40 mmHg), abdominal binders
- Timing: Put them on before getting out of bed, not after symptoms start

D. Fludrocortisone
- Function: Mimics aldosterone to retain sodium and fluid
- Side Effects: Possible low potassium, swelling, or increased BP
- Pro Tip: Monitor electrolytes regularly

E. Head-of-bed elevation
- Target: Raise the head of your bed by 6–10 inches using blocks, furniture risers, or a wedge

- Key Rule: Sleeping flat suppresses your RAAS (renin-angiotensin-aldosterone system); a slight incline helps maintain fluid balance overnight
- Tactic: Elevate the bed frame itself (not just extra pillows) to encourage salt and water retention while you sleep
- Bonus: May reduce morning dizziness, nausea, and the "I need to lie back down immediately" wake-up call

Science Snapshot

Sodium and mineralocorticoid therapy significantly improve orthostatic tolerance and cerebral perfusion in patients with POTS and OH.
　　　　　　　　　　　　　　— *Raj et al., 2005; Stewart et al., 2012*

Translation: Salt isn't indulgent. It's infrastructure.

Tilt Break: What's RAAS and Why Should You Care?

RAAS stands for Renin-Angiotensin-Aldosterone System — a hormone network that helps regulate blood pressure, sodium levels, and fluid volume. When your blood pressure drops or your kidneys sense low blood flow (like after standing up too quickly), RAAS kicks in to tighten your blood vessels and tell your body to hold onto salt and water.

But here's the twist: lying completely flat for hours can suppress RAAS overnight, making it less active in the morning — which is exactly when you need it most.

Head-of-bed elevation keeps just enough gravitational stress on your body to gently nudge RAAS into doing its job, helping you wake up a little less dehydrated and a lot less dizzy.

2. Vasoconstriction: Stop the Blood From Vacationing in Your Ankles

Goal: Improve vascular tone → prevent blood pooling → keep perfusion where it matters (brain, heart, muscles)

A. Midodrine
- Mechanism: Alpha-1 agonist that constricts blood vessels
- Timing: Take before high-risk situations (standing, meals, heat)
- Side Effects: Scalp tingling, goosebumps
- Caution: Avoid at night to prevent supine (ie. lying down) hypertension

B. Droxidopa
- Function: Converts to norepinephrine → raises BP, boosts energy
- Ideal For: Neurogenic OH or severe fatigue
- Monitor: Can raise both standing and seated BP

C. Pyridostigmine
- Mechanism: Boosts parasympathetic tone and slows HR
- Effect: Mild BP impact, often well-tolerated
- Bonus: Doesn't worsen supine hypertension

D. Cold Therapy
- Ice packs, cold foot baths, cooling vests
- Cooling skin tightens blood vessels, supporting perfusion

Science Snapshot
Midodrine and droxidopa significantly improve standing BP and reduce pre-syncope in autonomic failure.

— Freeman et al., 2011; Kaufmann et al., 2014

Translation: If your blood vessels won't cooperate, these meds will negotiate forcefully on your behalf.

3. Heart Rate Control: Because 145 BPM While Toasting Bread Is Absurd

Goal: Reduce inappropriate HR surges → stabilize energy → prevent over-activation of the sympathetic system

A. Beta-Blockers
- Examples: Propranolol (short-acting), metoprolol (longer-acting)
- Good For: Hyperadrenergic POTS
- Warning: Can lower BP — start low, go slow

B. Ivabradine
- Function: Slows heart rate without lowering BP
- Best For: Patients with isolated tachycardia or low BP
- Caveat: May interact with grapefruit juice, which blocks the enzyme (CYP3A4) responsible for clearing it — turning a normal dose into a biochemical tantrum with extra side effects

C. Clonidine
- Mechanism: Reduces sympathetic tone
- Side Effects: Drowsiness, low BP — use cautiously

D. Reconditioning
- Strategic, gradual exercise improves vascular tone and lowers resting HR (covered in Chapter 8)

Science Snapshot
Ivabradine improves symptom burden and HR control in POTS without lowering BP, making it ideal for patients with isolated tachycardia.
— Barzilai et al., 2019; McDonald et al., 2020

Translation: If beta-blockers are a blunt hammer, ivabradine is a polite whisper.

4. Neuromodulation: Calming a Nervous System That's Always Yelling

Goal: Reduce neuro-inflammation and over-activation; re-tune the autonomic system by quieting the internal electrical storm, one receptor at a time

A. Low-Dose Naltrexone (LDN)
- Use: Immune modulator; stabilizes microglia and tones down neuro-inflammatory volume
- Best For: Post-viral, autoimmune dysautonomia
- Pro Tip: Start with micro-doses and increase slowly

B. Vagal Nerve Stimulation
- Methods: Ear clips, neck patches, TENS-style gadgets
- Why It Matters: The vagus nerve is your internal chill button
- Extra Credit: Especially effective for GI issues, palpitations, and anxiety overlays

C. Cognitive Behavioral Therapy (CBT)
- To Be Clear: This is not because your symptoms are psychological
- Goal: Retrain your nervous system's threat response
- Strategy: Learn to identify "real danger" vs. "just standing up"

D. Psychotropic Agents (SSRIs, SNRIs, TCAs, Benzodiazepines)
1. **SSRIs** (e.g., sertraline, fluoxetine)
   - Use: Reduce sympathetic overdrive via serotonin modulation
   - Bonus: May help GI motility and discomfort

2. **SNRIs** (e.g., duloxetine, venlafaxine)
   - Use: Helpful for pain, mood, vascular tone
   - Caution: Can raise BP in some patients
3. **TCAs** (e.g., nortriptyline, amitriptyline)
   - Use: Sleep, migraines, GI hypersensitivity
   - Caution: Anticholinergic side effects and arrhythmia risks
4. **Benzodiazepines** (e.g., lorazepam, alprazolam)
   - Use: Sympathetic storms, anticipatory anxiety
   - Caution: Can lower blood pressure, worsen fatigue, and cause drowsiness.

Science Snapshot

Psychotropic agents such as SSRIs, SNRIs, TCAs, and benzodiazepines can modulate autonomic output by altering central sympathetic tone, dampening anxiety-linked surges, and improving comorbid symptom clusters like pain, insomnia, and nausea.

— Naschitz et al., 2006; Grubb et al., 2011; Raj et al., 2009

Translation: Your nervous system is using a bullhorn. These meds hand it a calming cup of tea. They don't fix the wiring, but they help your brain stop calling 9-1-1 every time you stand up.

Tilt Tip: Brain meds — Not just for feels, but for function

Psychotropic meds are not "just for mood." They're for modulating brainstem output, vagal tone, and sympathetic chaos. If your psychiatrist doesn't speak dysautonomia, bring them this chapter — and maybe a salty snack for morale.

5. Symptom-Specific Tools: Managing the Chaos in Chapters

Gastrointestinal
- Medications: Pro-kinetics (erythromycin, metoclopramide)
- Tactics: Small meals, low fiber, stay upright after eating
- Supplements: Ginger, peppermint, digestive enzymes

Neurologic
- Migraine preventives
- Modafinil or amantadine for brain fog (if BP tolerates)

Sleep
- Melatonin, low-dose doxepin
- Elevate head-of-bed 6–10 inches
- Tighten bedtime cues and routines

Menstrual Flares
- Hormonal regulation (oral contraceptives, IUDs)
- Increase salt and fluid in luteal phase
- Lower activity expectations

Heat Intolerance
- Cooling gear, cold beverages, shaded environments
- Prioritize air conditioning like it's medication

Daily Hacks That Actually Work

Hack	Why It Works
Morning salt/electrolyte	Primes volume before gravity arrives

Hack	Why It Works
Compression before standing	Prevents blood pooling
Recumbent exercise	Improves tone without provoking flares
Frequent salty snacks	Maintains sodium and glucose balance
Hydration alarm	Thirst is a late symptom, not a reliable guide
Foldable stool or seat cane	Sit anywhere, anytime — no apology necessary

Tilt Tip: Strategy Beats Stamina

Building a system that reduces flares isn't cheating. It's intelligent design. You're not supposed to "push through." You're supposed to manage. Systems over willpower — always.

Horizontal Summary -- Tilt Toolbox Overview

Objective	Tools That Help
Expand blood volume	Salt, fluids, fludrocortisone, elevate head-of-bed
Improve BP response	Midodrine, droxidopa, compression
Calm HR surges	Beta-blockers, ivabradine, strategic exercise

Objective	Tools That Help
Reduce nerve chaos	LDN, vagus nerve stimulation, CBT, SSRIs, SNRIs, TCAs, benzos
Symptom relief	GI meds, migraine control, sleep tools, heat strategies

Final Thought

This isn't about "pushing through." It's about precision. You're not managing dysautonomia by luck — you're managing it with salt, pharmacology, compression garments, and pure tactical brilliance.

The right treatment plan isn't a one-size-fits-all protocol. It's a neurovascular chessboard — and you're moving the pieces with scientific accuracy and lived expertise.

You're not just surviving flares. You're building infrastructure. And that makes you less of a patient — and more of a rebel commander in a salty, upright mech suit.

CHAPTER 5:
TRIGGERS, FLARES, AND THE PLOT TWISTS THAT TAKE YOU DOWN WITHOUT WARNING

A Field Guide to the Ambushes of Autonomic Dysfunction

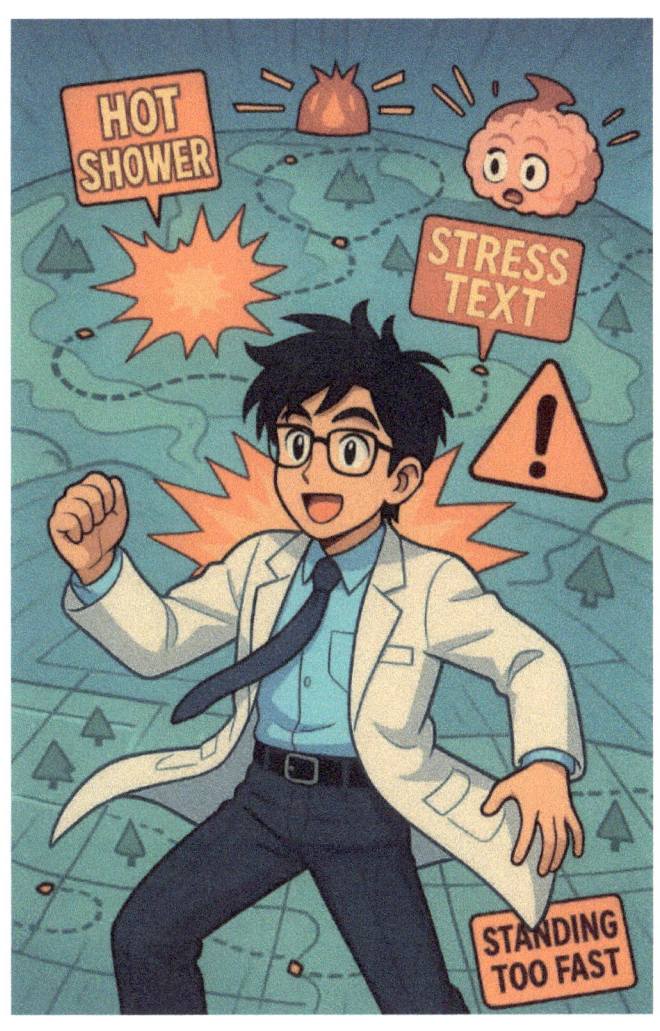

You finally found a rhythm — and then your body short-circuited because it was humid. Or loud. Or Tuesday. This chapter is about spotting the landmines before they take you down.

Managing dysautonomia isn't just about treatment — it's about terrain awareness. Because even with the right meds, salt, fluids, and compression, the wrong trigger can sideswipe you like a rogue shopping cart on a downhill slope.

These aren't random symptoms. They're physiological landmines: temperature, stress, standing still, hormones, noise, light, meals, dehydration, sitting too long, standing too long, existing too much.

If your symptoms fluctuate wildly, it's not inconsistency — it's interaction. Dysautonomia is a condition of thresholds. When your nervous system is already balancing on a tightrope, even a small push — a hot room, a large meal, a stressful phone call — can send it spiraling.

You're not unstable. You're exquisitely sensitive to internal and external feedback loops. Let's decode the landmines before they blow up your weekday.

Triggers, Mechanisms, and Countermoves: A Tilt Field Manual

Group 1: Physical Stressors

Trigger	Why It Happens	What to Do About It
Standing too long	Blood pools in legs → BP drops → HR spikes	Compression gear, counter-pressure maneuvers

Trigger	Why It Happens	What to Do About It
Sitting too long	Static position → reduced venous return	Set reminders to stand/move/stretch
Overexertion	Low perfusion = crash 12–48 hours later	Pacing, recumbent exercise, post-activity fluids
Showering	Heat + upright posture = vasodilation, volume loss	Cool water, sit if needed, pre-hydrate
Menstruation	Estrogen + fluid drop → autonomic disruption	Increase salt/hydration, adjust activity

Group 2: Environmental Triggers

Trigger	Why It Happens	What to Do About It
Heat	Vasodilation → reduced BP → HR surge	Cooling gear, hydration, avoid peak temps
Sunlight	Triggers heat response + visual overload	Sunglasses, shade, rest indoors
Loud noises/lights	Sensory overload = sympathetic activation	Headphones, tinted lenses, quiet breaks

Trigger	Why It Happens	What to Do About It
Crowds	Input + physical strain = overactivation	Plan exits, hydrate, pace social interaction
Travel	Altitude, activity, disruption → instability	Compression, fluids, preemptive meds

Group 3: Internal/Metabolic Triggers

Trigger	Why It Happens	What to Do About It
Dehydration	Lower blood volume = less perfusion	Electrolytes + water constantly throughout day
Skipping meals	Hypoglycemia → compensatory HR spike	Regular meals/snacks, avoid sugar crashes
Large meals	Blood diverted to gut → post-meal drop	Smaller meals, upright after eating
Alcohol	Vasodilation + fluid loss	Avoid or minimize; hydrate before/after
Illness/Infection	Fever, inflammation → autonomic disarray	Early intervention, hydrate, rest
Stress/Anxiety	Cortisol = HR/BP surges	Breathwork, CBT tools, vagus nerve stimulation

Trigger	Why It Happens	What to Do About It
Hormonal shifts	Estrogen drop = vascular instability	Track cycle, adjust salt/fluid intake
Sleep deprivation	HR variability decreases, reactivity increases	Prioritize consistent, high-quality sleep

Science Snapshot

In patients with POTS and orthostatic intolerance, triggers such as heat, large meals, prolonged standing, and emotional stress are associated with significant hemodynamic instability.

— *Stewart et al., 2006; Grubb & Karas, 2011*

Translation: Your system isn't fragile. It's finely tuned — but easily overwhelmed.

When Flares Happen Anyway

Even with perfect prep, some days still go sideways. That doesn't mean you failed. It means dysautonomia did what it does best: surprise flares, delayed crashes, and sudden U-turns.

Common Flare Signs:
- Tachycardia spike at rest
- Dizziness upon standing (more than usual)
- Fatigue disproportionate to activity
- Nausea, bloating, and bathroom stand-offs
- Cold hands/feet or sudden full-on sweat
- Brain fog thick enough to forget your own ZIP code

What to Do Mid-Flare:
- Lie down flat or elevate legs
- Hydrate with electrolytes (not just water)
- Use cold packs on chest, neck, or wrists
- Breathing techniques (slow inhale/exhale, box breathing)
- If safe, medicate: salt tabs, midodrine, beta-blocker, nausea meds
- Rest. Fully. Flare recovery is not optional downtime — it's recalibration.

Tilt Tip: Map Your Triggers

Keep a symptom log. Record meals, temperature, hydration, activity. Patterns emerge. And when they do, you can outmaneuver them. No, you can't avoid every trigger. But you can stop them from catching you off guard every time.

Horizontal Summary –- Tilt Trigger Recon

Trigger Type	Examples	Mitigation
Physical	Standing, exertion, menstruation	Compression, pacing, prep fluids
Environmental	Heat, noise, light, crowds	Cooling gear, plan exits, shade
Internal	Dehydration, meals, stress, sleep loss	Salt, snacks, pacing, CBT tools

Final Thought

Dysautonomia doesn't just affect what you feel — it dictates how you move through the world. The lights you avoid, the coats you carry in summer, the backup snacks in your bag, the seat you scan for at every event.

This isn't over-preparing. It's predictive medicine, patient-led. This is knowing your body well enough to intercept chaos mid-strike.

Flares are feedback. And every time you adapt, you teach your body — and the world — how to coexist with your uncooperative wiring.

CHAPTER 6:
DAILY TILT SURVIVAL GUIDE

Logistics, Life Hacks, and Low-Energy Wins That Actually Work

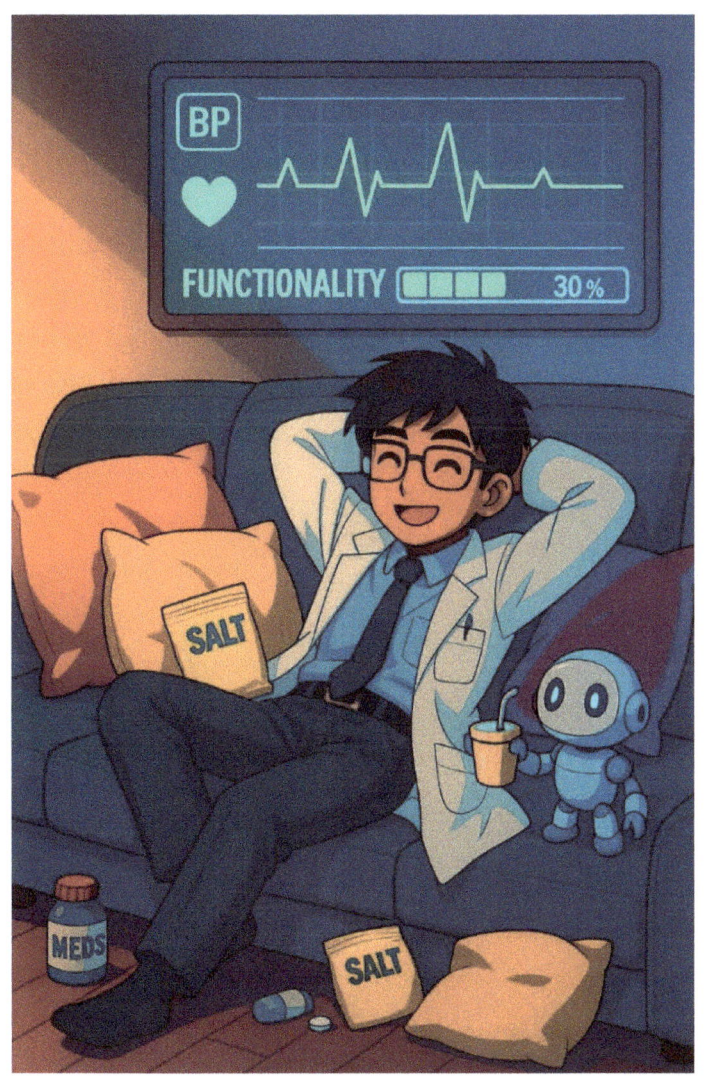

If Chapter 5 was about the landmines, this chapter is about the navigation system. Because avoiding flares is one thing — living well between them is another. This is where logistics meet physiology, and hacks meet strategy.

Every day is a game of pacing, predicting, and adjusting faster than your symptoms can. Welcome to the art of surviving the in-between. Your energy is limited. Your nervous system is dramatic. Your mission is to build a lifestyle that cooperates with reality without giving in to it.

You're not "just getting through the day." You're maintaining altitude with tools, habits, and tactical brilliance. Let's break it down.

Morning: The Battle Is Won Before You Stand

What you do in the first 30 minutes of your day determines how the next several hours go. Your system is dry, your blood vessels are slack, and gravity is already plotting its attack.

Build a Morning Launch Sequence:
- **Salt + Electrolytes immediately:** Not after breakfast. First thing. Salt shot, bouillon cube, or electrolyte drink.
- **Compression gear on before getting up:** If you wait, you've already lost half the benefit.
- **Elevated start position:** Sit up in bed for a few minutes before standing.
- **Hydration station at bedside:** Water + salt tabs + meds = ready launch pad. Always hydrate before you get out of bed. Trust me.
- **Snack before movement:** Something salty and protein-rich can soften the orthostatic transition.

Energy Budgeting: Time Is Money, but Energy Is Gold-Plated Cryptocurrency

Imagine your energy as a bank account that resets unpredictably and charges overdraft fees in dizziness, nausea, and crashing fatigue.

Tilt Energy Economy Rules:

- **Peak focus = first 3 hours:** Schedule high-effort tasks early, while BP and brain perfusion are best.
- **The 20-minute rule:** Sit or lie down for 10–20 minutes between tasks to reset perfusion.
- **Cycle focus, not multitask:** Brain fog punishes divided attention.
- **Batch tasks:** If you're upright once, knock out grouped tasks (e.g., kitchen → laundry → rest).
- **Use timers for rest:** Avoid the "accidental 4-hour nap" that turns into a full-system reboot.

Science Snapshot

People with dysautonomia often experience reduced cerebral perfusion, delayed cardiovascular recovery after standing, and exacerbated symptoms with sustained upright activity.

— *Stewart et al., 2010; Shibata et al., 2012*

Translation: Energy crashes aren't laziness — they're gravity tax plus neurologic lag.

Pacing ≠ Giving Up. It Means You Know the Terrain.

Strategic pacing lets you fly longer above the red zone. It's the opposite of fragility — it's neurological engineering.

Pacing Move	What It Does
Planned rest breaks	Prevent BP and HR from derailing
Symptom logs	Track patterns for intelligent adjustment
"Activity sandwiches"	High-effort task → low-effort task → rest
Task delegation	If someone else can do it — let them

Home Setup: Because Sitting Down Shouldn't Be a Project

Morning Setup:
- Elevated bed head: 6–10 inches reduces overnight pooling
- Compression zone: Socks, binders, gear in one location
- Hydration station: Kitchen or bedside; restock every night
- Medication tray: Timed doses, visual tracking, salt pairings

Midday Systems:
- Foldable stool in kitchen/bathroom: Sit while you prep or brush teeth
- Mini fan or cooling cloths nearby: For surprise overheating
- Task zones: Keep chores clustered (cleaning gear by trash, meds near food)

Emergency Kits:
- "Go bag" with salt tabs, meds, snacks, cold pack
- Pulse oximeter + BP cuff on-hand

- Symptom journal or phone app for flares
- Cooling vest/portable fan if venturing into the sun's death rays

Tilt Tip: Build Systems, Not Just Habits

You don't need more discipline. You need better defaults. When your tools are in reach, your body doesn't have to fight so hard. You win by design, not willpower.

Low-Energy Wins That Still Count

Win	Why It Matters
Changed clothes?	You engaged in autonomic challenge and survived
Made food, even snacks?	You nourished through the crash curve
Got outside, even briefly?	Sun + rhythm = brain benefit
Texted someone back?	Cognitive load = legit effort
Rested before you collapsed?	That's elite pacing strategy

Celebrate your 20-minute productivity streak like an autonomic gladiator. You're using a malfunctioning operating system with the grace of a hacker running five extensions on a glitching laptop.

Horizontal Summary –- Tilt Daily Logistics

Domain	Hacks & Tools
Morning launch	Salt, compression, snacks, fluid station

Domain	Hacks & Tools
Energy budgeting	20-min breaks, pacing, batching
Home flow	Cooling gear, seated stations, zone clustering
Wins that count	Meals, messages, movement, mindfulness

Final Thought

You don't need to prove you're trying. You're already doing the work of a full systems engineer just to stand, move, digest, and exist. That counts. That always counts.

You're not just surviving the day — you're managing a condition that never clocks out. And you're doing it with strategy, clarity, and unapologetic brilliance.

PART III:
FUNCTIONAL TILT LIVING

Meal Prep, Movement, and Making It Work From the Floor Up

CHAPTER 7:
FEEDING YOURSELF WITHOUT PASSING OUT

Nutrition, Nausea, and Tactical Meal Planning

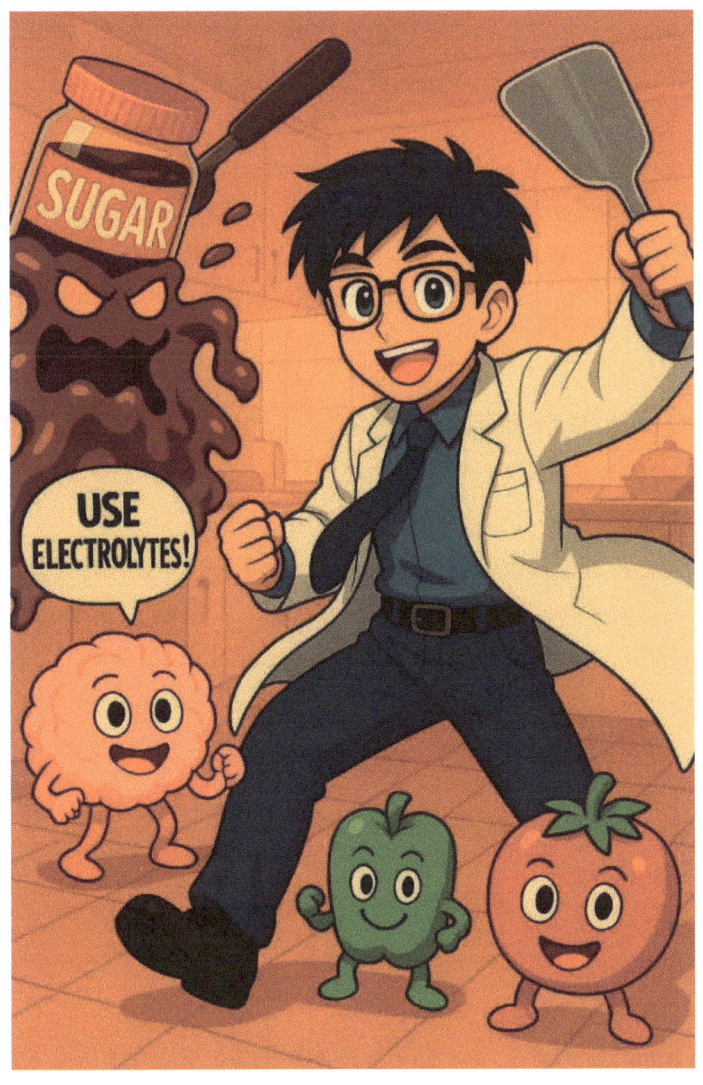

You mastered standing. Then you tried digesting. Meals shouldn't feel like cardiovascular events, but here we are. Food should be simple. You eat it, your body uses it, you move on.

But if you have dysautonomia, eating is more like negotiating with a moody houseguest who may or may not show up to digest. Meals can trigger dizziness, bloating, tachycardia, fatigue, and full-on collapses — especially when paired with upright posture, heat, or even the audacity to chew.

This isn't weakness. It's a direct result of how blood flow is redistributed during digestion — and how your autonomic system fails to reroute resources correctly. What should be a routine metabolic process becomes a tactical event requiring strategy, planning, and backup snacks.

Let's rebuild your relationship with food so it fuels you instead of flooring you.

Why Eating Makes You Crash: A Quick Gut-Brain Breakdown

- During digestion, blood is diverted to the GI tract.
- In healthy people, the body compensates with increased heart rate and vasoconstriction to maintain cerebral perfusion.
- In dysautonomia? That compensation flops.
- Blood pools in the gut, cerebral perfusion drops, and symptoms spike.

Common symptoms after eating:
- Fatigue
- Nausea
- Tachycardia
- Dizziness or near-fainting
- Bloating and slowed motility

You didn't "eat the wrong thing." Your nervous system mis-managed a basic assignment.

Science Snapshot
Postprandial hypotension and tachycardia are common in patients with autonomic failure, often leading to syncope or profound fatigue.
— *Hoeldtke et al., 1998; Freeman, 2008*

Translation: You didn't overeat. Your blood pressure ghosted you after lunch.

Tactical Meal Planning: Rewire the Ritual
General Strategy: Small. Salty. Frequent. Upright. That's the core. Think of meals like medication: dose, timing, tolerance.

Best Practices:

Rule	Why It Works
Smaller, more frequent meals	Prevents large blood shifts and glucose spikes
Add salt or electrolytes pre-meal	Preloads volume before digestion diverts it
Stay upright after eating	Aids gastric emptying and reduces pooling
Cool foods > hot foods	Less vasodilation, fewer crashes
Protein + fat with carbs	Slows glucose spikes and maintains BP longer
Hydrate before, not during	Water mid-meal may dilute acid and slow digestion

Tilt Tip: Eat Like You're Fueling a Spaceship, Not Sunday Brunch

You're not just feeding your body — you're stabilizing your blood pressure, appeasing your vagus nerve, and asking your digestive tract to behave for five whole minutes. That takes precision, not spontaneity.

Food Triggers to Know (and Navigate)

Not all foods are evil. But some provoke more rebellion than others.

Trigger	Why It's a Problem
Large, heavy meals	Huge volume = huge blood redistribution
Sugary snacks	Glucose spike → insulin drop → tachycardia
Alcohol	Vasodilation + fluid loss = double chaos
High-fiber meals	Slow motility = bloating, pressure, nausea
Hot soups or drinks	Heat = vasodilation = BP dip

You don't have to eliminate entire food groups. You just need to learn how and when your body tolerates them best. Timing, posture, temperature, and volume all matter.

Nausea: When Even Food Planning Feels Like a Battle

Sometimes the problem isn't food content — it's food proximity. Nausea is a frequent visitor in dysautonomia, often tied to vagus nerve dysfunction, slowed gastric motility, or low perfusion.

Nausea Survival Tools:

- Ginger (capsules, tea, chews)
- Peppermint (tea, oil, capsules)
- Acupressure wristbands
- Zofran, promethazine (Rx)
- Slow transitions in posture before meals
- Warm compress on abdomen or back to relax GI muscles
- Liquids > solids on flare days
- Pureed soups, smoothies, protein shakes when chewing feels feels unnecessarily ambitious

When You Can't Eat: Nutritional Workarounds

On days when food just isn't happening, aim for survival fuel.

Tool	Benefit
Oral Rehydration Solutions (ORS)	Sodium + glucose improves absorption and volume
Broths + bouillon	Salt + fluid without triggering fullness
Meal replacement shakes	Easy calories and electrolytes
Nut butter packets	Small, salty, calorie-dense
Electrolyte gummies	Chewable salt delivery for nausea days

These aren't meal replacements — they're autonomic patches. Use them wisely.

Science Snapshot

Gastroparesis and nausea are common in autonomic dysfunction and correlate with both sympathetic and vagal dysfunction.
— Camilleri et al., 2013; Tack et al., 2006

Translation: If your stomach feels like it's on strike, it probably is. That's not picky eating — it's autonomic neuropathy.

Horizontal Summary –- Tactical Tilt Nutrition Recap

Category	Strategy
Meal structure	Small, salty, upright, timed
Common triggers	Large meals, sugar, alcohol, hot/fibrous foods
Nausea plan	Ginger, peppermint, Rx meds, liquids first
Emergency fuel	Broths, ORS, shakes, nut butters

Final Thought

Your meals aren't just about calories. They're about chemistry, circulation, and control. You're not being difficult — you're navigating a digestive tract that misfires under pressure.

Every bite you tolerate, every snack you pre-load, every time you sit upright after eating instead of collapsing into a couch coma — that's resilience in action.

Feeding yourself is a high-performance feat. And you're doing it with the precision of a NASA flight director in a salted apron.

CHAPTER 8:
EXERCISING WHILE TILTED

Building Strength Without Collapsing in Public

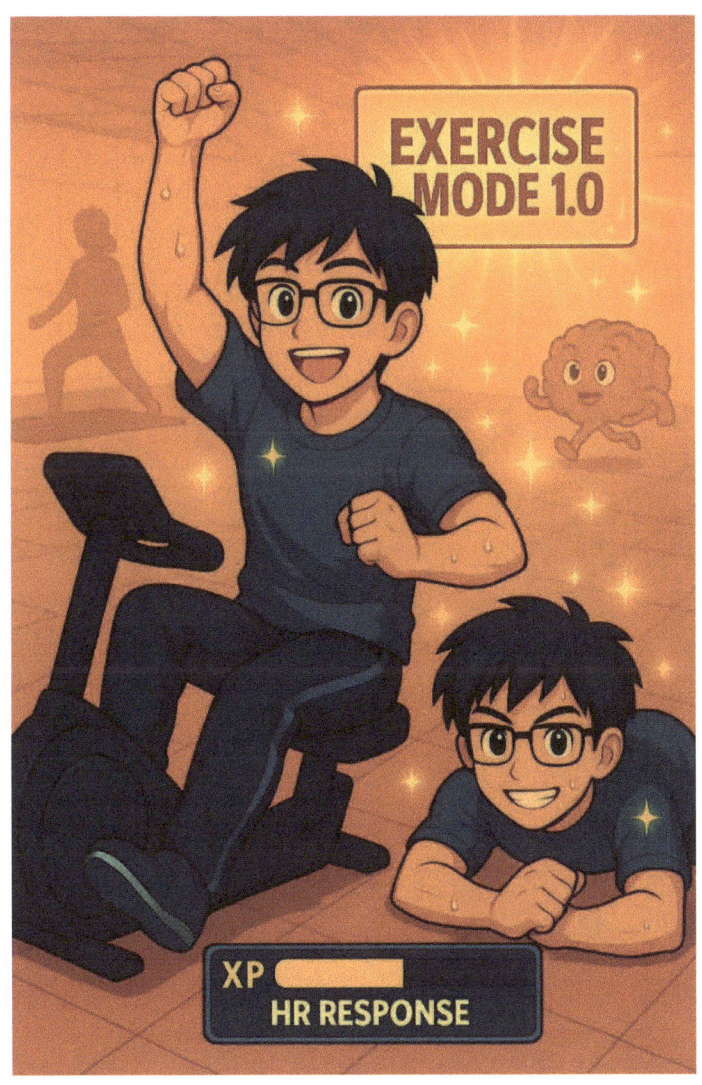

Movement helps — until it doesn't. If walking to the mailbox counts as cardio, you're not unfit — you're Tilted. This is how to build strength without picking a fight with gravity.

Exercise and dysautonomia sound like a mismatch. And in some ways, they are. You're dealing with a condition where upright posture itself is a stress test — so casually suggesting "just go for a jog" is like telling someone with a broken leg to take the stairs for healing.

But here's the twist — exercise, when done strategically, can recondition the autonomic system, improve blood volume, strengthen skeletal muscles, and reduce the severity of symptoms over time.

The key word: strategically. Because this is "Crash-Fit." And you're training not for medals, but for moments of autonomic stability.

Why Movement Helps (Even When It Feels Like the Enemy)

- Muscle contraction = vascular support. Stronger leg muscles reduce blood pooling.
- Regular movement = improved baroreflex sensitivity. This is the mechanism that keeps your blood pressure from doing interpretive dance.
- Increased plasma volume = better perfusion. More blood in the tank = fewer flares.
- Exercise improves autonomic tone over time. Slowly. Annoyingly slowly. But yes, it helps.

Science Snapshot

Exercise training in patients with POTS has been shown to increase plasma volume, decrease upright tachycardia, and improve quality of life and autonomic regulation.

— Fu et al., 2010; Shibata et al., 2012

Translation: Motion is medicine — as long as it's prescribed with the caution of a radioactive isotope.

The Levine Protocol (and How to Make It Work for You)

The **Levine Protocol** is a structured, multi-month exercise plan developed specifically for people with dysautonomia. It emphasizes:

- **Recumbent cardio** (think rowing, swimming, recumbent bike)
- **Gradual progression to upright activity**
- **Strength training** after cardio capacity improves
- **Daily salt and fluid intake** to support blood volume

It's one of the most well-researched and widely used exercise strategies for autonomic dysfunction, and many people have seen real improvements by following its principles.

But let's be honest — starting any structured plan when your body treats gravity like a personal threat can feel intimidating. That doesn't mean the protocol isn't helpful; it just means that real life often requires a little flexibility.

Here's the good news — you don't need to follow it perfectly to benefit. You can take the core principles — progressive movement, consistency, fluid support — and shape them to fit your current reality. No guilt. No gold stars. Just a plan you can actually do. Here's how.

Principles of Tilt-Compatible Movement

Principle	How It Works
Start horizontal	Rowing, swimming, floor Pilates, resistance bands
Keep it short	5–10 minutes is progress, not failure
Go slow	10% weekly increases max, no heroic jumps
Space it out	Alternate movement and rest days to avoid PEM (post-exertional malaise)
Track everything	HR, BP, fatigue levels, symptom trends

Stage One: Reclining Rebellion

For when your body throws a tantrum over standing still.

This stage is for those who can't tolerate upright activity without feeling like they're auditioning for a Victorian fainting couch.

Modality	Goal
Recumbent bike	Gentle, rhythmical cardio with minimal HR spikes
Rowing machine	Engage muscles while horizontal-ish

Modality	Goal
Supine resistance bands	Build strength without gravity's judgment
Lying-down yoga	Stretch and calm the nervous system without triggering it

- Start with **5–10 minutes, 3–4 times per week**
- Use **compression, salt, and hydration** before and after
- Rest like it's your job

Stage Two: Seated Survivors Club

You've graduated from lying down to sitting up without dramatic consequences. Congratulations.

Modality	Goal
Pedal exerciser	Gentle circulation boost
Seated resistance bands	Low-impact strength and tone
Chair yoga	Flexibility with stability
Light dumbbells (1–3 lbs)	Upper body tone without orthostatic insult

- Progress by adding **5 minutes every 1–2 weeks**, if recovery stays steady
- Mix upper and lower body to avoid overloading one system
- Keep salt and fluid onboard at all times

Stage Three: Upright, With Supervision (And Salt)

Once you can tolerate seated workouts without symptom spikes or next-day payback, it's time to flirt with verticality again.

Modality	Goal
Elliptical (slow pace)	Light cardio without pounding joints
Wall sits	Strengthen quads = improve venous return
Standing yoga	Control, breath, posture awareness
Flat-surface walking	Short walks with compression and hydration onboard

- Wear **compression gear**, hydrate in advance
- Keep walks under **10–15 minutes** to start
- Log your HR/BP before, during, and after

Strength Is Scaffolding, Not Showboating

If cardio is about conditioning your nervous system, strength training is about building structural support for your circulation.

Muscle Group	Why It Matters
Quads & glutes	Venous return = anti-fainting force

Muscle Group	Why It Matters
Calves	Your second heart — pump that blood back upward
Core	Helps with posture, balance, and HR modulation
Upper back	Carries your gear, your groceries, and your pride

Start with bodyweight or resistance bands. Then graduate to light weights. Always pair with rest days and hydration.

Tilt Tip: Build Muscle — Not Tolerance for Nonsense

Strong legs can help your blood pressure. Strong boundaries will help everything else. Resistance training isn't just for your quads — it's for your calendar, your relationships, and your sanity. Say yes to leg day, no to energy vampires, and watch both your systolic blood pressure and your self-respect stabilize.

Exercise Cautions: You're Not Training for the Olympics

Warning Sign	Translation
HR spikes > 40 bpm from baseline	Slow down. You're tipping into overexertion.
PEM (delayed crash)	You need more rest between sessions
Nausea/dizziness mid-workout	Your perfusion is tanking. Recline and rehydrate.

Warning Sign	Translation
Next-day cognitive fog	Back off by 25–50% next time
Chest pain or near-syncope	Stop. Reassess. This isn't a drill.

Science Snapshot

Graded exercise therapy improves plasma volume and vascular tone in POTS, but must be customized to prevent exacerbation of orthostatic intolerance and PEM.

— *Fu et al., 2010; Raj et al., 2009*

Translation: Go slow or go horizontal. Those are your two options.

Horizontal Summary –- Strategic Exercise Map

Phase	Activities	Tilt Strategy
Reclined	Rowing, supine bands, floor stretches	Salt + compression + short sessions
Seated	Chair yoga, pedal exerciser, light bands	Build up without provoking flares
Upright	Walking, wall sits, elliptical	Limit time, monitor HR, hydrate before/after
Strength	Legs, glutes, calves, core	Target support muscles to fight blood pooling
Recovery	Passive rest, hydration, leg elevation	Built-in. Non-negotiable.

Final Thought

You're not just "getting back into shape." You're hacking your nervous system. You're building vascular tone, cardiac resilience, muscular support, and systemic confidence. One slow, salty, strategic session at a time.

This isn't fitness for aesthetics or athleticism. This is mobility. This is independence. This is reprogramming your body with the gentlest rebellion possible.

And even on the days when you can't move at all? You're still in the game. Because every rest is a form of resistance. Every stretch is a flex. Every quiet adaptation is a win.

CHAPTER 9:
MANAGING YOUR ENVIRONMENT

Sensory Tweaks, Supportive Tools, and Setting Yourself Up to Function

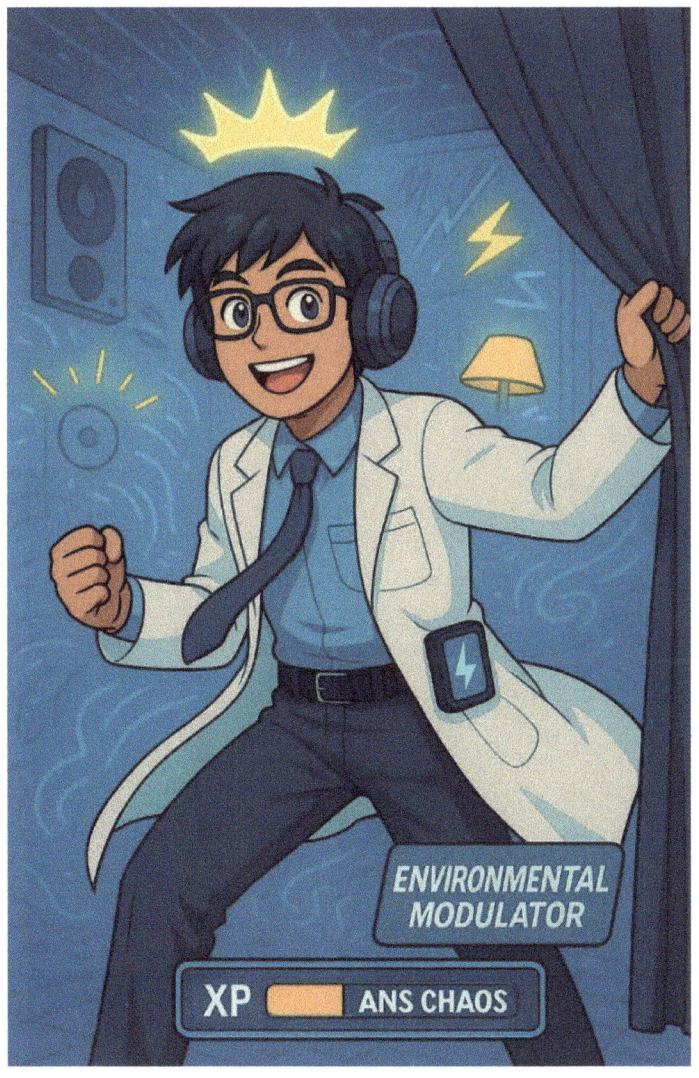

You may not control your blood vessels, but you can control your thermostat. When your surroundings work with you, everything else becomes easier. Let's redesign the battlefield.

In dysautonomia, your environment isn't neutral — it's an active participant in your symptoms. Bright lights? Sympathetic activation. Warm room? Vasodilation. Crowds, noise, smells, weird seating? Might as well be an autonomic minefield.

This isn't about being sensitive. It's about being in a body that responds to stimuli with the nuance of a smoke alarm in a candle store. Your sensory inputs are routed through a system already on edge, and your surroundings either support your function — or sabotage it.

Let's engineer your world to stop fighting your nervous system and start stabilizing it.

Why Environment Matters (More Than Most People Realize)

Your autonomic system processes external stimuli as part of its regulation process.

When those inputs become overwhelming or destabilizing, your body treats them as a threat. That means flares, crashes, and full-blown tilt attacks.

Input	Autonomic Impact
Bright or flickering lights	Overactivation of visual cortex → headache, nausea, fatigue
Loud or chaotic soundscapes	Activates fight-or-flight via auditory pathways

Input	Autonomic Impact
Heat	Vasodilation → lower BP → dizziness, fatigue
Standing room only	No muscular support = blood pooling, syncope risk
Scents and fumes	Vagal nerve irritation → nausea, migraines
Crowds	Sensory overload + physical exertion = Tilt time

Science Snapshot

Sensory hypersensitivity and environmental intolerance in dysautonomia patients correlate with increased sympathetic tone, reduced habituation, and heightened interoception.

— *Haensch et al., 2014; Allen et al., 2020*

Translation: You're not being dramatic. You're avoiding biological sabotage.

Sensory Domestication: Turn Down the Input, Turn Up the Function

Light Management
- **Tinted glasses:** Rose or FL-41 tint reduces photophobia
- **Dimmer switches:** Instant control over intensity
- **Blue-light filters:** Screens = stimulation. Use night mode 24/7.
- **Warm-toned lighting:** Less triggering than cold LED light
- **Room zoning:** Bright workspace, dark recovery zone

Sound Management
- **Noise-canceling headphones:** Reduce stress in stores, transport, waiting rooms
- **White noise machines:** Calm environment for brain breaks
- **Soft background music:** Avoid silence if it feels clinical
- **Earplugs:** Strategic use in overstimulating spaces

Temperature Control
- **Layering strategy:** Easy on/off garments to match sudden heat/cold shifts
- **Cooling vests, neck wraps, or fans:** Combat indoor heat ambushes
- **Heated blankets and hand warmers:** For winter vasoconstriction survival
- **Avoid hot baths and showers:** Use lukewarm water or sit to bathe

Home Base Optimization: Build a Supportive Habitat

Your home should reduce the friction of existing, not add to it.

Room	Tactic
Bedroom	Blackout curtains, wedge pillow, bedside fluids, elevated bed head
Bathroom	Shower chair, grab bars, dry shampoo, stool for brushing teeth
Kitchen	Prep while seated, store essentials at waist height, cooling towel nearby

Room	Tactic
Living Room	Recliner, fan, salt snack stash, dimmable lighting
Workspace	Ergonomic chair, footrest, wrist support, anti-glare screen filters

Outside the Home: Tilt-Proofing the World You Can't Control

Transportation

- Drive only when well-hydrated + rested
- Keep electrolyte drinks, cooling gear, and snacks in the car
- Request bulkhead or aisle seats when flying
- Use compression during travel and elevate legs when possible
- Wheelchairs or transport chairs for long distances are tools, not surrender

Social Events

- Pre-scout seating, bathrooms, exits
- Let hosts know you may need a quiet space
- Bring your own snacks, electrolytes, or seat cushion
- Arrive late, leave early. Zero apologies.

Workspaces

- Negotiate breaks and hybrid schedules
- Reframe accommodations as performance support
- Use sit-stand desks only if standing is safe
- Use symptom tracking to document disability accommodations if needed

Science Snapshot

Environmental modification—including lighting, sound reduction, thermal regulation, and physical accessibility—can significantly improve functional capacity and quality of life in dysautonomia patients.

— Garland et al., 2015; Benarroch, 2012

Translation: You're not babying yourself. You're designing your environment for nervous system compatibility.

Tools That Earn Their Keep

Tool	Purpose
Shower stool	Reduce BP drop and crash risk in hot water
Foldable cane chair	Sit anywhere, anytime — pure freedom
Wrist BP cuff / pulse oximeter	Quick vitals check = real-time adjustments
Salt packets / ORS	Emergency stabilization
Cooling vest / fan	Heat shield in human form
Compression wear	Blood volume support, fashion bonus optional
Noise-canceling headphones	Cancel chaos before it spikes symptoms
Emergency flare kit	Meds, ID, salt, instructions — ready in one pouch

Tilt Tip: Convenience Isn't Laziness — It's Survival

You're not "over-accommodating" yourself. You're recognizing that energy is a currency, and you're spending it where it counts. Every adaptation is a protest against autonomic dysfunction. Every modification is a vote for functionality.

Horizontal Summary -- Environmental Engineering for Autonomic Stability

Domain	Strategy
Light	Filters, dimmers, warm tones, anti-glare tech
Sound	Headphones, white noise, soundscaping
Temp	Layered clothing, cooling/heating gear
Home	Supportive furniture, layout tweaks, easy access storage
Out-and-about	Travel packs, pre-scouting, strategic exits
Tools	Shower stools, BP monitors, ORS, compression gear

Final Thought

You don't owe anyone an explanation for building a life that supports your nervous system instead of breaking it. You're not "overreacting."

You're pre-empting disasters with design, planning, and unapologetic environmental control.

The world may not be built for Tilted bodies. But that just makes your adaptations even more brilliant. You're not just managing dysautonomia. You're reshaping the world around it.

CHAPTER 10:
PARENTING WHILE CHRONICALLY EXHAUSTED

Tilted Adults Raising Small Humans Without Spontaneously Combusting

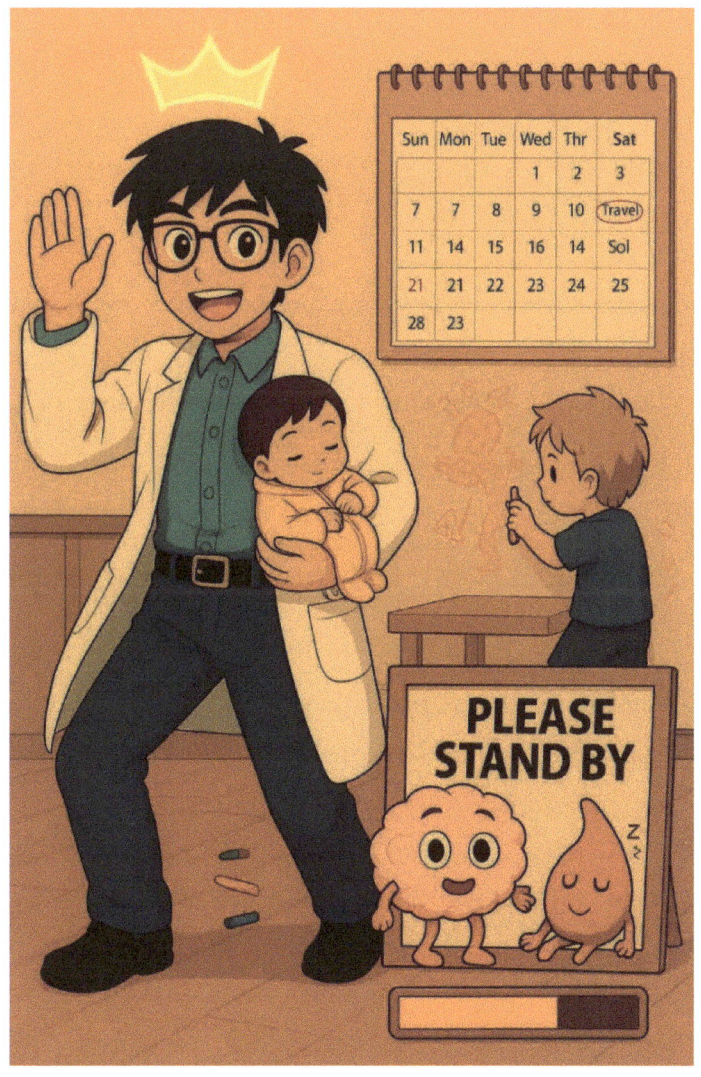

You made the house tilt-friendly — then a child ran through it with a juice box and a kazoo. Here's how to parent when you can't always be vertical.

Parenting is a total-body contact sport, even under ideal circumstances. Add dysautonomia into the mix, and congratulations: you've leveled up to playing life on expert mode with no pause button, limited stamina, and a team of tiny sentient tornados who think 5:00 a.m. is a great time to talk about dinosaurs.

This chapter is not about perfection. It's about survival. It's about parenting from the floor (sometimes literally), building systems that honor your limitations, and showing your kids that strength isn't about power — it's about persistence.

Let's redefine "showing up" so it actually reflects what you're doing.

First, The Truth: Parenting With Dysautonomia Is Legitimately Hard

You're navigating:

- Unpredictable symptoms
- Fatigue so thick you could nap standing up (but you can't stand)
- Brain fog during homework time
- GI flares during birthday parties
- Autonomic crashes mid-playdate

And yet, somehow, there's dinner on the table. Eventually. Maybe.

Parenting through a nervous system mutiny requires creativity, delegation, and grace. Mostly for yourself.

Science Snapshot

Chronic illness in parents is associated with increased physical and emotional strain, but children show higher resilience when caregivers model adaptability and communication.

— *van der Lee et al., 2007; Meltzer & Mindell, 2010*

Translation: Your kids don't need a superhero. They need a human who keeps showing up with love and logistics.

Tilted Parenting Tactics: What Actually Helps

1. Lower the Bar. Then Admire It.
- Let go of the social media parent trap
- "Good enough" is not only enough — it's sustainable
- Save energy for what really matters: connection, safety, snacks

2. Morning Prep While Horizontal
- Pack bags, set out clothes, prep breakfast while seated or the night before
- Keep morning options simple (yogurt tubes, pre-filled water bottles, checklists for the win)

3. Parenting from the Floor (Literally)
- Build play areas that don't require standing
- Make reading time, play time, or puzzle time horizontal bonding
- Lap parenting counts. So does couch supervision. Your presence is powerful, not posture-dependent

4. The Screen-Time Sanity Clause
- Screens are not the enemy. Guilt is.
- Educational, entertaining, or just a moment to let your heart rate drop — screen time is a bridge to survive the day
- Use it strategically. Schedule it like you would a medication dose

Delegation: Not a Luxury — A Lifeline
You cannot pour from an empty blood volume.

Task	Delegate To
Driving to school or activities	Partner, neighbor, carpool, ride service
Meal prep	Older kids, partners, grocery delivery, batch cooking days
Errands	Delivery services, list-based helpers
Household chores	Rotating chore chart, yes — even for toddlers

Communication With Kids: Say the Quiet Part Out Loud
You don't need to overshare, but you do need to talk.

Younger kids:
- "Even when I look okay, my body might be having a hard day."
- "I'm resting now so I can play with you later."
- "You can help by being my special assistant today."

Older kids:
- "This is a condition that affects my blood pressure and energy."
- "I may need to sit down quickly or cancel plans — it's not about you."
- "Your help really makes a difference."

Kids adapt best when they understand what's happening. You're not burdening them — you're modeling resilience with honesty.

Systems That Keep You Standing (Metaphorically)

Situation	Strategy
Homework time	Snacks + hydration station at the table for you, not just them
Bedtime	Seated reading rituals, audio books when your voice is gone
Meals	Reheatables, paper plates, family-style DIY dinners
Playdates	Host at your place = controlled environment, fewer flares
Outings	Keep go-bags stocked (salt, meds, snacks, wipes, charger)

Tilt Tip: Rituals Save Brainpower

The less you have to think about how to function, the more capacity you save for your kids.

- Weekly breakfast rotation = fewer decisions
- School clothes bins = less chaos
- "Quiet corner" = reset zone for them and you

Simplicity isn't laziness. It's neurologically protective design.

What to Say When Guilt Shows Up

Guilt Thought	Reframe
"I'm not doing enough."	You're doing the work of two systems — yours and your kid's world.
"They'll remember my limitations."	They'll remember your love, creativity, and courage.
"I miss how I used to parent."	That version of you was different, not better.
"They deserve more."	They have you — adapted, present, and resilient. That's enough.

Horizontal Summary –- Tilted Parenting Survival

Domain	Tools That Work
Daily function	Prep while sitting, simplify routines, keep go-bags stocked
Bonding	Floor time, couch rituals, lap parenting, screen time guilt-free
Delegation	Ask for help, use services, rotate responsibilities
Communication	Age-appropriate honesty builds trust and resilience
Emotional survival	Ditch perfection, reframe guilt, celebrate your endurance

Final Thought

You're parenting with a nervous system that misfires on standing, digestion, and emotion regulation — yet you're still here, still showing up, still offering love. Your kids don't need you vertical. They need you present. And you are. That's not just enough — it's heroic.

CHAPTER 11:
TRAVELING WHILE TILTED

Planes, Trains, Cars, and Salt Packets

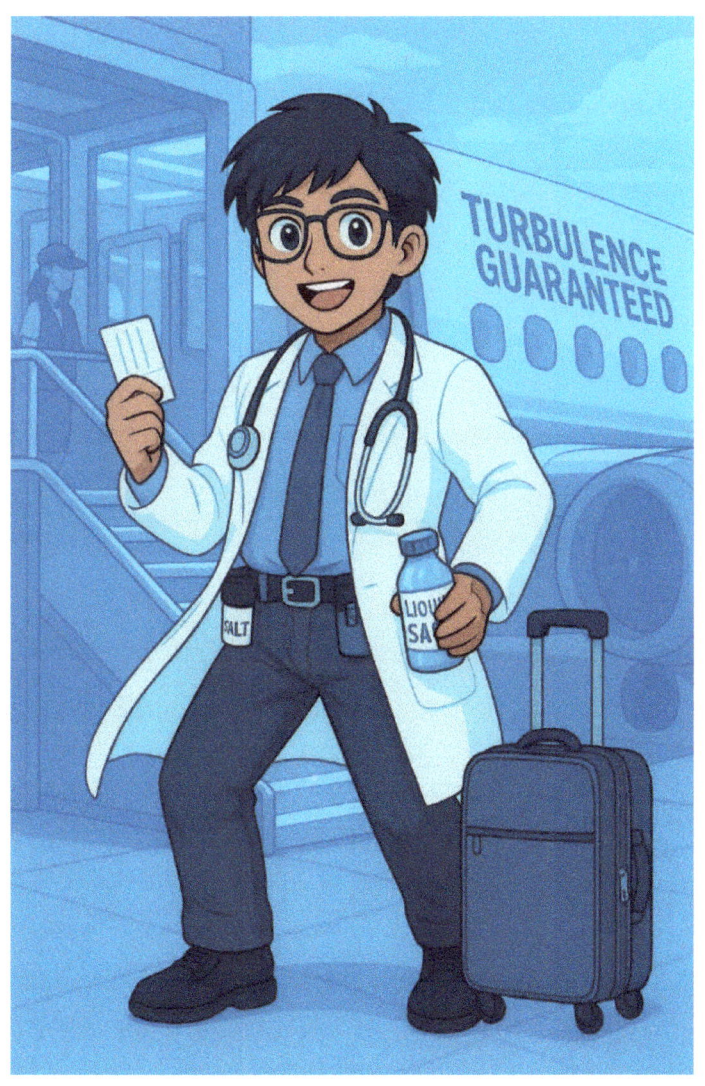

Home life is finally manageable. So obviously it's time to leave it all behind and wrestle compression socks onto a moving train. Here's how to take your condition on the road without sacrificing function (or snacks).

Travel is the gladiator arena of autonomic dysfunction. It's the perfect storm of dehydration, upright time, overstimulation, temperature shifts, unpredictable food, inaccessible bathrooms, schedule changes, and strangers who have opinions about your cooling vest.

But here's the thing: it's possible. Tilted bodies can travel — it just takes more prep, more gear, more hydration, and way more salt than you'd find in a normal carry-on.

This isn't about "pushing through." It's about plotting every leg of the trip like a neurologic heist movie. Let's get tactical.

Pre-Trip Planning: Hydration Begins Before the TSA

Task	Timeline
Increase fluids and electrolytes	Start 24–48 hours before travel
Prep meds	Organize by dose, time zone, and emergency extras
Compression gear	Pack + wear during transit days
Cooling/heating tools	Neck wraps, vests, portable fans, hand warmers

Task	Timeline
Documentation	Travel letter for TSA, meds, mobility gear, and disability assistance
Route planning	Know where elevators, bathrooms, and exits are ahead of time
Request accommodations	Wheelchair service, pre-boarding, aisle seats, hotel room with fridge

Tilt Tip: Ask for Help Early — You Deserve It

Airport wheelchair assistance isn't about weakness. It's about efficiency. You can walk. You just shouldn't waste all your blood pressure doing it before a three-hour flight in an aluminum cylinder with no leg room and a cabin pressure that thinks you're at 8,000 feet.

Packing for the Tilted Traveler

The "If I Don't Pack This, I Will Definitely Regret It" List:

- Salt packets, ORS (oral rehydration solution), electrolyte powders
- Meds + extras (plus a printed list in case of emergency)
- Neck fan, cooling cloths/vest, or heating pads
- Compression socks or abdominal binder
- Snacks: high-protein, salty, non-perishable
- Refillable water bottle
- Documentation for mobility aids, meds, and any official diagnoses

- Change of clothes (sweat + travel delays = wardrobe drama)
- Pulse oximeter, BP cuff, or smartwatch with vitals tracking
- Sunglasses, earplugs, noise-canceling headphones
- Foldable cane seat or travel stool
- Distraction tools: books, movies, playlists, anything to keep your nervous system entertained and mildly sedated

Transit Strategy by Mode of Travel
Road Trips

Challenge	Tilt Solution
Sitting too long	Schedule stops every 60–90 minutes to stretch, lie down, hydrate
Heat and sunlight	Sunshades, cooling vest, ice packs under thighs
Dehydration	Salt snacks + electrolyte drinks — sip constantly
Fatigue crash	Rotate drivers, don't fight flares — rest as needed for the win

Air Travel

Phase	Tilt Strategy
Check-in	Use mobility services, ask for early boarding
Security	Bring a TSA letter if you're bringing meds or devices

Phase	Tilt Strategy
In flight	Compression gear, hydration, salty snacks, neck support
Mid-air flares	Recline if possible, breathe slow, cold compress on chest/neck, portable O2 concentrator (yes, really; don't be shy)
Arrival	Hydrate immediately, give yourself rest time — not straight to activity

Tilt Break: Airplanes, Oxygen, and That Thing Where You Can't Sit Upright

So you're 36,000 feet in the air, trying to look like a normal traveler, but your autonomic nervous system has other plans. Why? Because airplane cabins are pressurized to the equivalent of about 8,000 feet of altitude — meaning lower oxygen saturation levels even for people without chronic illness. For those of us with dysautonomia, that mild hypoxia can be the straw that breaks the baroreceptor's back.

Translation: The air's thinner, your blood volume's already sketchy, and your body's trying to run uphill on fumes. Add in dehydration, prolonged sitting, and that delightful cabin air dryer than your humor, and you've got a recipe for lightheadedness, tachycardia, and the sudden need to be horizontal immediately.

Trains & Public Transit

- Pick seats near bathrooms or exits
- Use folding stool if standing is required

- Hydrate continuously but cautiously (bathroom access matters)
- Avoid rush hour crowds whenever possible
- Wear a sign if you're feeling spicy: "Ask me about my low blood pressure."

Accommodations: Make Hotels Work for You

Feature	Why It Helps
Fridge/microwave	Meds, electrolyte drinks, snacks = lifeline
Elevator access	Obvious reasons
Near front of building	Less walking = more blood in your brain
Climate control	You need thermostat power — non-negotiable
Blackout curtains	Sensory control, sleep, and recovery

Tilt Tip: Strategic hospitality with a side of self-respect

Ask ahead for early check-in or late checkout. Explain your medical needs without shame. You're not being difficult — you're protecting your function.

Science Snapshot

Postural intolerance during travel is common in dysautonomia due to prolonged seated time, hypovolemia, and environmental stressors. Prehydration and compression reduce in-transit symptom severity.

— Raj et al., 2005; Grubb et al., 2008

Translation: You need salt, compression, and the power to recline on demand.

What to Expect Post-Travel: The Flare Tax

You may feel okay during the trip — adrenaline is tricky like that. The crash usually comes 12–48 hours after arrival. Plan accordingly.

- Block recovery time into your itinerary
- Schedule low-effort days on either side of travel
- Don't put away your salt-stained compression gear yet — you'll need it

Horizontal Summary –- Tilted Travel Toolkit

Phase	Strategy
Before	Pre-hydrate, pack gear, request assistance, plan routes
During	Compression, salt, hydration, break up movement
After	Build in rest days, monitor flares, replenish fluids

Final Thought

You're not a high-maintenance traveler — you're a high-efficiency strategist with a malfunctioning autopilot and a talent for packing enough salt to season an entire cruise buffet.

Tilted travel is an act of rebellion. You're not staying home just because your nervous system is annoying. You're taking your dysfunction on tour — strategically, salty, and gloriously unbothered by side-eyes at the airport.

CHAPTER 12:
ROMANCE, DATING, AND OTHER FORMS OF CARDIOVASCULAR EXERCISE

*Tilted Hearts, Real Talk, and Managing Love
When You're Managing Flares*

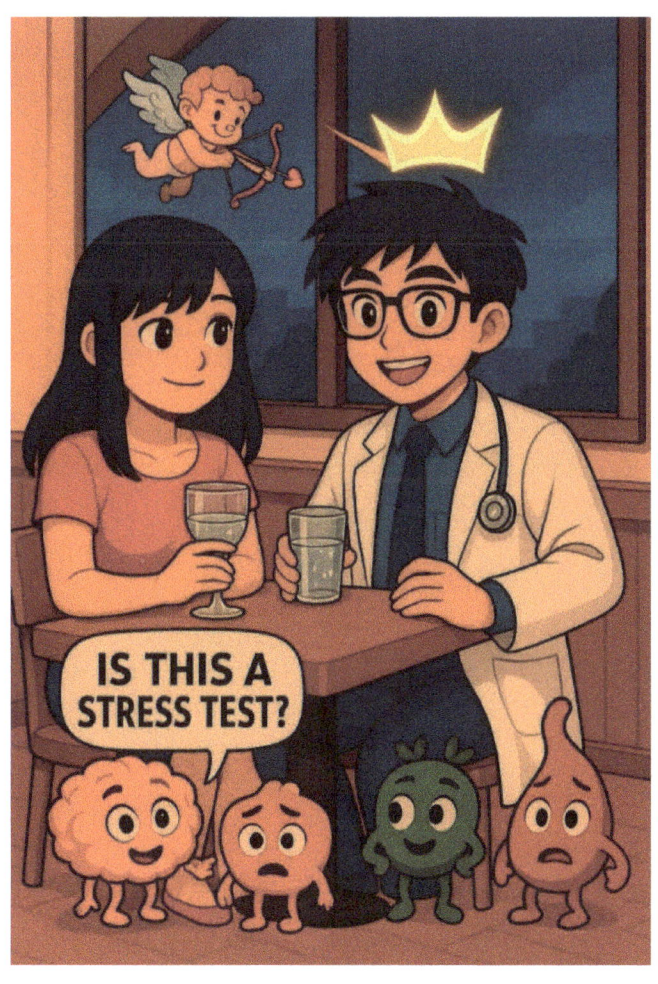

You've explained your condition to family, friends, doctors, and flight attendants. Now it's time to explain it to someone you'd like to share more than just your electrolyte packets with. Spoiler: it's possible — and maybe even worth it.

Dysautonomia doesn't just affect your circulation. It affects your relationships. When your nervous system declares mutiny, your social life, romantic partnerships, and confidence often get caught in the crossfire.

Because let's be honest: it's hard to connect when your vagus nerve might stage a protest mid-sentence. And date night gets a little complicated when standing in line gives you tachycardia, your GI tract schedules surprise performances, or your energy budget evaporates after putting on socks.

This chapter isn't about fixing your love life. It's about navigating your social circles with honesty, humor, and the knowledge that connection doesn't require perfection. It requires presence, boundaries, and maybe an emergency salt packet in your wallet.

Let's Start With the Truth: Chronic Illness Changes the Rules

Romantic or otherwise, every relationship you maintain while managing dysautonomia asks you to communicate better, expect flexibly, and love yourself radically.

You're not a burden. You're a person with a high-maintenance nervous system — and a whole lot of insight.

Science Snapshot
Chronic illness often leads to role redefinition in relationships, requiring explicit communication, recalibration of expectations, and adaptive intimacy.
— *Martire et al., 2010; Rolland, 1994*

Translation: Love with dysautonomia isn't less than. It's just built differently.

The Tilted Dating Landscape
Dating while Tilted is like trying to schedule a moon landing using a calendar and your own blood pressure.

Common Challenges:

Challenge	Tilt Translation
Unpredictable energy	"Let's hang out — unless my heart rate says no."
Weird symptoms	"I promise I'm interested. I'm just sweating through my shirt while seated."
Standing in lines / venues	"Can we skip standing and go straight to the part where we sit and talk forever?"
GI flares mid-date	"I'd love to get dinner, as long as my stomach isn't staging a rebellion."
Flirting with brain fog	"Sorry, I blanked on your name. Again. Not because I'm aloof. Because — neurons."

Tips for Dating While Managing Dysautonomia

1. Be Clear — Not Apologetic

"Hey, just so you know, I have a condition that makes heat, standing, and sudden movements… complicated. I promise I'm not a diva. I'm just trying to keep my blood pressure out of the dirt."

You're not being high-maintenance. You're offering a user manual.

2. Choose the Right Environments

- Sit-down cafes > crowded clubs
- Daytime hangs > late-night fatigue crashes
- BYO snacks and salt if needed — no shame
- "Binge-watching and low-stim lounging" is a totally legitimate first date

3. Schedule Around Your Autonomic Curve

Plan dates during your best-functioning hours. Don't let social norms dictate nighttime romance if your body clocks out at 7:30 p.m. with a migraine and tachycardia.

Communication Is the Relationship Hack

Even in long-term partnerships, Tilt requires communication that's frequent, clear, and ego-free.

Topic	How to Talk About It
Flares	"When I suddenly need to lie down, it's not personal. It's tactical."
Sexual health	"I may need breaks, different pacing, or alternate forms of intimacy. Let's figure that out together."

Topic	How to Talk About It
Energy	"If I cancel, I'm not flaking. I'm preserving function."
Support	"You don't need to fix me. Just be with me while I manage this."

Sex and Dysautonomia: Yes, We're Going There

Because surprise syncope isn't exactly romantic.

Sex can be affected by:
- Fatigue (sometimes even before clothes are off)
- Tachycardia (not the fun kind)
- BP drops (horizontal is helpful, but not always enough)
- GI issues (bloating and nausea are rarely foreplay)
- Pain, dryness, or sensory overload

Solutions? Yes. Creativity is your co-pilot here.

Concern	Adaptation
Position-related dizziness	Lying on your back with legs elevated (romantic and practical)
Overexertion	Take breaks, hydrate before/after, slow pacing
Vaginal dryness or pain	Lube, hormonal support, pelvic floor therapy
Low libido	Address fatigue, meds, and mood before blaming interest
Dysautonomic flares during sex	Pre-load salt/hydration, communicate, pause if needed

Tilt Tip: Intimacy Isn't Just Physical

Touch, conversation, shared space — these are all forms of closeness.

Redefine intimacy on your terms. Sex is one tool, not the full relationship toolbox.

Horizontal Summary –- Tilted Relationship Survival

Domain	Strategy
Dating	Choose calm venues, communicate early, schedule smart
Communication	Be honest, don't apologize, frame things clearly
Intimacy	Adapt, hydrate, slow down, redefine
Support	Offer presence, flexibility, and snacks
Self-Compassion	You're not too much — you're just neurologically complex

Final Thought

Love, connection, and intimacy aren't off-limits just because your nervous system is running a side rebellion. You don't need to be symptom-free to be desirable, lovable, or enough. Tilted love isn't weaker. It's wiser. It's slower, deeper, and forged in the fires of flexibility and radical communication.

You are a masterpiece in motion, with a nervous system that writes its own love story. You're a romantically-inclined autonomic acrobat. And if that's not sexy, we don't know what is.

CHAPTER 13:
RELATIONSHIPS, BOUNDARIES, AND THE PEOPLE WHO LOVE YOU (EVEN WHEN YOU'RE HORIZONTAL)

Social Survival Strategies for the Tilted Life

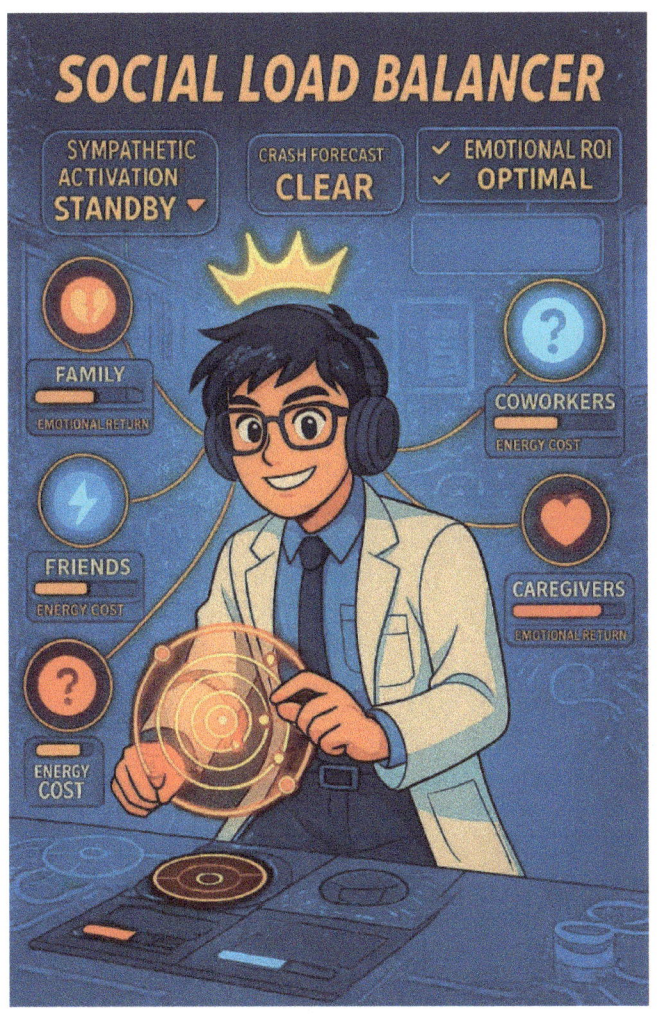

Chronic illness doesn't just change your heart rate. It changes your social velocity. You cancel plans. You pace conversations like workouts. You spend an hour psyching yourself up to return a text, and another recovering from the effort. Welcome to Tilted Social Engineering — where connection meets cardiovascular compromise and relationships are filtered through a new gravitational algorithm. But make no mistake: this isn't about loss. It's about curation.

This chapter is about friendship, family, caregiving, work dynamics, and finding your crew when your energy is on a rationed drip and your social calendar looks like a defragmented hard drive.

The Energy Cost of Being a Person

Relationships take stamina. You, strategically speaking, are on a different energy economy. When other people swipe a card, you're trading a rare crystal.

Everything has an energetic cost:

- Answering a text = one salt tab.
- Small talk at a party = two units of brain fog.
- Hosting a friend = pre- and post-exertional malaise with a social hangover garnish.

You can absolutely maintain deep, meaningful relationships. You just have to be smarter, faster, and more tactical about it than most people ever need to be. Welcome to the advanced class in Tilted connection management.

Tilted Translation — What You Say vs. What You Mean

You Say	You Mean	They Often Think
"I'm having a low-energy day"	My body is rerouting blood to stay conscious	You're flaking again
"I need to cancel"	I hit a physiological red line and I'm saving the crash	You don't care about this plan
"I'm managing some symptoms"	I just navigated autonomic sabotage without an ambulance	You're being dramatic
"I'm fine"	I have a 3-hour recovery plan and an ice pack under this hoodie	You're totally better now, right?

Helping people understand your reality is generous. Repeating yourself to those who refuse to listen is not your job.

Family: The Original Tilted Support Group (Terms and Conditions Apply)

Families can be wonderful. They can also be relentless, confused, patronizing, or missing entirely. Sometimes all at once. They are your genetic fan club, but that doesn't mean they come with a user manual for dysautonomia.

Common Family Archetypes

Character Type	Defining Behavior	Your Move
The Fixer	Sends 47 articles about turmeric and vagus nerve resets	"Thanks for caring—my treatment is already in progress"
The Skeptic	"You don't look sick"	"Invisible ≠ imaginary. Here's a journal article"
The Over-Helper	Hovers, pities, takes over basic tasks	"I appreciate the help, but I still need to function"
The Vanisher	Drops off the map when things get real	Let them go. Invite those who show up
The Rock	Listens, learns, adapts	Clone immediately if possible

You're not here to perform wellness for their comfort. You're building boundaries, not resentment.

Friends: Who Gets a Seat on the Tilt Couch?

Illness clarifies friendship faster than a holiday group trip in a shared rental cabin. Some will rise to the occasion. Some will politely fade. A few will imply you're ghosting them when your blood pressure is the one doing all the disappearing.

Tilt-Compatible Friend Green Flags:
- "Want to hang out horizontally and eat salty snacks?"
- Understands you're not canceling *on them*, you're canceling *for survival*.
- Doesn't make your condition the center of every interaction.

Friendship Upgrades That Work:
- Low-pressure invites: "Drop by if you're up for it."
- Parallel play: side-by-side scrolling, crafting, or binge-watching.
- Long text gaps with zero guilt.

Social Energy ROI Audit

Interaction Type	Energy Output	Emotional Return	Worth It?
Group dinner (upright)	High	Mixed	Rarely
Movie night on couch	Low	High	Yes
Video chat with closed captions	Medium	High	Often
Friendship check-in via meme	Minimal	Moderate	Absolutely

The key is not to isolate. The key is to design your social life like a mobility aid — with precision and personal engineering.

Caregivers: Support Without the Side of Guilt

Caregivers, bless them, are often unpaid emotional paramedics. Whether it's a spouse, a sibling, or a friend-turned-medical-logistics-officer, this role gets complicated quickly.

Keep it mutual. Keep it transparent. Keep it adult.
You can need help and still be in charge of your life. You can accept assistance and still define the terms. Communicate early and often:

- "I need support, not control."
- "It helps when you ask before stepping in."
- "Please don't narrate my symptoms to other people. Especially at brunch."

They don't need to be perfect. They need to be consistent. And you both need space to not talk about dysautonomia sometimes.

Tilt Tip: Supporting a Tilted Partner — A Mini-Guide for the Normotensive

To the loved ones reading this: You don't need to be a hero. You need to be curious, calm, and willing to adjust the plan when gravity does something rude.

Support Move	Why It Helps
Ask, don't assume	"What would help right now?" is gold
Offer seating, shade, snacks	Makes a Tilted person feel safe and seen

Support Move	Why It Helps
Don't minimize symptoms	"You don't look sick" is not a compliment
Learn their rhythms	Know the crash times, the triggers, the tells
Make space for adaptation	Flexibility is the language of love in dysautonomia

Workplace Realities: Functioning in Public with Tactical Stealth

You've got choices:

- Disclose your condition and request accommodation.
- Say nothing and juggle the aftermath in a bathroom stall.
- Somewhere in between, with a modulated persona and a contingency plan.

Reasonable Accommodations to Consider:
- Flexible schedules
- Remote work or hybrid setups
- Rest breaks for recumbence
- Modified lighting or seating

Tilt Tip: You don't owe capitalism your nervous system

Your productivity doesn't define your worth. But strategic adjustments can help you be more productive with fewer crashes.

Accommodations That Aren't Special Treatment — They're Standard Engineering

Issue	Accommodation Example	Justification
Fatigue spikes	Flexible work hours	Prevent post-exertional crashes
Temperature sensitivity	Personal fan, seat near AC	Thermoregulation failure is real
Orthostatic intolerance	Sit/stand desk, reclined breaks	Blood pooling, cognitive drop
Cognitive fog	Written follow-ups after meetings	Retention lags ≠ comprehension failure

Needing support doesn't mean you're fragile. It means you're proactive.

Building Community Without Burnout

You don't need a dozen friends. You need the right two. Maybe three. And if one of them is your physical therapist and the other is a dog, that still counts.

Connection Strategies That Respect Tilted Capacity:
- Set recurring "low-energy" hangouts with no pressure.
- Join a support group with clear moderation rules.
- Create your own Tilt Crew: people who understand your needs and show up anyway.

You are allowed to be selective. That's not withdrawal — it's curation.

Science Snapshot

High-quality relationships correlate with lower inflammatory markers, improved parasympathetic tone, and better emotional regulation in chronic illness. Social stress, on the other hand, activates the same sympathetic pathways as physical illness, compounding autonomic symptoms.

— Uchino, B.N. (2006). Social support and health: Physiological processes underlying links to disease outcomes. Journal of Behavioral Medicine, 29(4), 377–387.

Translation: Stressful people trigger sympathetic surges. Supportive ones act like medicine. Choose accordingly.

Horizontal Summary -- Relationship Engineering for the Tilted

Guiding Principle	Practical Strategy
Boundaries are healthy	Clarify limits without apology
Fewer people, deeper roots	Choose quality over obligation
Honesty protects energy	Share your reality once, then conserve explanations
Inter-dependence > independence	Accept help without surrendering control
Connection = strategic medicine	Invest where the return outweighs the crash

Tilt Break: Who Stays, Who Fades, and What That Tells You

Chronic illness has a brutal way of auditing your contact list. The good news? The ones who stay are the real deal. They'll pivot, check in, and learn how to love you on the days when "love" looks like bringing compression socks and not expecting you to stand up while wearing them.

The rest? Let them fade. Your nervous system isn't the only thing recalibrating — your standards are too.

Final Thought

You are managing a system-wide protocol with precision, grit, and social intelligence most people never need to develop. Your people will find you — through the pauses, the missed events, the recalibrated invitations. And they'll stay, not in spite of your reality, but because they recognize your strength. This is your network. Not built in speed, but built in trust. Tilt-tested and top-tier.

PART IV:
SYSTEMIC TILT DISRUPTION

Healthcare Systems, Bureaucratic Red Tape, and You, the Glorious Outlier

CHAPTER 14:
CHRONIC ILLNESS IN THE AGE OF ALGORITHMS

Online Myths, Misinformation, and the Tyranny of the Wellness Influencer

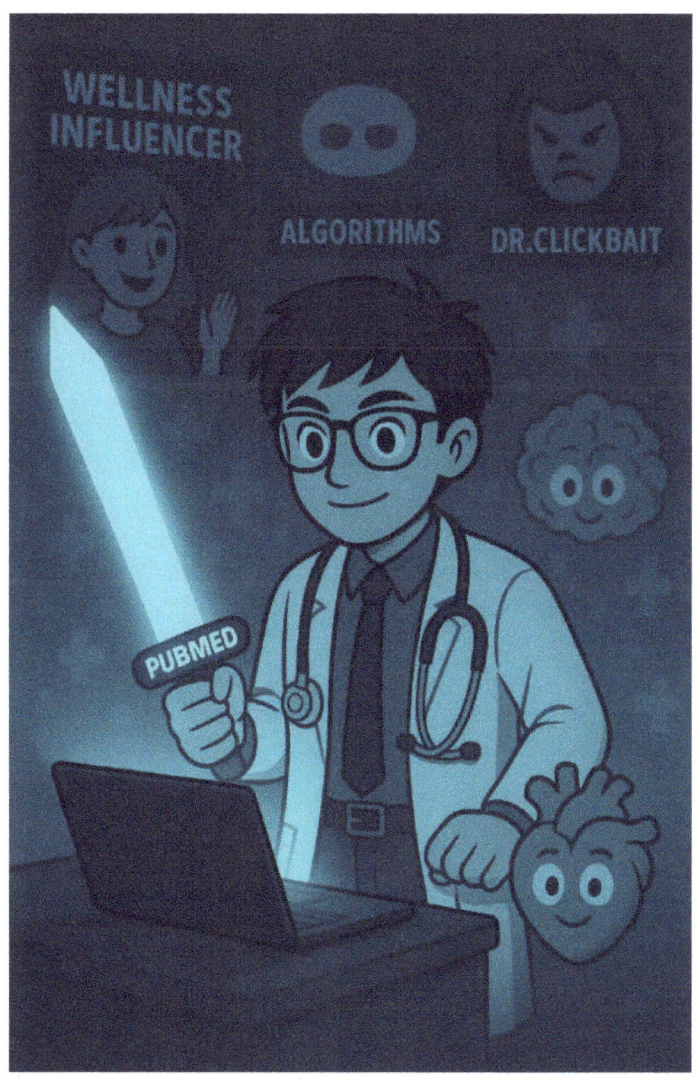

You've curated your lifestyle with care. Then the algorithm offered an endless parade of strangers recommending smoothies, saunas, and spiritual detox. Let's talk about filters — both digital and mental.

Once upon a time, managing chronic illness meant listening to your doctor, reading the occasional medical journal, and exchanging weary nods in waiting rooms.

Now? You log onto social media and immediately encounter:

- An influencer selling Himalayan salt lamps to "reset your vagus nerve"
- A random social media post claiming Amla extract cures POTS
- A subreddit full of medical refugees diagnosing each other with esoteric gene mutations
- And at least three people telling you it's all trauma, vibes, or candida

Welcome to the algorithmic age of illness. Where search engines think "natural cure for dizziness" means "drink celery juice," and everyone with a ring light is an expert.

Let's break down what's helpful, what's harmful, and how to stay grounded when your social media page looks possessed.

Why the Internet Is a Tilted Minefield

- **Information overload** = constant contradiction
- **Algorithmic bias** = the loudest (not the most accurate) gets seen

- **Conflicting advice** = "Try everything" becomes "Trust nothing"
- **Wellness culture** = sells shame disguised as empowerment
- **Medical trauma** = makes people vulnerable to pseudoscience

You're not paranoid. You're navigating a landscape built to sell, not to serve.

Science Snapshot

Digital health misinformation, particularly around chronic illness, increases emotional distress and decreases adherence to evidence-based care. Social media amplifies health anxiety and confounds decision-making for complex conditions.

— Chou et al., 2018; Wang et al., 2021

Translation: You're not failing. You're being bombarded with bad advice framed by good lighting.

Spotting Tilted Misinformation in the Wild

Red Flag	What It Usually Means
"Cures all chronic illness"	Marketing, not medicine
"Doctors don't want you to know this"	Weaponized mistrust
"It's all trauma"	Oversimplification that ignores physiology
"You just need to detox"	Translation: expensive supplements incoming
"One protocol for everyone"	Dysautonomia is not a one-size disaster
"Eliminate 43 food groups"	Orthorexia disguised as health

But… What About Patient Communities?

They're real. They're valuable. They're lifesaving.

Online communities can:

- Validate your experience
- Offer workarounds and hacks
- Share provider recommendations
- Provide data in the absence of research
- Be the only place where someone gets it — and gets *you*, too

Just remember — shared experience is not universal expertise. Your body still gets the final vote.

The Wellness-Industrial Complex: Profits, Not Progress

There's a whole industry that thrives on your desperation.

They sell:

- Overpriced magnesium sprays
- Unregulated cleanses
- Genetic tests that explain nothing but sound important
- Fancy vagus nerve devices that might as well be dog shock collars
- "Health coaches" who read half a blog and now want to charge $400/hour for energy alignment

Tilt Tip: Your mitochondria don't need a brand ambassador

If the cure fits in a bottle, costs $199.99, and promises detox, optimization, and rebirth — walk away. You're not a marketing target. You're a person.

When Influencers Get It Right
Some folks are legit. You'll know them because they:

- Acknowledge nuance
- Share their personal journey without making it gospel
- Cite science or link to reputable sources
- Encourage dialogue, not dogma
- Say "this worked for me" instead of "this will work for you"

Bookmark them. Follow them. Send them salty appreciation messages.

How to Vet Health Info Online Without Going Full Tinfoil Hat
Ask these five questions:

1. Who is this person, and what are their credentials?
2. Are they selling something?
3. Do they cite actual research or only anecdote?
4. Does this advice sound like it supports your autonomy — or shame you for being sick?
5. Is it too good to be true? (Spoiler: it probably is.)

Tilt Tip: Your Lived Experience Is Valid, But Not Infinitely Transferable
Just because something helped someone on social media doesn't mean it will help you. And just because something didn't work for you doesn't mean you did it wrong. You're not the glitch. You're a complex system experimenting under pressure.

How to Use the Internet Without Getting Flattened

Goal	Smart Strategy
Find providers	Use support groups + clinic reviews, then cross-check credentials
Research meds/treatments	Use PubMed, Mayo Clinic, Medscape, academic centers
Find community	Join disease-specific groups, forums, Discord servers
Avoid burnout	Set time limits, unfollow high-drama accounts, unplug periodically
Log symptoms	Use trusted apps — not a post on your ex's cousin's essential oils blog

Horizontal Summary –- Algorithm Armor

Threat	Countermove
Bad advice	Vet sources, verify with clinicians
Overwhelm	Limit exposure, curate your feed
Toxic positivity	Choose realistic support, not perfection theater
Medical mistrust	Channel it into better questions, not conspiracies
Pseudoscience	Ask for citations, not testimonials

Final Thought

The internet is not your doctor. It's not your therapist. And it's definitely not your autonomic nervous system whisperer. But it can be a lifeline — if you use it like a tool, not a truth oracle.

Stay skeptical. Stay informed. Stay curious. You're not closed-minded for protecting your peace. You're being strategic in a world that monetizes your confusion.

You're not here for clicks. You're here to survive. And survive you shall — one algorithm-proof boundary at a time.

CHAPTER 15:
INSURANCE, PAPERWORK, AND BUREAUCRATIC GASLIGHTING

Why the System Isn't Built for Tilted Bodies

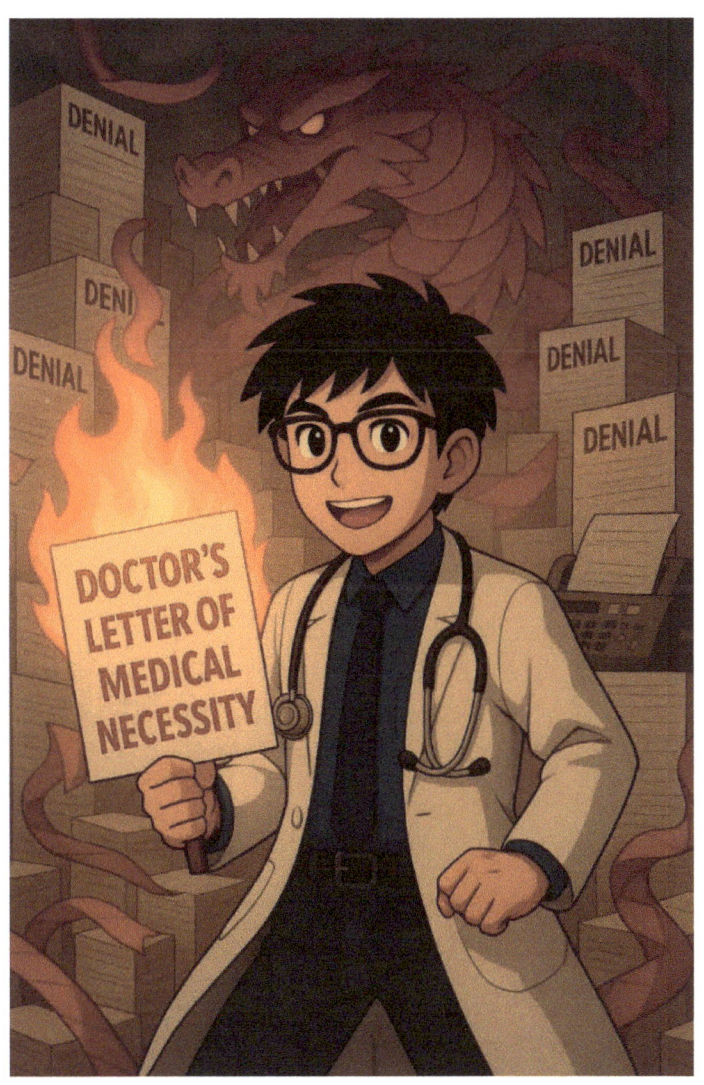

Your symptoms are real. The system just wants proof in triplicate, faxed from a machine last used in 1997. Bureaucracy isn't just paperwork — it's its own chronic condition.

To be clear — it's not just your nervous system malfunctioning. The health care system, insurance industry, and disability process are also structurally dysautonomic — chaotic, unsupportive, prone to collapse under pressure, and riddled with delays and non-responses.

This chapter isn't here to fix the system (you're managing enough revolutions as it is). It's here to equip you with tactical armor — because when the paperwork pile is taller than you and your claim was denied because "you looked fine in your chart," you need more than patience. You need power.

Why It Feels So Personal (Even Though It's Not)
- Invisible illness ≠ visible urgency
- Complex diagnoses ≠ easy CPT codes
- Intermittent function ≠ consistent support
- Fluctuating symptoms ≠ stable forms
- Multi-system flares ≠ single-specialty boxes

You're not being "difficult." The system was built for neat rows of symptoms, rapid recoveries, and binary logic. You are none of those things.

Science Snapshot
Chronic illness patients report higher rates of delayed diagnoses, treatment denials, and administrative burden compared to acute illness patients, leading to worsened outcomes and care avoidance.

— Himmelstein et al., 2015; Zia et al., 2020

Translation: You're not imagining the red tape. It's actively tangling you on purpose.

The Insurance Maze: Why They Always Say No First

Their Move	What It Means
"We don't cover that medication"	Try three cheaper ones that won't work first
"It's not medically necessary"	We don't understand your condition, so we default to denial
"Request more documentation"	We're hoping you'll get tired and stop trying
"Your labs are normal"	We don't know what dysautonomia is, and we didn't ask

This isn't about logic. It's about stalling. Insurance companies don't share their rules upfront — they wait for you to apply, deny you, and then act shocked you didn't meet their invisible criteria. They count on fatigue, confusion, and overwhelming paperwork to save them money.

Your Tools: Words, Records, and Weaponized Organization
1. Medical Records = Receipts
Keep everything:
- Test results
- Visit summaries
- Letters from specialists
- Diagnosis codes
- Vital signs logs
- ER visit summaries
- Tilt test printouts
- Photos of flares (if appropriate)

Keep both digital and physical backups. Name your files like a CEO. Color-code your binders like a survivalist.

2. Letters Matter (Even When No One Reads Them)
Request these:

- Letter of medical necessity (for meds, mobility aids, accommodations)
- Detailed diagnosis letters (for work, school, insurance)
- Provider notes listing specific functional impairments
- List of failed prior treatments (for appeal leverage)

Navigating Disability Claims Without Losing Your Will to Function
Whether it's short-term leave, long-term disability (LTD), or Social Security Disability Insurance (SSDI), the process is built to confuse you.

Concept	Translation
"You're applying for function loss, not a disease"	"Dysautonomia" is not enough — describe what you can't do
"Assume initial denial"	It's not about you. It's about the system testing attrition
"Documentation is everything"	The more objective data, the harder they have to work to say "no"
"Language matters"	"Fatigue" sounds subjective. "Inability to sustain upright posture for >30 min without syncope" sounds like a limitation they can't ignore

When Doctors Don't Understand the Forms (or You)

Some doctors are amazing. Others?

Their Response	What It Signals
"I don't do disability paperwork"	They don't understand your condition or your needs
"But you're so articulate"	Classic gaslighting — intelligence ≠ function
"You don't look sick"	Their diagnostic lens is broken
"Let's wait and see"	They don't understand how fast this impacts your life

Solution: Ask clearly, calmly, and with prepared templates. Bring them example language. Offer to send documentation to copy. Make it easy for them to say "yes."

Tilt Tip: Drag Your Doctor Into the Future (Gently)

With the advent of AI, there is no reason your physician can't complete forms and/or write letters specifically tailored to your situation. You may need to remind them the internet has evolved a lot since dial up modems.

How to Appeal Like a Tilted Lawyer

- Request written denial with specific reasons
- Gather counter-evidence (labs, notes, letters, HR logs)
- Write an appeal that rebuts each denial point with data
- Have your doctor co-sign if possible
- Submit by certified mail or portal with confirmation
- Use the magic phrases: "functional impairment," "objective clinical findings," and "risk of exacerbation without treatment"

Tilt Tip: You're Not Begging — You're Documenting a Dysfunction.

There's no shame in requesting what you need to survive. The only shame is in how hard they make you fight for it.

When to Hire Help

- **Social Security Disability:** Consider legal assistance early
- **Long-Term Disability (LTD):** Many policies have traps — get advice before applying
- **Health insurance appeals:** Patient advocates or case managers can help
- **School accommodations:** Ask for a 504 plan or IEP if relevant

You don't have to know the law. You just have to know when to outsource the battle.

Horizontal Summary -- Tilted Bureaucracy Survival Kit

Battle	Tool
Insurance denial	Letters, documentation, repeat appeals
Disability claim	Detail function loss, not diagnosis alone
Doctor confusion	Educate, bring templates, don't apologize
Burnout	Pace yourself, get help, rest between rounds
Organization	Binders, folders, app-based trackers

Final Thought

You're not crazy for being frustrated over a denial letter. You're exhausted. You've been navigating a system that rewards opacity and punishes honesty. And you're still in the fight.

This is not just paperwork. It's access to care, to medication, to mobility, to basic human dignity. And every form you submit, every appeal you write, every binder you assemble is an act of defiance.

You're not just surviving dysautonomia. You're surviving bureaucracy — with receipts, stamina, and righteous rage.

CHAPTER 16:
HOW TO TALK TO DOCTORS WITHOUT LOSING YOUR MIND

Translating Tilt Into Medicalese
Without Primal Screaming in the Parking Lot

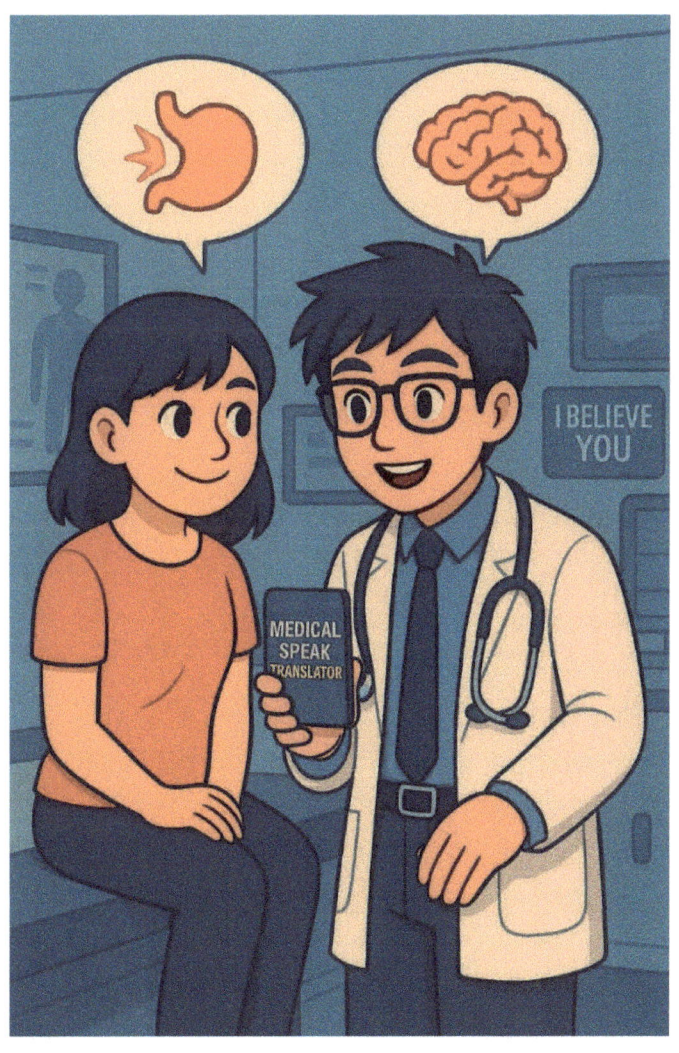

You've got notes, a list, and three minutes of polite stamina. They've got one hand on the doorknob and a checklist. Here's how to speak fluent autonomic dysfunction with calm efficiency.

Talking to doctors about dysautonomia is a bit like speed-dating in a foreign language. You get ten minutes to summarize a lifetime of symptoms, translate your lived experience into jargon, and hope the person in the white coat doesn't mistake your vocabulary for wellness.

You've likely already heard the classics:

- "Your labs are normal."
- "It's probably anxiety."
- "But your heart looks fine."
- "Try more water and exercise."

And after the third shrug and second specialist dismissal, you start questioning your sanity.

Let's fix that. Not the broken system — but your ability to navigate it without losing your grip on dignity, salt, or the last shred of your executive function.

Why It's Not Just You: The System Isn't Designed for Dysautonomia

Reality	System Bias
Multi-system illness	Referral ping-pong to disconnected specialties
Normal labs	Assumed wellness, not invisible dysfunction

Reality	System Bias
Smart articulate patient	"Too functional" to be truly ill
New symptoms each visit	Labeled as inconsistent or somatic

You're not "difficult." You're uncontainable in a 15-minute office visit box.

Science Snapshot

Patients with chronic, complex, or invisible conditions report higher rates of diagnostic delay, dismissal, and psychologizing by providers, especially when female, nonwhite, or neurodivergent.

— Werner & Malterud, 2003; Blease et al., 2017

Translation: If it feels like you're being gaslit, it's because you probably are.

What Doctors Hear vs. What You Mean

Let's rewrite your symptoms into phrases that make the clinician's diagnostic radar ping instead of flatlining.

What You Say	What They Hear	What To Say Instead
"I feel weird when I stand up."	Vague, non-specific	"My heart rate jumps 40 bpm when I stand for more than a minute."

What You Say	What They Hear	What To Say Instead
"I'm dizzy all the time."	Possibly psychogenic	"I experience orthostatic lightheadedness that resolves when lying down."
"I'm so tired."	Lifestyle issue	"I experience non-restorative fatigue and post-exertional crashes that last 24–48 hours."
"Everything hurts."	Fibromyalgia trope	"I have widespread pain that flares with temperature, stress, and activity."
"Nothing helps."	Helplessness	"I've tried X, Y, Z. Here's what's worked slightly, and here's what worsens it."

You're not being dramatic. You're building clinical credibility. One pre-phrased sentence at a time.

Tilt Tip: Bring a Script — Literally

If your brain fogs in the clinic, bring notes. Bullet points. Symptom timelines. Vitals logs. Your words don't need to be spontaneous — they need to be accurate. Bonus points if you print them out and hand them over with the impenetrable calm of a cat watching a house burn that it definitely set on fire.

How to Build a Productive Appointment

- **Have a clear agenda.** Know what you're there for. Prioritize 1–2 key goals.
- **Bring your data.** Logs, test results, BP/HR charts, med trials, symptom trackers.
- **Open strong.** "I'm managing a form of dysautonomia. I've tracked my symptoms and responses. I'd like to share a brief summary."
- **Redirect when dismissed.** "I've been evaluated for anxiety. These symptoms persist despite management. May I walk you through the pattern I've tracked?"
- **End with a plan.** "What are the next steps? Is there a specific goal you're using to monitor improvement or response?"

Scripts for Difficult Moments

When they say "But your tests are normal…"
"Many forms of dysautonomia don't show on routine labs. The dysfunction is in regulation, not structural damage. That's why I brought this HR/BP log to illustrate the pattern."

When they suggest anxiety — again
"I understand why that comes up. But I've experienced panic attacks, and this is different. The onset is positional, not emotional, and improves with fluid and salt — not Xanax."

When they suggest more exercise
"I've tried upright cardio and it triggered a multi-day crash. I'm following a recumbent, graded protocol now. I'd appreciate guidance on pacing and monitoring."

If You're Masking Too Well

Some of us show up too coherent. Too clean. Too dressed. Too composed. If your function is inconsistent but your communication is sharp, consider saying:

"I tend to perform well in short bursts, especially in structured environments. But I crash after appointments and need hours — or days — to recover. Please take that into account when assessing my functional baseline."

Tilt Tip: You're Allowed to Fire a Doctor

If someone makes you feel dismissed, disrespected, or gaslit — Leave. You are not a difficult patient. You have a complex multi-system illness. And that deserves partnership, not condescension.

How to Find a Dysautonomia-Literate Provider

- Start with patient networks, forums, and support groups
- Look for specialties: Autonomic Neurology, Electrophysiology (EP) cardiology, Complex Internal Medicine, Integrative Physiatry
- Don't be afraid to email ahead and ask if they're familiar with POTS, OH, or autonomic testing
- Telehealth expands your options — use it
- Once again — insert that shameless plug for our clinic right here.

Horizontal Summary -- Tilted Clinic Survival Tactics

Challenge	Strategy
Dismissal	Reframe symptoms in clinical language
Brain fog	Bring notes, data, bullet points
Time crunch	Prioritize top 1–2 concerns
Bad fit	Leave. Fire. Replace. Repeat as needed
Success	Clear goals, clear language, empowered plan

Final Thought

You don't need to impress your doctor. You need to partner with them. You need someone who listens with both ears, thinks beyond the lab orders, and respects your lived expertise.

Until you find that? You show up with notes, science, salt, and the steely calm of someone who's had to explain their existence more times than they've explained their resume.

You're not just navigating medicine. You're translating survival into strategy — and you're doing it with style.

CHAPTER 17:
LIVING WITH CHRONIC UNCERTAINTY

Making Peace with Plot Twists You Didn't Ask For

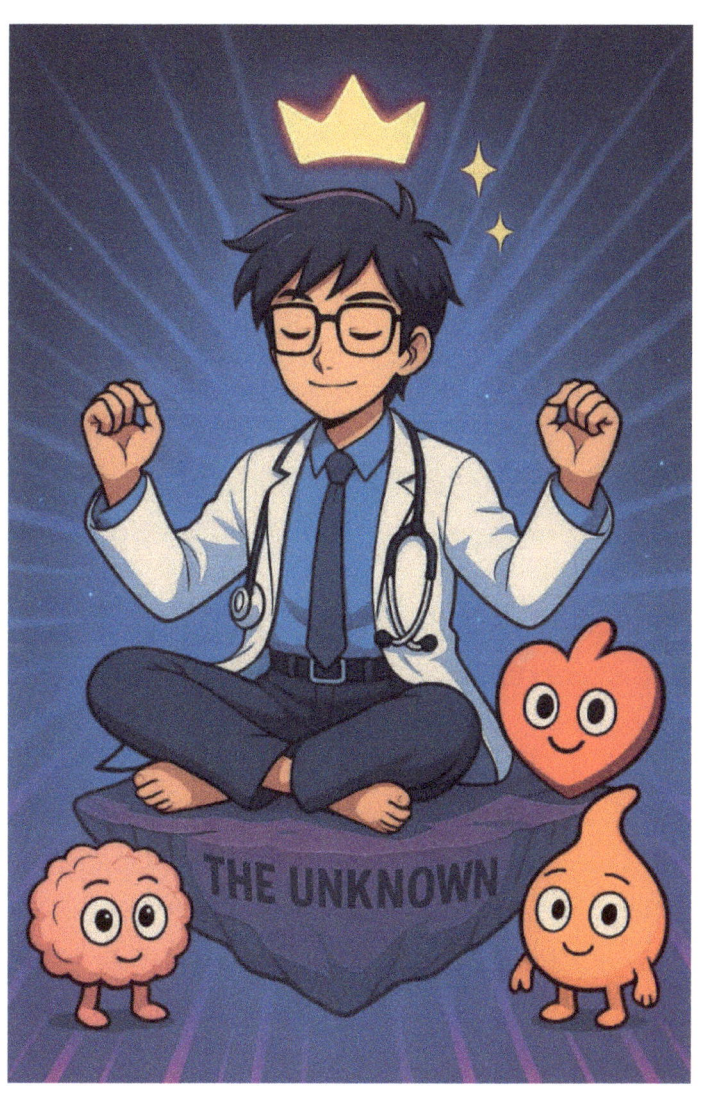

You've followed every plan, ruled out every possibility, and still landed in "we don't know." That's not a setback — it's the starting point for living anyway. This chapter is about moving forward when clarity isn't coming.

There's no sugar-coating this — one of the hardest parts of living with dysautonomia isn't the tachycardia, the nausea, or the inconvenient fainting episodes. It's the not knowing.

Not knowing when the next flare will hit. Not knowing if today will be functional or horizontal. Not knowing if this medication will help — or backfire. Not knowing what the future looks like with a body that won't commit to consistency.

Chronic uncertainty is a full-time co-pilot. And while you can't evict it, you can learn to live beside it — without letting it drive.

This Is the Part No One Prepares You For

Medicine talks a lot about symptoms. It talks less about ambiguity.

There's no set timeline for recovery. No roadmap for how long you'll feel like this. No contract that says, "If you do everything right, your nervous system will behave."

Which means: your new skill set isn't just medical. It's emotional.

You're learning to function without clarity. To rest without guilt. To celebrate stability without fearing relapse. To make plans knowing you may cancel them.

That's resilience in its rawest form.

Science Snapshot

Uncertainty in chronic illness correlates strongly with emotional distress, but psychological flexibility—acceptance, reframing, and adaptive behavior—is associated with reduced anxiety and improved quality of life.

— Mishel, 1990; Kashdan & Rottenberg, 2010

Translation: You can't always predict the crash, but you can buffer your emotional whiplash.

Let's Reframe This: Uncertainty Isn't Defeat — It's Flux

Your nervous system doesn't follow a linear healing arc. It's not a staircase. It's a scatter-plot. With flares, rebounds, plateaus, and "Why am I dizzy while eating crackers in a recliner?" moments.

Myth	Reality
"If I find the right treatment, I'll get better and stay better."	Some days will be better. Others will be chaos. The trend matters more than the moment.
"Everyone else has this figured out."	They don't. They're just quieter about their confusion.
"My progress is too slow."	If you're still showing up, you're progressing. Even at 0.5 mph.
"This is all in my head."	Your symptoms are real. Your frustration is real. Your uncertainty is evidence of awareness, not imagination.

Building a Life With Moving Goalposts

Step 1: Ditch the Timeline
There is no fixed recovery date. There is no "normal" to return to. There's only this version of you and what you can build around it.

Step 2: Define Success by Function, Not Fantasy
- "I cooked dinner without crashing" > "I went to a party for 5 hours"
- "I managed my energy well today" > "I did everything on my list"
- "I said no before the crash" > "I pushed through"

Step 3: Separate Your Identity From Your Instability
You are not a flare. You are not your worst day. You are a person with a condition — not a condition with a person trapped inside it.

Tilt Tip: Ritual Beats Routine
Routines rely on predictability. Tilted life doesn't offer that.

Rituals — small, repeated acts of stability — can replace the illusion of control with the comfort of rhythm.

- Morning tea
- Afternoon journaling
- Evening leg elevation + reality show streaming
- Weekly symptom log + reward
- "I showed up" dance party in pajamas

Things You're Allowed to Do Even If You Don't Know What's Next

- Make plans (and cancel them later)
- Laugh (even when things are messy)
- Rest (without "earning" it)
- Ask for help (and ask again)
- Change your mind about treatment, tools, or tactics
- Call it a win just for getting out of bed

When the Fear Creeps In (Because It Will)

Fear Thought	Reframe
"I'll never get better."	Healing doesn't always look like cure. It looks like adaptation.
"I can't live like this forever."	You don't have to. You just have to live today.
"I'm falling behind."	You're running a different race. On a different course. With different rules.
"I don't know what's next."	That's hard. And also true. And you're still here. That's enough.

Horizontal Summary -- Coexisting With Chaos

Strategy	Tool
Accept nonlinear progress	Track patterns, not perfection
Build rituals	Repeat small wins, not rigid routines

Strategy	Tool
Redefine success	Based on capacity, not comparison
Hold space for uncertainty	Journal, therapy, support groups
Stay present	Ground in today, not the forecast

Tilt Break: The Power of "No" (A Full Sentence)

Saying no isn't quitting. It isn't rude. It isn't selfish. It's capacity management, and it's what keeps your nervous system from flipping the emergency switch mid-day. You're not declining because you don't care — you're declining because you *do* care: about your health, your energy, and your ability to function tomorrow.

You're allowed to say:

"No, I can't make it."
"No, I don't have the bandwidth."
"No, I'm not explaining it again."

Permission granted — to cancel plans, to guard your recovery, to not justify your needs. "No" is not a dirty word. It's a survival tool — and it works even better when you say it without apologizing.

True friends won't flinch. The people who matter will still be there — after the flare, after the nap, after you've rehydrated and questioned every life choice that led to standing upright.

If someone walks away because you set a boundary, they weren't actually part of your support crew. They were just orbiting your energy like a satellite that didn't pay rent.

Final Thought

Uncertainty is exhausting. But it's also a weird, uninvited teacher. It educates you to pay attention. To stay flexible. To soften your grip on the version of yourself that existed before all this began.

You are living in a body that doesn't always follow the rules — and you're still showing up, adapting, and writing your own damn manual. That's not just survival. That's resilience under pressure.

CHAPTER 18:
WHAT I WISH I KNEW SOONER

Lessons From the Tilt Trenches From Someone Who Lives It Every Day

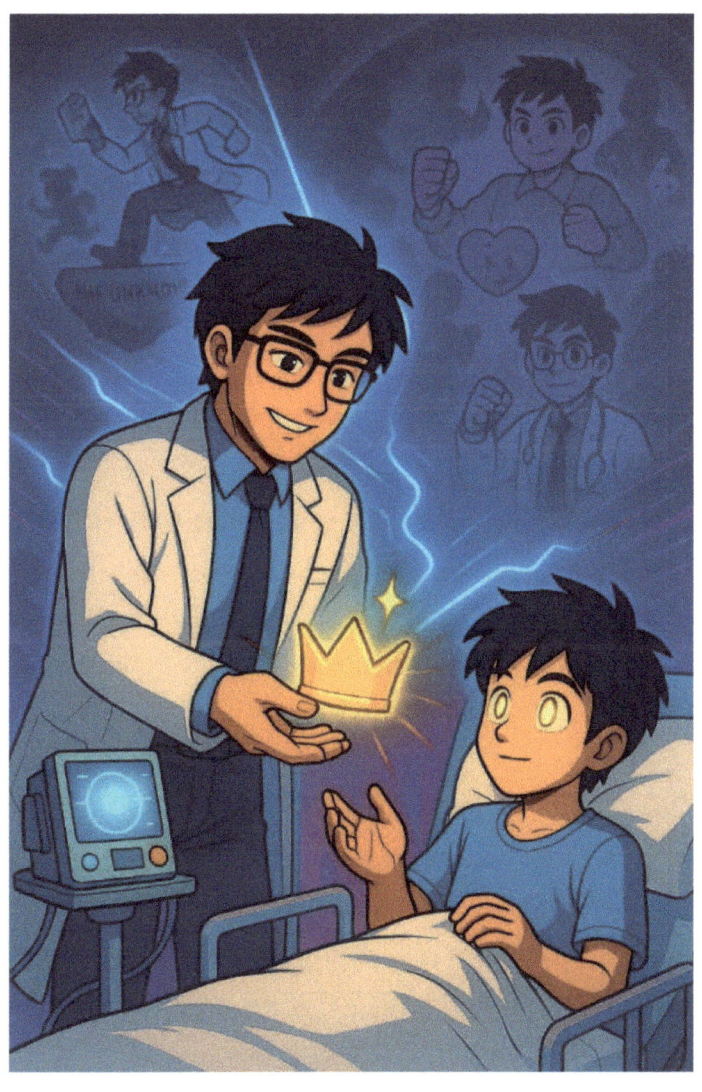

Tilt doesn't give you time to prepare. So you figure it out in real-time — with trial, error, and humor you weren't planning on needing. Here's what would've helped earlier.

If you've made it this far, congratulations. You've waded through symptoms, science, salt, strategies, side-eyes, and systemic gaslighting — and you're still standing. Or seated. Or reclining with dignity.

This final chapter isn't a summary. It's a confessional. A collection of hard-earned truths that might've saved some flares, some tears, and a few thousand milligrams of sodium had someone whispered them to me earlier.

So consider this your time machine. These are the things I wish someone had told me — not gently, but urgently — before I learned them the hard way.

1. You're Operating on a Different Rulebook

What may look like weakness from the outside is actually hyper-vigilant adaptation. You're recalibrating in real time. Every time you rest early, snack strategically, or cancel preemptively — you're not giving up. You're giving yourself a chance to stay upright tomorrow.

2. It's Not "Just Anxiety" If Salt Fixes It

If your heart rate calms after electrolytes, it's not emotional distress — it's autonomic instability. Anxiety can coexist with dysautonomia, sure. But don't let anyone reduce you to a trope when your physiology is trying to conduct a jazz ensemble with no sheet music, no rhythm, and a rogue saxophone.

3. Symptom Journals Are Gold, Not Guilt Traps
You will forget how bad it was. You'll gaslight yourself. Write it down. Track your HR, BP, crashes, meals, meds. Not to obsess — but to gather intel. You're not documenting illness. You're building a case file for liberation.

4. Compression Socks and Salt Are Not Optional Accessories
They are assistive devices. Like glasses, but for your blood pressure. Stop pretending you can power through without them. You can't. And you shouldn't have to. Nothing says "chronic illness couture" like 30 mmHg compression thigh-highs and a shaker of Himalayan sea salt in your fanny pack.

5. You Can Still Laugh While Lying Flat
Your sense of humor will save you. Not because this is funny — but because sometimes, the only thing left to do when you faint on your cat or cry over pre-cut fruit is to laugh before the tears dry. Find the absurdity. Make the memes. Weaponize the irony. Comedy is cardiovascular rehab for the soul.

6. You're Allowed to Outgrow Doctors
If someone makes you feel small, confused, or invisible, you do not owe them continued access to your body, mind, and spirit. Medical credentials do not guarantee emotional safety. Fire with flare. Replace with precision. Keep the good ones, educate the curious ones, and walk away from the ones who write "anxious" more quickly than they order a tilt table test.

7. Resting Is a Treatment, Not a Moral Flaw
Autonomic recovery mode is mandatory. You are implementing a horizontal intervention for circulatory preservation and neurologic stabilization. That's clinical. That's strategic. That's science, baby.

8. Flare Days Don't Erase Progress

One bad day doesn't mean you're regressing. It means your body had to renegotiate terms. And that's fine. This isn't a staircase. It's a dance-floor. You'll merengue back and forth. That's still moving forward.

9. Not Every Battle Needs Fighting. But the Ones That Do? Choose Rage + Receipts

Some systems aren't worth your energy. But when you do need to fight — insurance, disability, discrimination — come armed. With your binder, your logs, your letters, and your fury. This is survival. You get to be loud.

10. You Are Still You — Even in a Recliner

You haven't lost your value because you lost your standing time. You're still smart. Still fierce. Still creative. Still lovable. Still full of purpose. Your worth isn't on hold while your nervous system recalibrates. You don't have to wait for a recovery arc to reclaim your identity. You're already whole. Tilted. Complicated. Glorious.

Horizontal Summary –- Tilted Wisdom in Hindsight

Truth	Takeaway
You're not fragile	You're neurologically advanced
Salt + compression are tools	Not negotiable lifestyle "choices"
Humor is therapy	Laughing is survival chemistry
Rest isn't quitting	It's strategy
Progress is non-linear	Dance through it
You are enough — right now	Not "once you're better." Now.

Final Thought

There's no perfect ending here. No magic recovery montage. No sudden return to "normal." That was never the goal.

The goal was this — To understand your body. To adapt without apology. To survive with systems, humor, science, and salt. And to reclaim your life — not by erasing your illness, but by expanding your definition of possible.

So if no one else tells you today, let me be the one:

You're doing this. You're brilliant at it. And you're not alone — not in the Tilt, not in the chaos, and definitely not in the revolution.

FINAL TILTED THOUGHTS — LOOKING BACK, TILTING FORWARD

How to Stay Tilt-Defiant — Resist. Recline. Repeat.

You've made it to the end — not just of a book, but of a conversation I wish someone had with me years ago.

When my own body started misfiring in ways that didn't line up with textbooks or tidy diagnostic algorithms, I did what doctors are trained to do — I investigated. I tracked symptoms. I ran labs. I tried to out-think physiology. But this wasn't a board exam question. It was my life.

I was the patient now. And let me tell you — nothing rewires your perspective faster than going from the white coat to the waiting room.

This book was born from that dual view — from the exam room *and* the lived-in recliner. From the need to understand a condition that doesn't play by the usual rules, and the stubborn refusal to accept "just anxiety" as a diagnosis when my heart rate was doing acrobatics from brushing my teeth.

Tilt-defiance came out of necessity. But it's become something much more.

Being Tilt-defiant™ means understanding your nervous system well enough to support it, guide it, and — on some days — negotiate gently with it. It's not about pushing through. It's about pacing with purpose. It's building systems instead of relying on willpower. It's learning when to rest, when to move, and when to pull out the salt packet like a seasoned professional.

You're not waiting for permission. You're leading with precision.

Tilt-defiance means:

- Planning your day like a cardiovascular engineer.
- Showing up for yourself with consistency, not force.
- Learning how to adjust, recharge, and re-engage — on your terms.
- Trusting that a horizontal pause can be just as powerful as any heroic effort.

My experience — both as a physician and a patient — has taught me autonomy isn't just about nervous system function. It's about reclaiming control over your story. Whether you're lying down with a cooling towel, walking with intention, or meal prepping with compression socks on — this is your blueprint. And you built it.

So no, this journey isn't a detour. It's a masterclass in awareness, adaptability, and alignment.

You've read the chapters. You've seen the data. You've felt the resonance. Now carry that forward — not as pressure, but as possibility.

You are Tilt-defiant.

With knowledge. With clarity. With the audacity to lead your care like the expert you are — because you are.

Keep adjusting. Keep innovating. Keep moving in ways that honor your nervous system and elevate your life.

And remember — rising doesn't always require standing.

Khalid Saeed, D.O.
Physician|Dysautonomia Guru|Tilt-defiant

ABOUT THE AUTHOR

Dr. Khalid Saeed, D.O. is a board-certified physician, patient advocate, and reluctant member of the Autonomic Dysfunction Club — where the first rule is "Don't stand too fast" and the second rule is "Seriously, don't."

He doesn't pass out (usually), but he *does* live with dysautonomia — and all the symptom roulette, salt rituals, and cardiovascular drama that come with it. After navigating his own diagnostic maze while practicing medicine, Dr. Saeed realized that most resources for patients were either wildly inaccurate, depressingly dry, or written as if people with chronic illness had infinite energy and zero sarcasm. So he wrote the book he wished someone had handed him — blunt, funny, evidence-based, and just sarcastic enough to be honest.

By day, he works with real patients, real symptoms, and the occasional diagnostic plot twist. By night, he translates medical jargon into something functional (and occasionally entertaining). He believes in empowering patients, challenging medical gaslighting, and defending the constitutional right to lie down in public without explanation.

When he's not writing, doctoring, or managing his own nervous system like an unpredictable sidekick with commitment issues, you can find him enjoying stillness, spreadsheets, and the subtle joy of stable blood pressure.

He lives in Florida, where he works to make complex medicine accessible, patient stories audible, and outdated medical dogma re-hydrated, re-educated, and respectfully dismantled.

You can reach Dr. Saeed at TampaBayConciergeDoctor.com or on Instagram @dr.khalid.saeed

REFERENCES

Peer-Reviewed Validation for Your Salty Lifestyle

In-text Citations

Benarroch, E. E. (2008). The clinical approach to autonomic failure in neurological disorders. *Nature Reviews Neurology*, 4(12), 673–684.

Camilleri, M., Park, S. Y., & Carlson, P. (2011). Autonomic dysfunction in gastroparesis and functional dyspepsia. *Neurogastroenterology & Motility*, 23(9), 856–862.

Freeman, R., Wieling, W., Axelrod, F. B., et al. (2011). Consensus statement on the definition of orthostatic hypotension, neurally mediated syncope, and the postural tachycardia syndrome. *Clinical Autonomic Research*, 21(2), 69–72.

Fu, Q., VanGundy, T. B., Galbreath, M. M., et al. (2010). Cardiac origins of the postural orthostatic tachycardia syndrome. *Journal of the American College of Cardiology*, 55(25), 2858–2868.

Garland, E. M., Celedonio, J. E., & Raj, S. R. (2015). Postural tachycardia syndrome: Beyond orthostatic intolerance. *Current Neurology and Neuroscience Reports*, 15(9), 60.

Goldstein, D. S. (2013). Dysautonomia in Parkinson's disease: Neurocardiological abnormalities. *The Lancet Neurology*, 12(5), 429–440.

Grubb, B. P., & Karas, B. J. (2011). Clinical disorders of the autonomic nervous system associated with orthostatic intolerance: An overview of classification, clinical evaluation, and management. *Pacing and Clinical Electrophysiology*, 34(5), 602–614.

Kaufmann, H., Norcliffe-Kaufmann, L., & Palma, J. A. (2014). Droxidopa in neurogenic orthostatic hypotension. *Expert Review of Cardiovascular Therapy*, 12(7), 855–866.

Low, P. A., Sandroni, P., Joyner, M., & Shen, W. K. (2003). Postural tachycardia syndrome (POTS). *Journal of Cardiovascular Electrophysiology*, 14(3), 280–287.

Raj, S. R. (2006). The postural tachycardia syndrome (POTS): Pathophysiology, diagnosis & management. *Indian Pacing and Electrophysiology Journal, 6*(2), 84–99.

Raj, S. R., Black, B. K., Biaggioni, I., et al. (2009). Propranolol decreases tachycardia and improves symptoms in the postural tachycardia syndrome: Less is more. *Circulation, 120*(9), 725–734.

Raj, S. R., & Robertson, D. (2007). Blood volume perturbations in the postural tachycardia syndrome. *The American Journal of the Medical Sciences, 334*(1), 57–60.

Shibata, S., Fu, Q., Bivens, T. B., Hastings, J. L., & Levine, B. D. (2012). Short-term exercise training improves the cardiovascular response to exercise in the postural orthostatic tachycardia syndrome. *Journal of Physiology, 590*(15), 3495–3505.

Stewart, J. M., Boris, J. R., Chelimsky, G., et al. (2018). Pediatric disorders of orthostatic intolerance. *Pediatrics, 141*(1), e20171673.

Stewart, J. M. (2012). Common syndromes of orthostatic intolerance. *Pediatrics, 131*(5), 968–980.

Uchino, B. N. (2006). Social support and health: Physiological processes underlying links to disease outcomes. *Journal of Behavioral Medicine, 29*(4), 377–387.

General Dysautonomia & Epidemiology

Cleveland Clinic. (2024). *Success of POTS treatment reduced by concurrent anxiety.* Consult QD. https://consultqd.clevelandclinic.org/success-of-pots-treatment-reduced-by-concurrent-anxiety/

Grubb, B. P., & Kanjwal, Y. (2007). Postural orthostatic tachycardia syndrome: A heterogeneous and multifactorial disorder. *Cardiology in Review, 15*(4), 211–217.

Wikipedia contributors. (2025, May). *Dysautonomia.* Wikipedia. https://en.wikipedia.org/wiki/Dysautonomia

Wikipedia contributors. (2025, June). *Postural orthostatic tachycardia syndrome.* Wikipedia. https://en.wikipedia.org/wiki/Postural_orthostatic_tachycardia_syndrome

Diagnosis & Testing

Haensch, C. A., & Jörg, J. (2014). Autonomic dysfunction in neurological disorders. *Journal of Neurology, 261*(7), 1413–1421.

Raj, S. R., Guzman, J. C., Harvey, P., Richer, L., Peltier, A., Abdollah, H., ... & Sheldon, R. S. (2013). Canadian Cardiovascular Society position statement on POTS and related disorders. *Canadian Journal of Cardiology, 29*(5), 557–564.

Stewart, J. M., Medow, M. S., Messer, Z. R., & Hensel, K. (2012). Autonomic testing in the young: Clinical relevance. *Seminars in Pediatric Neurology, 19*(1), 3–9.

Pharmacologic Management

Grubb, B. P., Kanjwal, Y., & Kosinski, D. J. (2011). The use of midodrine and other pressor agents in the treatment of orthostatic hypotension and POTS. *Cardiology in Review, 19*(4), 192–198.

Kaufmann, H., Norcliffe-Kaufmann, L., Palma, J. A., & Biaggioni, I. (2014). Droxidopa in neurogenic orthostatic hypotension: A randomized, controlled trial. *Neurology, 83*(4), 328–335.

Raj, S. R., Arnold, A. C., Barboi, A., Claydon, V. E., Limberg, J. K., Lucci, V. M., ... & Vernino, S. (2024). Oral pharmacotherapy for postural tachycardia syndrome: A systematic review. *Frontiers in Neurology, 15*, 1515486.

Exercise & Deconditioning

Fu, Q., Vangundy, T. B., Shibata, S., Auchus, R. J., & Levine, B. D. (2010). Exercise training versus propranolol in the treatment of the postural orthostatic tachycardia syndrome. *Hypertension, 56*(2), 286–293.

Shibata, S., Fu, Q., Bivens, T. B., Hastings, J. L., Wang, W., & Levine, B. D. (2012). Short-term exercise training improves the cardiovascular response to exercise in the postural orthostatic tachycardia syndrome. *Journal of Physiology, 590*(15), 3495–3505.

Autoimmunity & Mechanisms

Vernino, S., Stiles, L. E., & Low, P. A. (2018). Autoimmune basis for POTS: Evidence and implications. *Journal of the American College of Cardiology, 72*(12), 1430–1437.

Qing, X., Jin, H., & Raj, S. R. (2023). Autoantibodies in postural orthostatic tachycardia syndrome: Diagnostic value and therapeutic implications. *Autonomic Neuroscience, 241*, 103035.

Geddes, J., Ottesen, J. T., Mehlsen, J., & Olufsen, M. S. (2021). Postural Orthostatic Tachycardia Syndrome explained using a baroreflex response model. *arXiv Preprint*, arXiv:2109.14558.

Geddes, J., Mehlsen, J., & Olufsen, M. S. (2019). Characterization of blood pressure and heart rate oscillations of POTS patients via uniform phase empirical mode decomposition. *arXiv Preprint*, arXiv:1910.10332.

Long COVID–Related Dysautonomia

Johnson, M. M., Aranda, J. A., & Shaw, D. M. (2025). Long-COVID dysautonomia: Mechanisms, symptoms, and clinical approaches. *medRxiv*. https://doi.org/10.1101/2025.03.24.25324564

Zhu, W., Wong, R., & Lee, D. H. (2024). Long COVID and the autonomic nervous system: What we know and what we need to learn. *OSF Preprints*. https://osf.io/preprints/osf/2tvmk_v1

Washington Post. (2025, March 27). Long-COVID brain: New studies show lingering effects two years later. *The Washington Post*. https://www.washingtonpost.com/wellness/2025/03/27/long-covid-brain-cognition/

National Library of Medicine. (2024). Long-COVID–related autonomic dysfunction. *PubMed Central*. https://pubmed.ncbi.nlm.nih.gov/38585346

Cognitive & Imaging Correlates

Nelson, T. M., & Stewart, J. M. (2024). Functional brain changes in postural tachycardia syndrome: A review of imaging evidence. *Journal of Neuroimaging, 34*(2), 221–229.

SetPT USA. (2024). What's new in POTS research: A look at the latest studies changing the game. https://setptusa.com/blog/research/whats-new-in-pots-research-a-look-at-the-latest-studies-changing-the-game

SUGGESTED READING & TOOLS

Because You Can't Fight a Dysfunctional Nervous System With Vibes Alone

Books That Educate, Validate, and Occasionally Prevent a Breakdown

The Dysautonomia Project – Dr. Blair Grubb & colleagues
A clinician and patient guide that *actually* explains dysautonomia without burying it in jargon. Clinician-approved, patient-understandable.

POTS: Together We Stand – Jodi Epstein Rhum
A patient-centered survival manual that's part memoir, part rally cry. Comforting, empowering, and doesn't blame you for needing three chairs and a hydration IV just to grocery shop.

The Invisible Kingdom – Meghan O'Rourke
A lyrical, literary deep dive into chronic illness, diagnostic limbo, and the existential slap of realizing your body and the system are both glitchy.

How to Be Sick – Toni Bernhard
Written by a Buddhist law professor with chronic illness, this guide is equal parts philosophical and practical. May reduce rage-spiraling when your symptoms say "nope" again.

The Body Keeps the Score – Bessel van der Kolk
Trauma, physiology, and the mind-body split — If your dysautonomia showed up after illness or trauma, this helps decode the "why am I like this" loop.

The Deepest Well **– Dr. Nadine Burke Harris**
Explores the connection between early life stress, chronic illness, and the long arc of healing. Short, readable, and occasionally infuriating (in a good way).

Tilt-Taming Tools, Apps, and Tactical Gadgets

Heart Rate Monitor – Chest Strap Preferred
The Polar H10 is the gold standard. Your wristwatch might lie to protect your feelings. A chest strap won't. Use it for tilt tracking, exercise, and proof that, yes, your heart rate does hit 140 when you're brushing your teeth.

Blood Pressure Monitor – Automatic Arm Cuff
Go for models that store readings or sync to your phone. Skip the wrist cuffs unless you want erratic nonsense numbers. Bonus: provides actual data to hand your doctor, not just vague descriptions.

Pulse Oximeter
Great for when you feel like you're about to pass out and want to confirm it's not low oxygen — or when it is, and you'd like someone to believe you.

Electrolyte Packets
Options include LMNT, Liquid I.V., DripDrop, Nuun, and Hydralyte. Rotate to avoid flavor fatigue. Sugar-free options are available. Avoid "low sodium" versions unless you enjoy defeat.

Compression Gear
Socks, leggings, sleeves, abdominal binders — aim for 20–30 mmHg minimum. Brands like Jobst, Sigvaris, and Juzo are solid. Not cute, but neither is fainting.

Cooling Vests and Neck Wraps
If heat makes you tilt, these are essential. Try Torcool, Ergodyne Chill-Its, or Mission. Also: fans. Neck fans. Desk fans. Fan yourself like the dramatic protagonist you are.

Cooling Towels
Frogg Toggs or Mission HydroActive towels can turn you into a mildly damp but upright human in hot weather.

Salt Capsules
For those who can't stomach salted everything: Thermotabs, SaltStick FastChews, or Buffered Electrolyte Salts. Monitor your labs. Overcorrection is real.

Reclining/Wheelchair Mobility Aids
Brands like Karman, Permobil, and Bounder offer reclining chairs designed for those with orthostatic intolerance. Not everyone needs one, but if you do — you're not "giving up." You're adapting like a boss.

Shower Chair + Handheld Showerhead
If upright hygiene is impossible, these make verticality optional. Combine with a waterproof fan and you're basically in a spa. A very medicalized spa.

Apps to Track, Tame, and Translate Your Tilt
Bearable
Tracks symptoms, meds, mood, energy, triggers, and sleep in a clean interface. Bonus: exportable graphs for doctor visits.

CareClinic
A health journal and medication tracker with integration options. Accommodates complex regimens and supplement chaos.

Waterlogged
Because hydration math is hard. Visuals make it easy to see when you're behind.

MyFitnessPal
Not just for dieting. Use it to track sodium, fluids, and calories if POTS is messing with your appetite or digestion.

Symple Symptom Tracker
Minimalist and fast. Good for tracking a few things without getting overwhelmed.

Flaredown
Made for chronic illness. Log flares, symptoms, triggers, and treatments without losing your mind or your formatting.

Websites That Won't Gaslight You

Dysautonomia International
Advocacy, awareness, research funding, provider resources, and an annual conference where carrying salt packets is normal.
https://www.dysautonomiainternational.org

DINET (Dysautonomia Information Network)
Forums, guides, patient stories, and support from people who truly understand "I stood up too fast" as a medical event.
https://www.dinet.org

The Dysautonomia Project
High-quality provider education, practical patient handouts, and resources to educate your doctor without needing a professional slideshow presentation.
https://www.thedysautonomiaproject.org

SUGGESTED READING & TOOLS

NIH Genetic and Rare Diseases Information Center (GARD)
Deep-dive medical information, subtype descriptions, and alphabet soup acronyms for those who like their reading dense and verified.
https://rarediseases.info.nih.gov

POTS UK
A UK-based nonprofit with educational videos, handouts, and global perspective. Particularly useful for comparing international care models.
https://www.potsuk.org

Standing Up to POTS
Research-focused nonprofit offering resources for families, schools, and clinicians. Especially strong for pediatric and adolescent POTS.
https://www.standinguptopots.org

GLOSSARY OF TERMS

For the Tilted, the Curious, and the Clinically Confused

Active Stand Test
A homegrown version of the tilt table test. You lie down, then stand up and record your vitals. Bonus points if you don't pass out.

Adrenaline
Also known as epinephrine, this fight-or-flight chemical floods your body when your ANS panics — like when you stand up or think about your inbox.

Amla
Also known as Indian gooseberry. Packed with vitamin C, antioxidants, and enough hype to make kale jealous. Claimed to boost everything from immunity to hair growth.

Autonomic Flare
A sudden worsening of symptoms, often triggered by heat, stress, dehydration, food, loud noises, or the audacity of existing.

Autonomic Nervous System (ANS)
The autopilot system that runs things like heart rate, blood pressure, digestion, temperature, and bladder control. Except when it doesn't.

Baroreceptors
Pressure sensors in the cardiovascular system that regulate blood pressure. In dysautonomia, they're like a GPS that says, "turn left" into oncoming traffic.

Beta-Blockers
Medications that lower heart rate and blunt the body's stress response. Like emotional Novocaine for your cardiovascular system.

Blood Pressure (BP)
A measurement of the force of blood against your vessel walls. In dysautonomia, it's more of a mood than a number.

Brain Fog
A cloud of confusion, memory lapses, and slowed thinking. Often mistaken for low motivation, when it's actually low perfusion.

Bradycardia
A heart rate that's too slow. The opposite of POTS, and just as inconvenient.

Cerebral Hypoperfusion
Low blood flow to the brain, often responsible for dizziness, brain fog, and questioning your life choices.

Cognitive Behavioral Therapy (CBT)
A form of mental health therapy that helps people reframe their thinking. Can be helpful for managing chronic illness, especially when the system gaslights you.

Compression Garments
Elastic clothing that helps blood move back to your heart and brain. Not cute, but effective. Think medical-grade hugs for your circulatory system.

Constipation
Sluggish bowels caused by autonomic dysfunction. May require a team effort and a support group.

Deconditioning
Loss of physical fitness from prolonged inactivity. Often blamed for dysautonomia even when it's a symptom, not the cause.

Droxidopa
A medication that boosts norepinephrine to help regulate blood pressure. Sometimes magical, sometimes meh.

Electrocardiogram (EKG/ECG)
A test that measures your heart's electrical activity. Usually normal in dysautonomia, unless you've had five energy drinks.

Electrolytes
Sodium, potassium, magnesium, and chloride — essential for nerve and muscle function, and your new best friends.

Exercise Intolerance
An inability to exercise without worsening symptoms. Not laziness — just your body filing a protest.

Fludrocortisone
A steroid that helps retain salt and water, boosting blood volume. Side effects may include swelling, cranky kidneys, and a love-hate relationship with pickles.

Gastrointestinal (GI) Dysmotility
When your gut operates at a sloth's pace. May include bloating, nausea, constipation, or mystery cramps.

Heart Rate (HR)
The number of times your heart beats per minute. In POTS, it spikes like it's trying to break a record just from standing.

Heat Intolerance
An inability to regulate temperature properly. May result in dramatic exits from summer events.

Hypovolemia
Low blood volume. Like trying to run a hydraulic system on a half tank of fluid.

Hypoxia
Low oxygen levels in your body. Not enough to knock you out, just enough to make you dizzy, foggy, and question all your life choices at cruising altitude.

Ivabradine
A medication that slows heart rate without dropping blood pressure. A rare gem for some POTS patients.

Levine Protocol
A cardiovascular conditioning plan that teaches your body to stand without staging a coup. Involves science, sweat, and salt — not necessarily in that order.

Lightheadedness
Feeling faint or woozy. The prequel to actual fainting.

Low Blood Pressure
A common feature of dysautonomia. The reason you sit down while waiting in line, lie down in the elevator, and nap after showering.

Merengue
A high-energy dance style from the Dominican Republic with fast steps, hip action, and a tempo that's probably too optimistic for someone with orthostatic intolerance. Attempt at your own risk — or while seated.

Glossary of Terms

Midodrine
A vasoconstrictor that tightens blood vessels to raise blood pressure. Side effects may include scalp tingles and sudden ambition.

Nausea
The unofficial mascot of dysautonomia. Triggered by food, heat, stress, smells, motion, air, or nothing.

NCS (Neurocardiogenic Syncope)
A type of fainting caused by a reflex that drops heart rate and blood pressure. Basically your ANS's version of rage quitting.

Neurotransmitters
Chemical messengers like norepinephrine and acetylcholine that keep your nervous system humming. Or in this case, stuttering.

Orthorexia
An obsessive fixation on "eating clean." It's not about weight — it's about purity, control, and demonizing anything that isn't organic kale.

Orthostatic Hypotension (OH)
A drop in blood pressure upon standing. More dramatic than a soap opera exit.

Orthostatic Intolerance (OI)
Your body's refusal to function properly in an upright position. Standing — not your strong suit.

Palpitations
The sensation of a fast, pounding, or irregular heartbeat. Often real, sometimes terrifying, usually benign in dysautonomia.

Parasympathetic Nervous System (PNS)
The "rest and digest" branch of your autonomic nervous system. In dysautonomia, it's either ghosting or gaslighting you.

Post-Exertional Malaise (PEM)
A flare of symptoms following even mild activity. Your reward for doing too much.

Postural Orthostatic Tachycardia Syndrome (POTS)
A form of dysautonomia where standing causes a dramatic rise in heart rate. Like your body yelling "Mayday!" every time you get vertical.

Pre-syncope
The phase before fainting. You don't hit the floor, but you think about it really hard.

RAAS (Renin-Angiotensin-Aldosterone System)
A hormonal system that regulates blood pressure and fluid balance. Dysautonomia's favorite malfunctioning feedback loop.

Salt Loading
Deliberate high sodium intake to increase blood volume. Finally, a medical excuse to drink pickle juice.

Sensory Overload
When lights, sounds, or motion overwhelm your nervous system. Common at concerts, airports, and fluorescent-lit waiting rooms.

Small Fiber Neuropathy (SFN)
Damage to small nerve fibers that regulate things like sweating, pain, and temperature. Because you needed more drama.

Stress Response
Your body's hormonal overreaction to perceived danger. Dysautonomia turns this up to 11, even when the threat is a houseplant.

Supine
Lying flat on your back. Often the position of least resistance for Tilted people.

Sympathetic Nervous System (SNS)
The "fight or flight" side of the ANS. In dysautonomia, it fights even when you're just trying to digest lunch.

Syncope
The medical term for fainting. You'll get used to it. Hopefully.

Tachycardia
A heart rate that's too fast, typically over 100 bpm. In POTS, it's your daily standing greeting.

Thermoregulatory Dysfunction
When your body forgets how to heat or cool itself. Think broken thermostat in human form.

Tilt Table Test (TTT)
A diagnostic test that tilts you upright while strapped to a table. If it sounds medieval, that's because it kind of is.

Tilt Zone
The realm of dysautonomia where symptoms reign, salt is sacred, and being vertical is optional.

Vagus Nerve

The wandering nerve that controls heart rate, digestion, and more. A frequent saboteur in the Tilted community.

Valsalva Maneuver

That classy move where you hold your breath and bear down like you're bracing for a bowel movement — except it's a medical test. Used to mess with your heart rate, not your dignity.

CREDITS

Who Helped, Who Tolerated, and Who Had No Idea They Were Enlisted

Cover Design, Interior Layout, and Visual Mischief
By Dr. Khalid Saeed, D.O., who learned just enough design software to be dangerous and who now sees text boxes in his dreams.

Editing and Sanity Preservation
Thanks to the early readers, medical misfits, and grammar loyalists who caught typos, logic errors, and the occasional sentence that tried to be funny but sounded like a caffeine crash in a thesaurus. You know who you are — and your red pens are deeply appreciated.

Medical Sources and Scientific Street Cred
Gratitude to the researchers whose data helped build this book's backbone — especially those who've studied POTS, autonomic dysfunction, and the neuro-humoral circus without blaming anxiety. Their citations live in the References section, but their impact lives in every footnote, joke, and rebuttal to "just hydrate."

Snarky Peer Review
To the invisible council of chronic illness rebels, late-night message thread co-conspirators, and meme-generators who tested metaphors like stress-tests for the soul — your ability to translate suffering into sarcasm is a public service.

Technological Chaos Containment
Thank you to every device, app, and cloud backup system that didn't crash during this project. And to the ones that *did* — I see you, and we are no longer on speaking terms.

Inspirational Fuel
Salt. Adrenaline. Texts from friends that said "Gravity won again but I'm fine — anyway, loved that paragraph on the vagus nerve." Also, rage at bad advice and a surprisingly resilient adrenal system.

Spouse, Family, and Innocent Bystanders
Thanks for putting up with test paragraphs read out loud during dinner, late-night rewriting rants, and living inside a home where "baroreceptor" was said more often than "please pass the remote."

To Dysautonomia Itself
You've been the worst kind of uninvited guest — disruptive, exhausting, and devoid of anything resembling self-awareness. But in the chaos, you accidentally created a sarcastic author with vertical dysfunction and a horizontal sense of humor. Nice move, genius.

www.ingramcontent.com/pod-product-compliance
Lightning Source LLC
Chambersburg PA
CBHW052029030426
42337CB00027B/4924

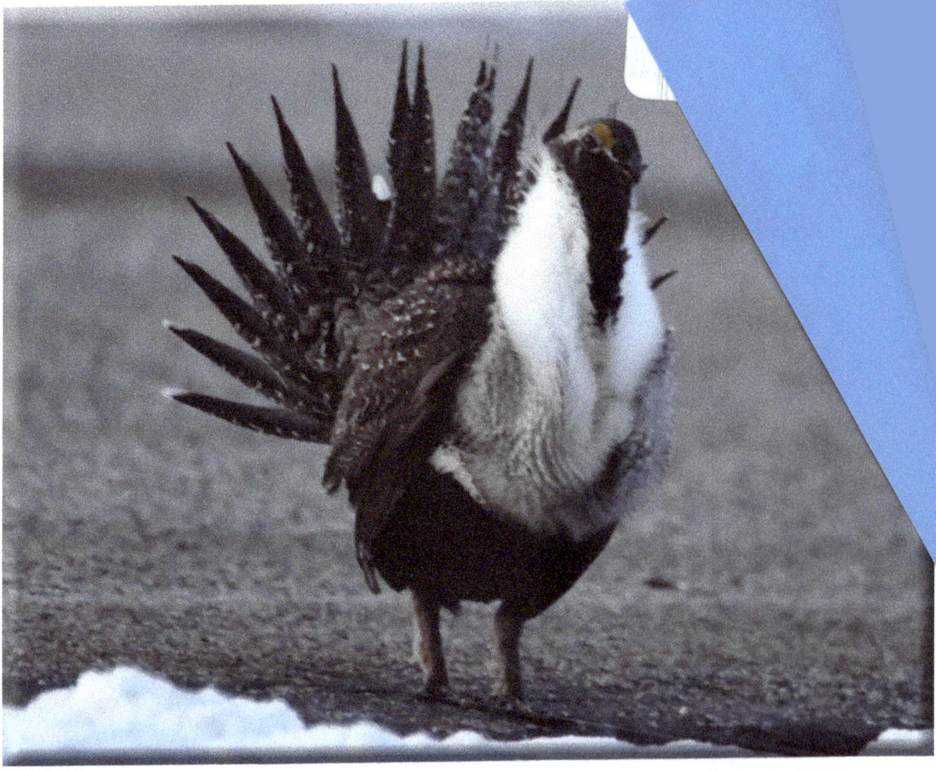

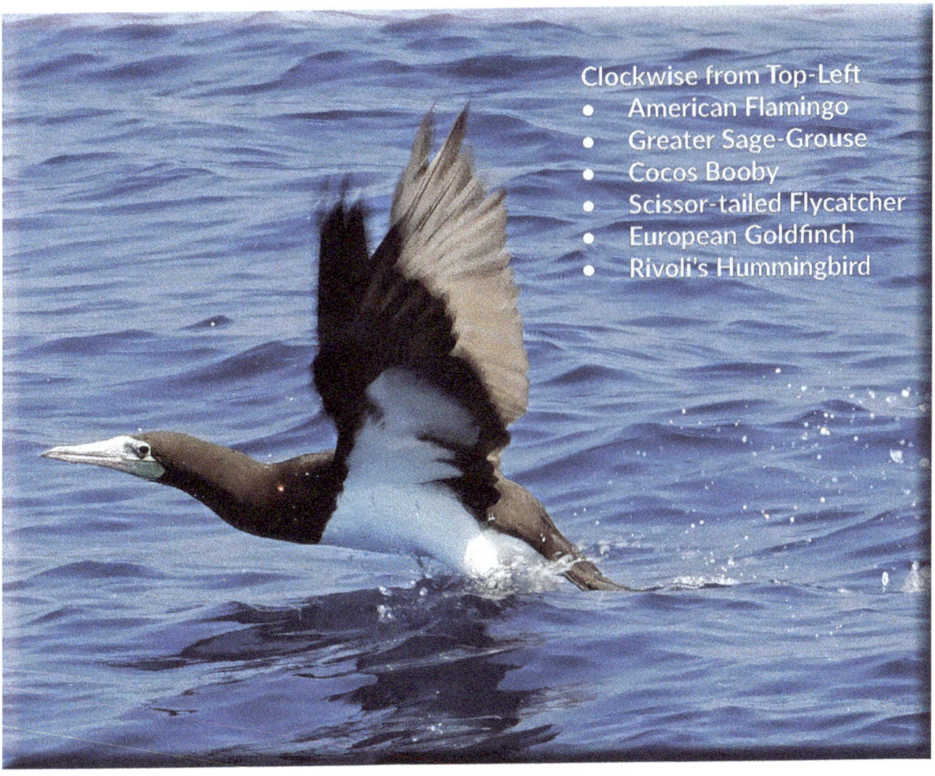

Clockwise from Top-Left
- American Flamingo
- Greater Sage-Grouse
- Cocos Booby
- Scissor-tailed Flycatcher
- European Goldfinch
- Rivoli's Hummingbird

Magnificent Frigatebirds

What is a Big Year?

A Big Year is a personal challenge in which birders aim to see or hear as many bird species as possible in a calendar year within a defined area. It's a popular endeavor in birding circles, drawing those with a passion for tracking down rare species and expanding their life lists. The official rules vary depending on the organization and scope, but generally, a bird seen or heard must be identified without question, using any legal and ethical means. Birders typically report their sightings to an established birding organization such as eBird, which verifies records.

There are several types of Birding Big Years:

• The most famous type is the ABA Area Big Year, where birders attempt to see as many species as possible within the American Birding Association (ABA) region, which includes the contiguous United States, Canada, and offshore waters. Birders go to great lengths, traveling across vast landscapes to spot difficult or rare species and spending considerable resources to maximize their count.

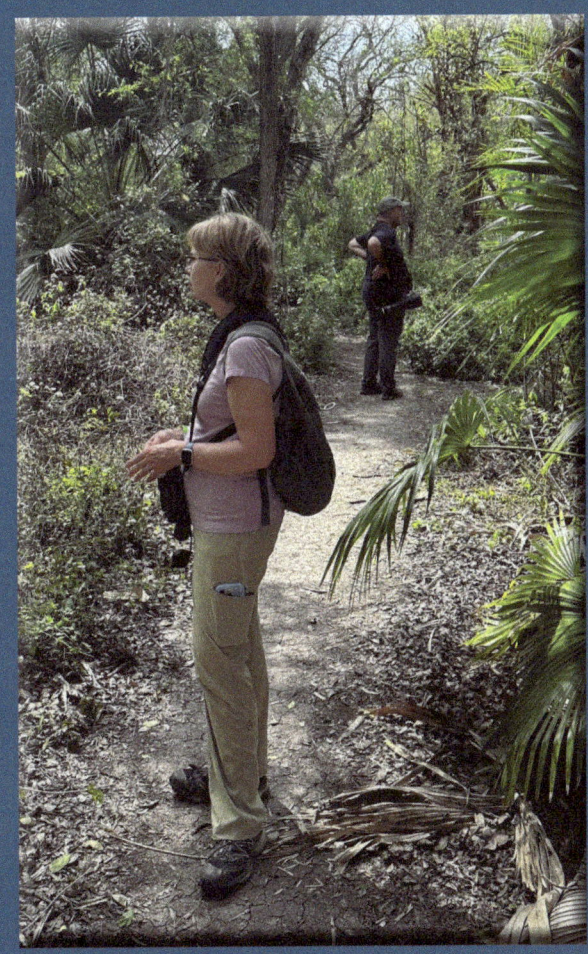

• A Lower 48 State Big Year focuses on spotting as many bird species as possible within the contiguous United States, excluding Alaska and Hawaii. This version offers a significant challenge without requiring the extreme logistical demands of an ABA Area Big Year. Birders tackling a Lower 48 Big Year must still cover diverse ecosystems and climates, from coastal areas and deserts to mountain ranges and wetlands, as they chase both migratory and resident birds across seasons.

• For a more local approach, birders often attempt a State Big Year or County Big Year, limiting their efforts to a specific state or county.

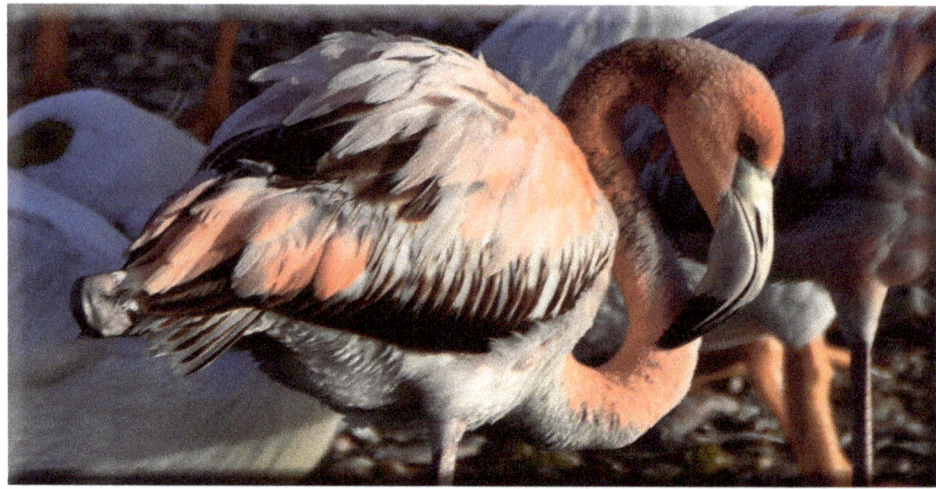
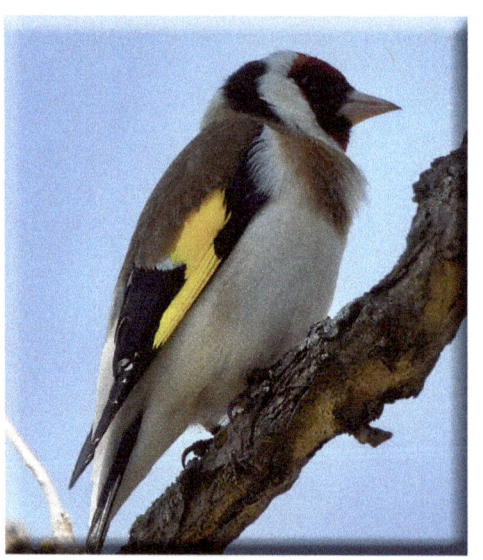
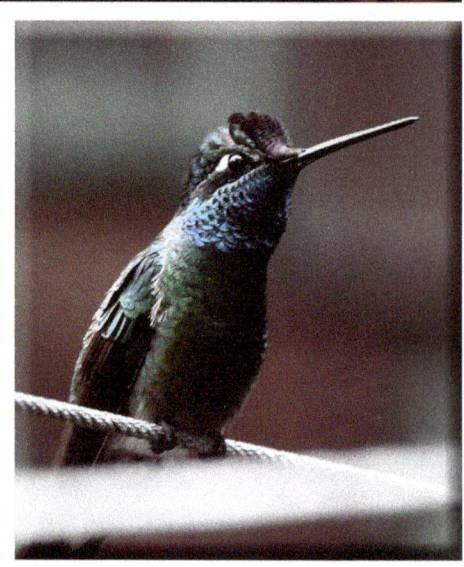
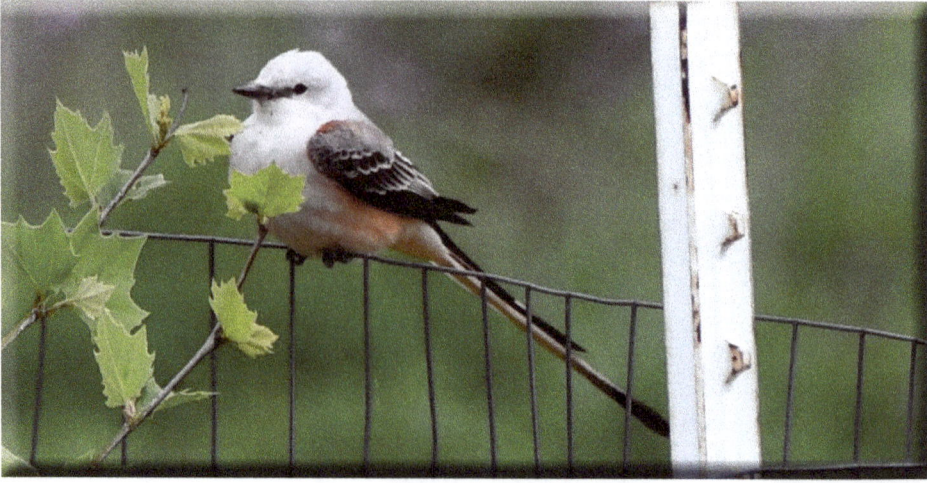

EVERY BIRD FROM SEA TO SHINING SEA

ONE COUPLE'S BIG YEAR IN BIRDING
A PHOTOGRAPHIC ADVENTURE ACROSS THE LOWER 48 STATES

BY ETHAN & INGRID WHITAKER

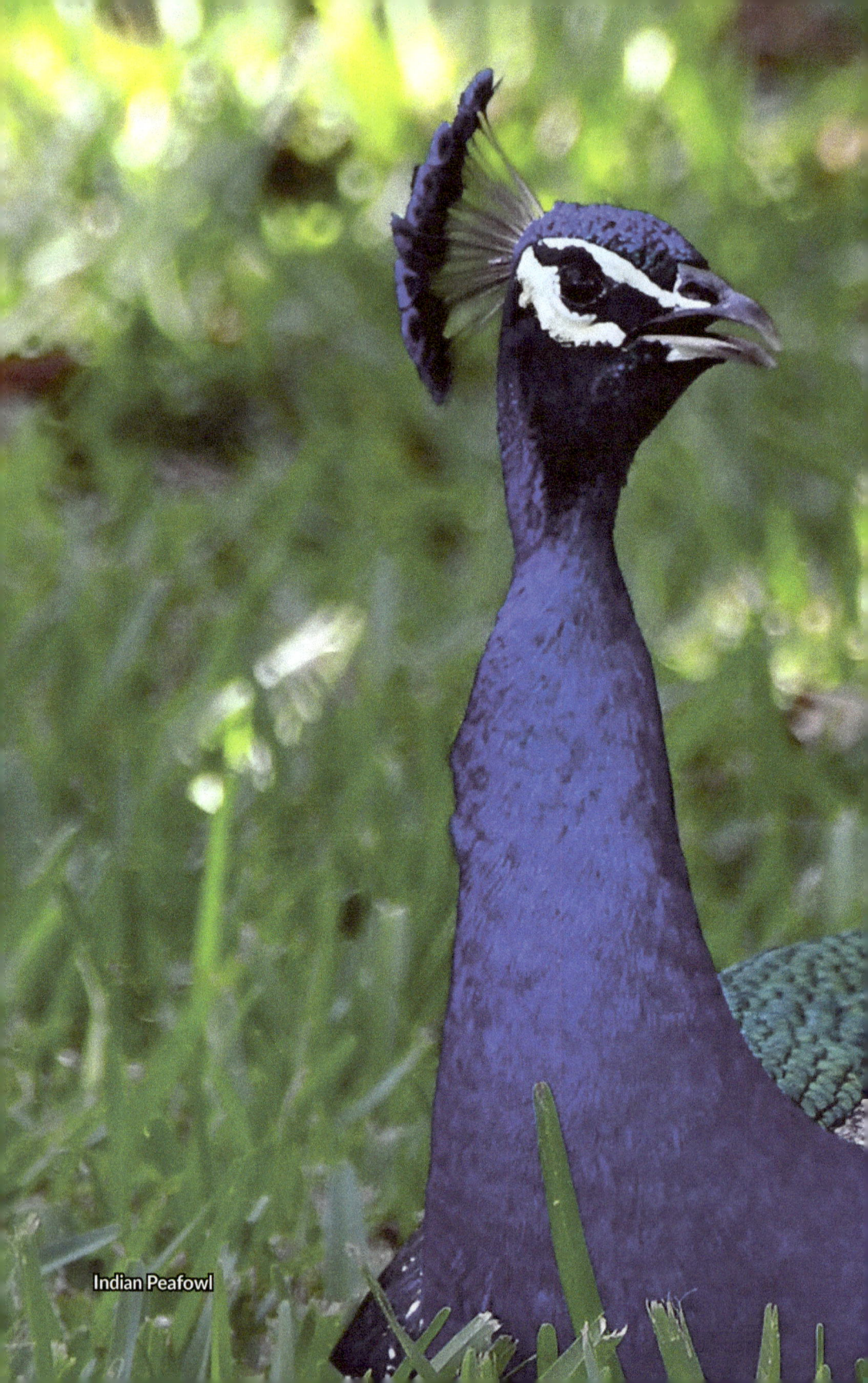
Indian Peafowl

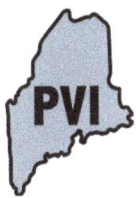 An imprint of PVIMaine LLC

Every Bird From Sea to Shining Sea

One Couple's Big Year in Birding
A Photographic Adventure Across the Lower 48 States

By Ethan J. Whitaker & Ingrid J Whitaker

Copyright © 2025 by PVIMaine LLC

ALL RIGHTS RESERVED. No part of this book may be reproduced in any form or by any electronic of mechanical means, including information storage and retrieval systems, without written permission of the publisher, except by a reviewer who may quote passages in a review.

Library of Congress Cataloging-in-Publication Data

ISBN: 979-8-9856205-8-0 (paperback)
ISBN: 979-8-9923804-1-5 (hardcover)
ISBN: 979-8-9856205-9-7 (kindle)
ISBN: 979-8-9923804-0-8 (epub)

Requests for Information and/or speaking engagements:
Mail: PVIMaine LLC
attn: Ethan Whitaker
117 Cushman Point Rd
Wiscasset, Maine 04578

Phone: 1-207-671-2006

E-Mail: ewhitaker@PVIMaine.com

To Anna, Marita and Bradley:

Who not only watched us spend down their inheritance ... but cheered us on!

We love you!

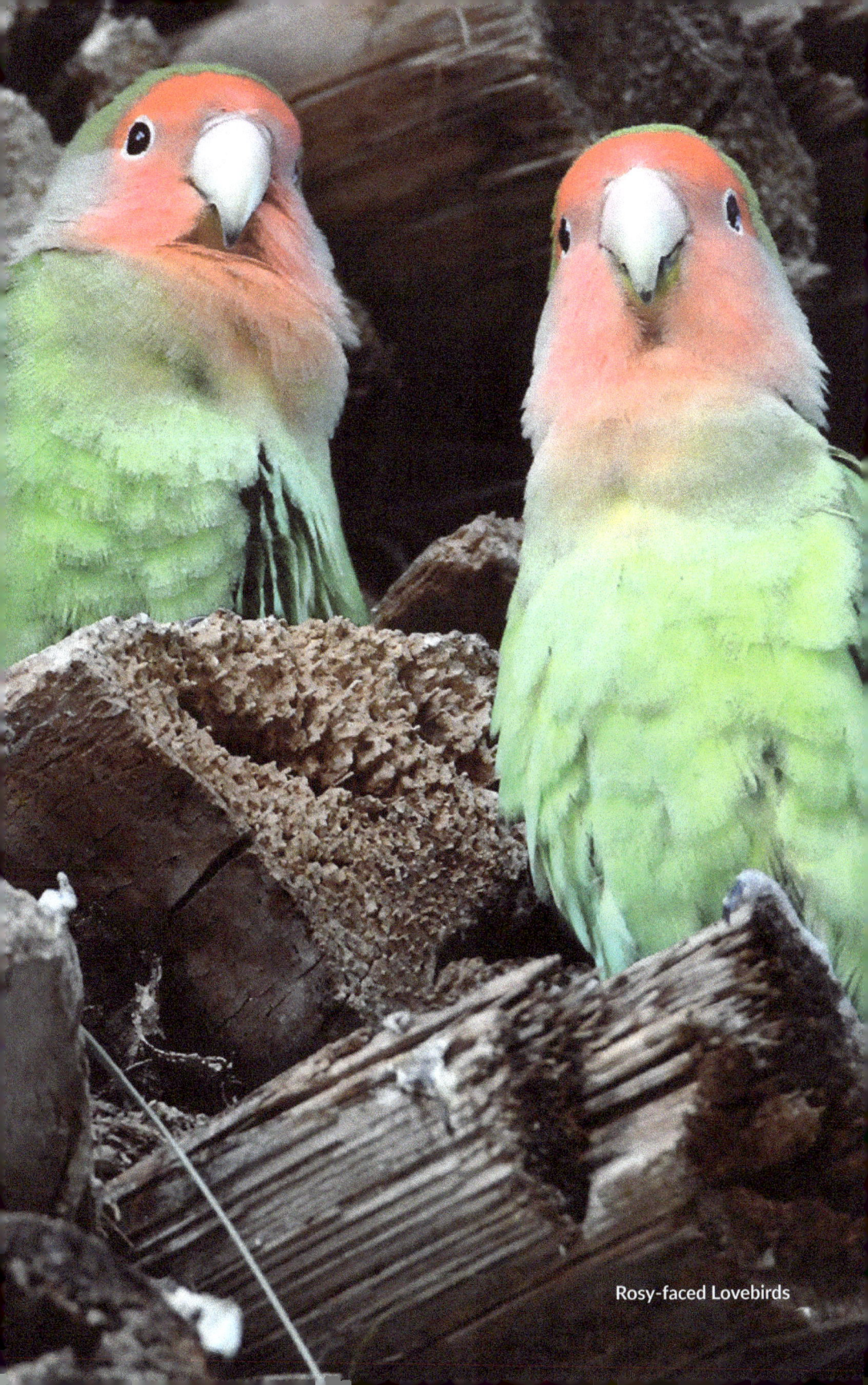
Rosy-faced Lovebirds

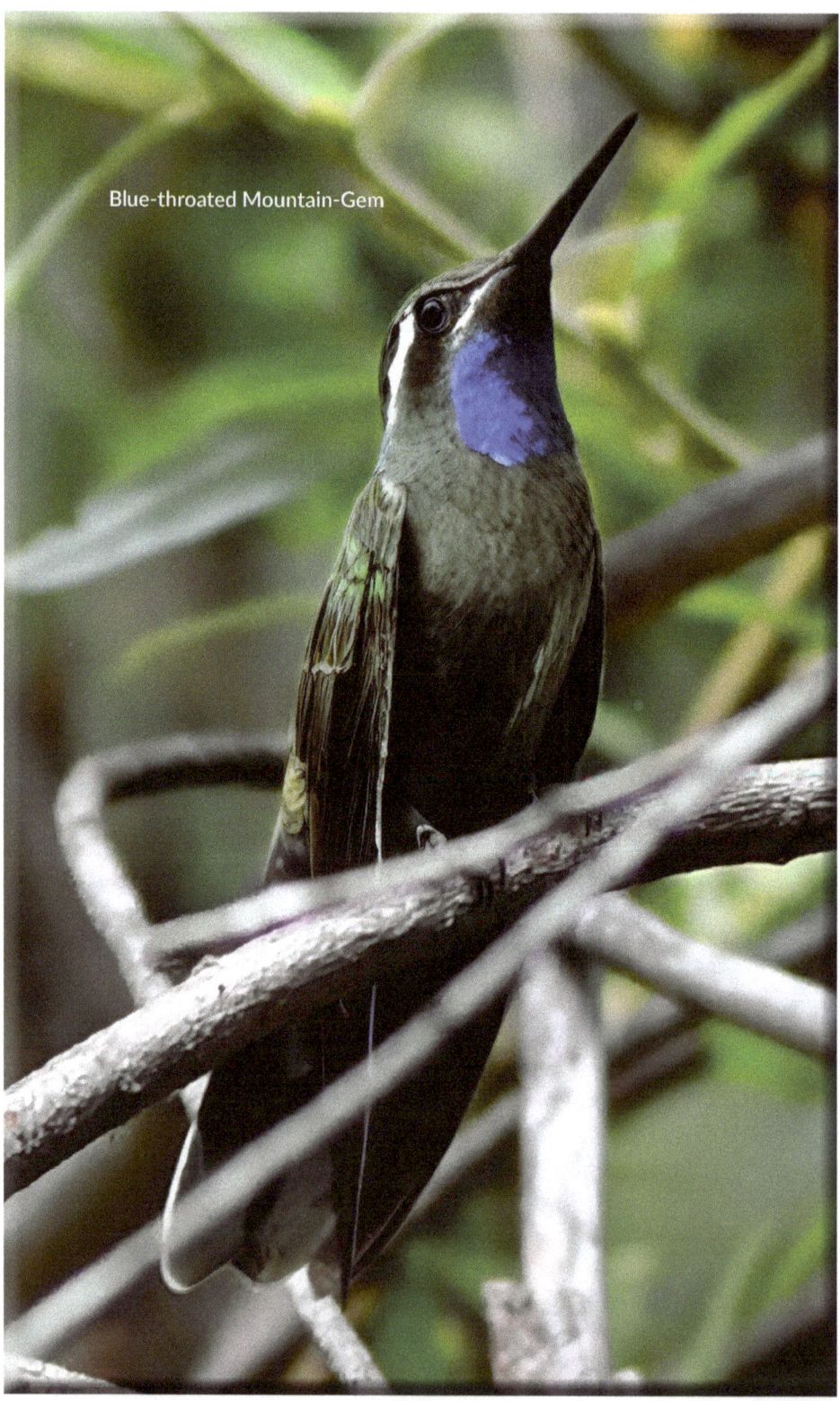
Blue-throated Mountain-Gem

Contents

1	What is a Big Year?	99	Spruce Grouse
11	Contents	100	Pacific Northwest
12	Every Bird? Why?	102	Dipper Day
14	Our Plan	102	Ingrid's Journal - Jun 22
16	**January**	103	600th Bird of the Year
17	And So It Begins …	107	A Bird By Any Other Name
18	Winter in Maine	108	The Patagonia Picnic Table Effect
22	Sax-Zim Bog	109	Weekly Recap
26	Lifer Pie	**110**	**July**
27	Driving the Atlantic Coast	110	Florida Again
28	Ingrid's Journal - Jan 31	113	Return to Dumpster Watch
30	1st Bird of the Year	114	Little Gull
30	50th Bird of the Year	117	The Birds We Skipped
30	100th Bird of the Year	118	Sapsuckers
30	150th Bird of the Year	**120**	**August**
32	Scrub-Jays	121	Arizona in August???
34	**February**	122	Ingrid's Journal - Aug 8
34	Florida	123	Southeast Arizona Birding Festival
35	Ingrid's Journal - Feb 1	125	Ingrid's Journal - Aug 10
37	Exotics	127	Hudsonian Godwit
38	Ingrid's Journal - Feb 11	127	Cape Cod
39	Texas	128	Mammals
42	Santa Margarita Ranch	**132**	**September**
44	200th Bird of the Year	133	California
44	250th Bird of the Year	134	650th Bird of the Year
44	300th Bird of the Year	134	San Diego Pelagic
44	350th Bird of the Year	138	Finishing Up in California
47	**March**	139	Ingrid's Journal - Sep 11
47	Back in Maine	140	Ingrid's Journal - Sep 12
48	Winter Birds	141	Connecticut Warbler
50	Sandia Crest	**143**	**October**
51	Ingrid's Journal - Mar 27	144	Waiting for Vagrants
52	Drive to Arizona	144	Long Island Ferry
53	400th Bird of the Year	146	Colorado
54	Ingrid's Journal - Mar 29	149	Arizona
56	eBird	151	700th Bird of the Year
58	**April**	152	The Birds That Got Away
59	Hummingbirds and Owls	154	Orioles
60	Ingrid's Journal - Apr 4	**156**	**November**
62	450th Bird of the Year	157	Common Gull
62	Grand Canyon and Prairie Chickens	158	Snowy Owl
67	Big Year Assistant	160	Texas for the Third Time
69	Driving from Missouri to Maine	161	Thank You
70	Packing	162	Groove-billed Ani
72	New England Birding	**166**	**December**
73	Spring Migration	167	All Good Things …
76	Chickadees	168	Final Bird of the Year
78	**May**	168	Ezekiel Dobson
78	The Dry Tortugas	169	Points of the Compass
80	500th Bird of the Year	170	Woody Had It Right
85	Massachusetts	**172**	**Big Year Overview**
85	Ingrid's Journal - May 8	**173**	**Superlatives**
87	Atlantic Puffins	**174**	**Year Bird Map**
87	550th Bird of the Year	**177**	**Gallery**
89	Mt. Washington	**214**	**Index**
95	**June**		
96	Hatteras Pelagic		

Every Bird? Why?

While birding did not cause them to meet, it has been a big part of their lives since their first date, twelve years ago. Ingrid had been birding for many years, while Ethan only knew the birds that came to his yard feeders in coastal Maine.

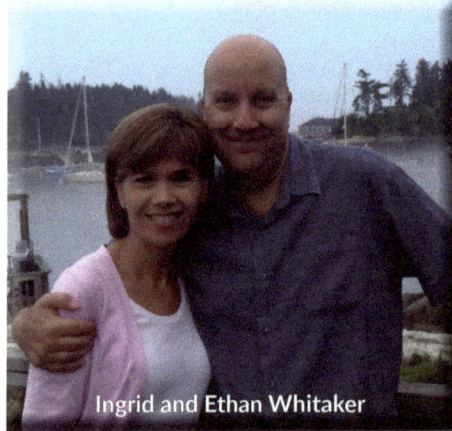
Ingrid and Ethan Whitaker

On that infamous first date, the subject of birds came up, and Ethan attempted to impress Ingrid by promising to show her a place near his home where he swore Snowy Egrets could be found…in February…in Maine. Intrigued but dubious, Ingrid played along. Needless to say, there were no Snowy Egrets to be found, but Ethan's effort was charming and opened the door to all that was to come.

In 2011, 20th Century Fox released *The Big Year*, a comedy starring Steve Martin, Owen Wilson and Jack Black. The movie was a box office failure and was quietly retired to the rear of various movie streaming services. One evening, Ethan stumbled across *The Big Year* and introduced Ingrid to the movie not long after meeting her. They thoroughly enjoyed the story of three 'competitive' birders striving to see the highest number of North American bird species in a calendar year.

Ingrid quickly became Ethan's birding mentor, buying him a decent pair of binoculars, taking him to birding festivals and slowly creating a birding addict. They vacationed at birding hot-spots in Texas, California and Arizona and began to talk a bit about what it might be like to do their own Big Year once they were both done working.

Ethan retired from the insurance

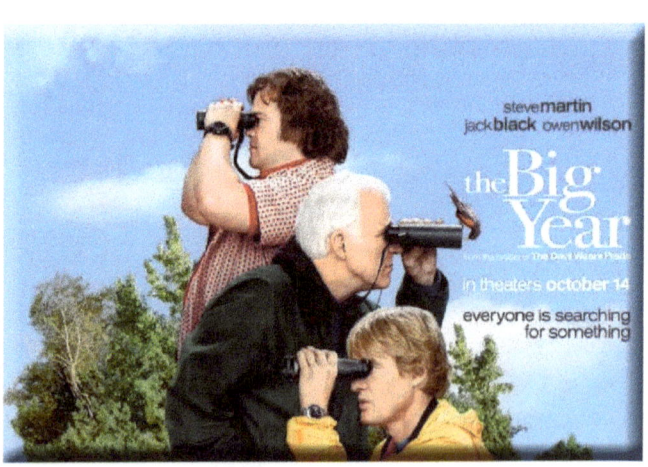

software business in 2020 and enjoyed the freedom of being able to rush out the door whenever a rare bird was spotted and spending his time in marshes, bogs and shorelines. This soon led to Ethan's Maine Big Year in 2021, when he clocked 60,000 miles on his car and established a new state record for most birds seen in a calendar year in the state, 324. He chronicled his adventures in *Every Bird in Maine*, published in 2022.

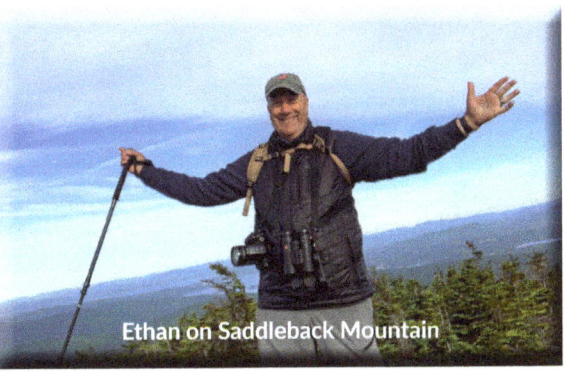
Ethan on Saddleback Mountain

With Ingrid's retirement approaching, it was time to start planning their couple's Big Year. Should they do an ABA Region Big Year or a Lower 48 Region Big Year? How would they decide where to go and when? How long would they stay in each location? Would they drive or fly or do a combination of the two? What about their pets? Should they get a camper van and bring them along, or find a house-sitter they could trust with their care? Where would they need the help of a guide, and where would they be fine on their own? These were some of the many things they needed to consider and plan for. Ethan made this his primary job for the next year.

Ingrid retired from teaching in 2023, and on January 1 2024, their Lower 48 Region Big Year plan was set in motion. Could they see 500 birds? 550? 600 or more? Join their journey - the birds, the places, the people, the highs and the lows. They are excited to share it with you.

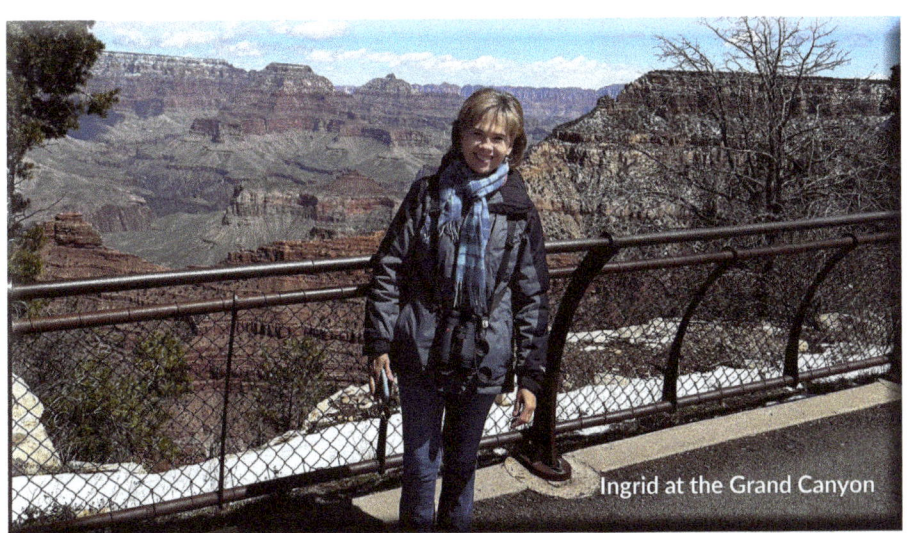
Ingrid at the Grand Canyon

Every Bird??? WHY??? 13

Our Plan

The most famous of Big Year birders was the late Sandy Komito, who broke the ABA Big Year record twice, once in 1987 and again in 1998. The latter effort was the subject of Mark Obmascik's 2005 Book, *The Big Year: A Tale of Man, Nature, and Fowl Obsession*, and later *The Big Year* film. The movie's Kenny Bostic character, portrayed by Owen Wilson, was loosely based on Komito.

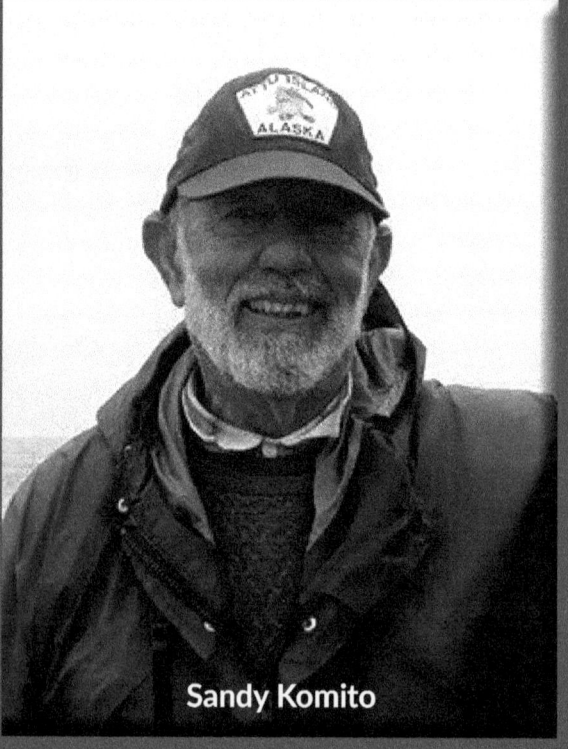

Sandy Komito

Komito's strategy was aggressive ... spending 75% of the year on the road and immediately chasing every rarity when they were seen. He would not stop for coffee or to look at the bird on the wire. He would push until he got the rare bird.

While we wanted to see as many birds as possible, the idea of spending the equivalent of nine months on the road was too much.

Ethan came up with an alternative strategy. Being a retired software developer, he designed a computer model that crunched publicly available eBird data and devised a plan to see as many species as possible while traveling as efficiently as possible.

Komito's strategy of "chase the rarities and the common birds will take care of themselves" was turned on its head. The Whitakers would try to be in the vicinity of common birds as they moved through the lower 48 states ... and the rare birds would take care of themselves.

In addition, Ethan developed an iPhone App that looked at our Big Year needs list and in real time updated maps and tables, making us aware of nearby birds as we moved across the country. [see page 67]

Instead of being on the road for 270 days like Komito, we were shooting for something closer to 140. We wouldn't challenge the Lower 48 State Record (751), set in 2022 by Ruben and Victor Stoll, but we hoped our high-tech approach would get us a commendable 600 and maybe in the top 15 birders nationally.

Not bad for a couple of 60 something retirees.

As you'll see on the following pages ... the plan worked far better than we had hoped.

January

Travel	#
Plane Flights	4
Rental Cars	2
Nights Away	9
Boat Trips	1

State	Year Birds
Connecticut	8
Delaware	1
Illinois	1
Massachusetts	41
Maryland	10
Maine	56
Minnesota	13
North Carolina	22
New Hampshire	1
New Jersey	12
Total	165

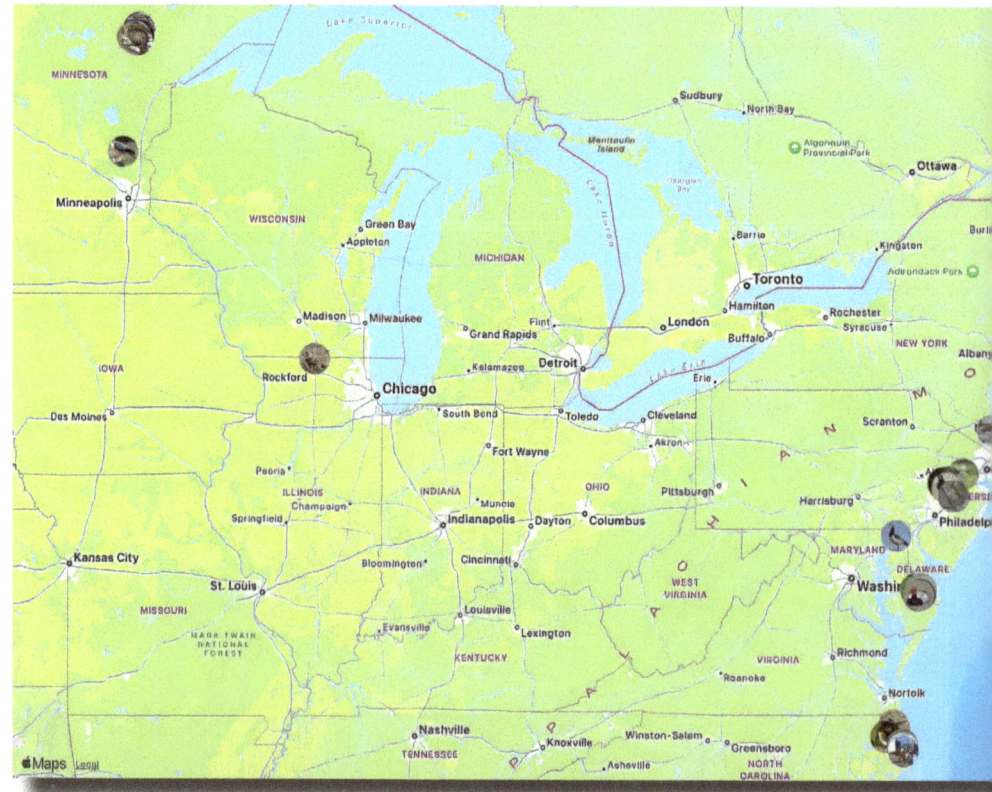

And So It Begins ...

Many birders begin their Big Years in states with a high diversity of species. While getting dozens of birds on our lists quickly would have been fun, we had a different strategy.

In the Northeast, there are birds that are most easily found in winter - Thick-billed Murre, Dovekie, and White-winged Crossbills. Our plan was to spend the first couple weeks of the year in Maine getting these birds out of the way. But as we all know, plans are made to change.

Plan deviation #1 occurred on New Year's Eve, when we spent the night in Newburyport, MA near the location of a Long-eared Owl that a birding friend had alerted us to. A Long-eared Owl is not easy to get, and we could not pass up this opportunity.

On New Year's Day, the owl was right where reported but hidden behind a pine branch ... in a hollow ... made from pine branches. In other words, very hard to see.

Fortunately, we had better views of an Eastern Screech-Owl that was also in the area. Incredibly, she was sleeping contentedly in a tree cavity in the middle of town surrounded by beautiful sea-captains' homes.

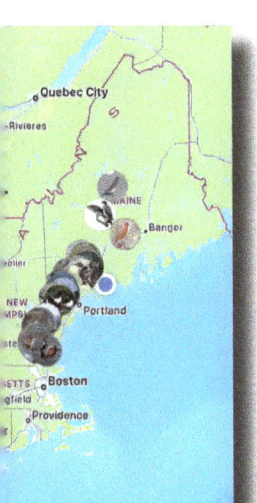

Our Day One total was 44 species, which put us in 2,666th place among Lower 48 State Birders. Not exactly an auspicious start.

We returned to our initial plan on January 2 ticking off several Maine winter birds, many of which head north into Canada and the Arctic once spring arrives. The Purple Sandpiper, one of our favorite such birds, lives on frosty, wave tossed rocks under terrible winter conditions.

On the 3rd, we deviated from our plan once again and piled into our Subaru Outback, aptly named the 'Touring Edition'. A road trip to New Jersey was called for and a quest for the Red-flanked Bluetail, a thrush-like bird. This Eurasian species, common from Great Britain to Taiwan but extremely rare in North America, had been hanging around a suburban condo community for several weeks. The homeowner was graciously allowing birders to stand in her yard and wait for the Bluetail to visit. Birds being birds, it might not stick around, so we decided we'd better try while we could.

When we arrived at the "Red-flanked Bluetail Stakeout", the bird was very cooperative, making several brief visits between a holly bush and water dish, seemingly ignorant of the dozen birders standing 30 feet away. We watched it for an hour before rushing out to see a couple of Trumpeter Swans in the next town over.

This trip proved to be an unexpectedly productive one for us, adding several more birds to our year list on our trek to and from New Jersey: Tufted Duck, Black-headed Gull (both European birds that had been blown off course), Tundra Swan and Common Gull (in of all places, a Connecticut Walmart parking lot!).

Back home, we continued to work on our list of hard-to-find Maine birds.

On a beach in York we endured miserable cold and wind, working our way through an enormous flock of gulls (400+) milling about on the sand. The flock consisted of our omnipresent Herring Gulls, Great Black-backed Gulls and Ring-billed Gulls. We hoped to find two gull species that appear in Maine each winter in very small numbers.

Trying to sort through that many birds while searching for two similar species that may or may not be there, with the wind making your eyes water and the neighborhood Irish Setter periodically rushing into the maelstrom of birds sending them all into the air, was difficult.

Incredibly though, we found both an Iceland Gull and a Glaucous Gull. Two more birds off of our must-find list.

We ended the week with a total of 89 species. Birders in Florida, Texas and Arizona had exceeded that number on January 1. It was a little embarrassing as we had publicized our Big Year effort, and now we were so far behind.

We just kept telling ourselves that Big Years are a marathon ... not a sprint.

Winter in Maine

To make matters worse, 3 nasty storms hit in the second week of the year making travel around Maine challenging. This did not stop us from pursuing a tip about a very difficult to find Northern Hawk Owl in a remote agricultural field two and a half hours from our house. We searched power lines, checked trees, stopped and walked around periodically.

After an hour and a half of searching, covering more than 9 miles, we had not found the Owl, were getting unhappy looks from adjacent landowners, and all we had to show for it was one new year bird ... a tiny Horned Lark. Our Big Year was not going well.

We decided to cut our losses and drive 90 minutes to the coast to see if the Hepatic Tanager that was frequenting a residential feeder last December was still there, and it was. We expected to see a Hepatic Tanager in Arizona in the spring, but it is remarkable that this warm weather bird, the first one ever seen in New England, was surviving a Maine winter.

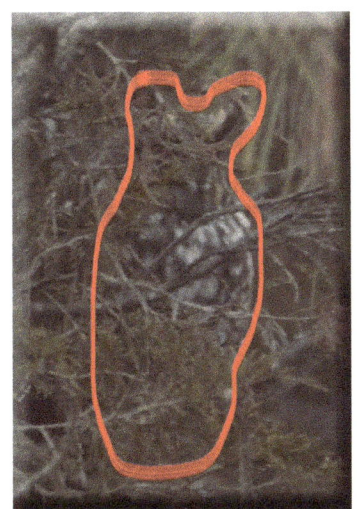
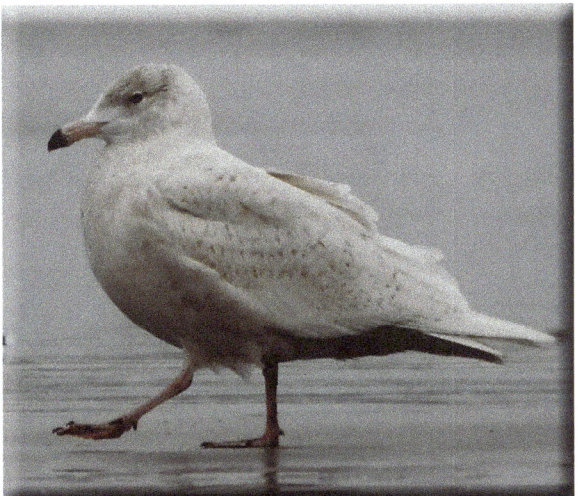
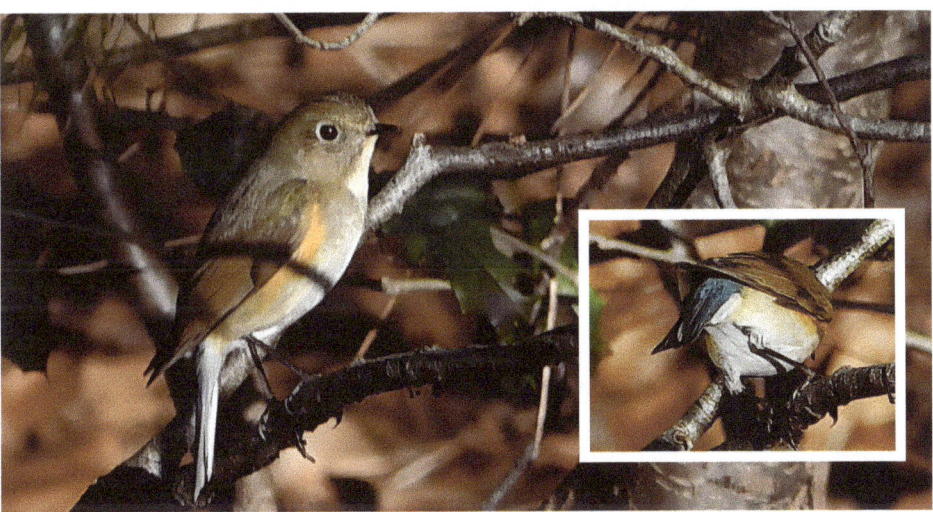
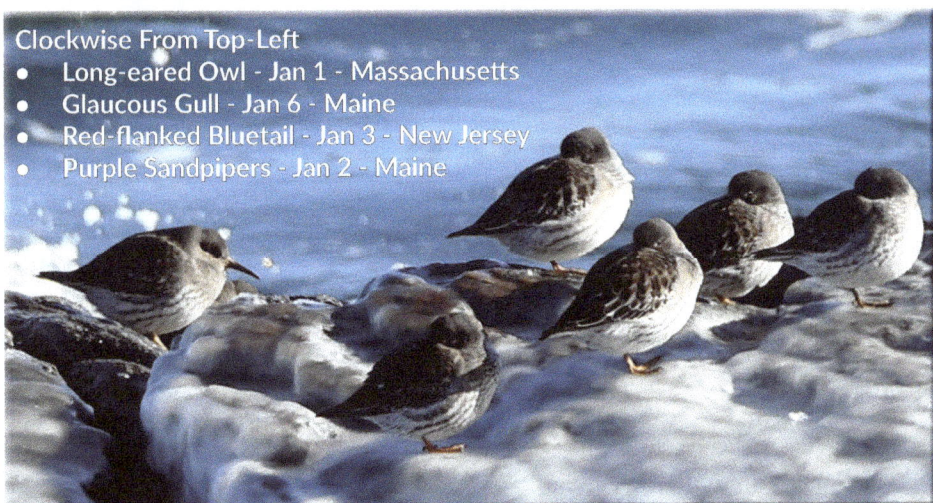

Clockwise From Top-Left
- Long-eared Owl - Jan 1 - Massachusetts
- Glaucous Gull - Jan 6 - Maine
- Red-flanked Bluetail - Jan 3 - New Jersey
- Purple Sandpipers - Jan 2 - Maine

JANUARY 19

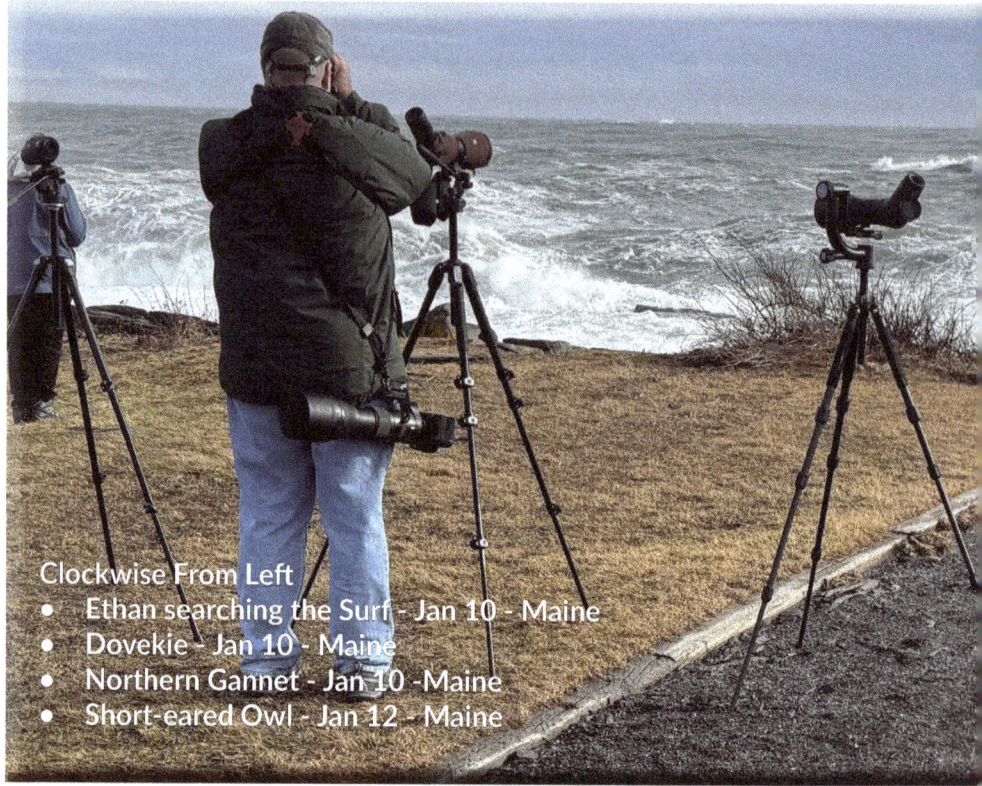

Clockwise From Left
- Ethan searching the Surf - Jan 10 - Maine
- Dovekie - Jan 10 - Maine
- Northern Gannet - Jan 10 - Maine
- Short-eared Owl - Jan 12 - Maine

Later in the week we were delighted to find a Western Tanager in Portland. A few of our local birding friends were there when we arrived, and we enjoyed their company as we waited for the bird to visit a residential feeder.

That evening, Maine was hit by another huge storm. This time we didn't get 10 inches of snow but two inches of rain with 50 to 60 mile per hour winds coming in from the ocean. We knew this wind would push seabirds toward shore, but many of the ideal locations to see these birds were closed due to severe flooding and road damage.

Fortunately, Dyer Point in Cape Elizabeth was open, despite the intimidating and dangerous surf. After our eyes adjusted to the waves, we began to see birds - lots and lots of birds – some navigating the rough waters, many more wheeling in the air. These included:

- A Northern Gannet, a bird we don't see too often in the winter.
- A handful of Dovekie ... a pigeon sized sea bird that generally stays far out to sea but was pushed toward shore by the storm.
- A couple of Razorbills, which look like a football with wings.
- And a half dozen Black-legged Kittiwakes, an uncommon gull.

When all these birds started appearing, we posted to a birding chat board, and our

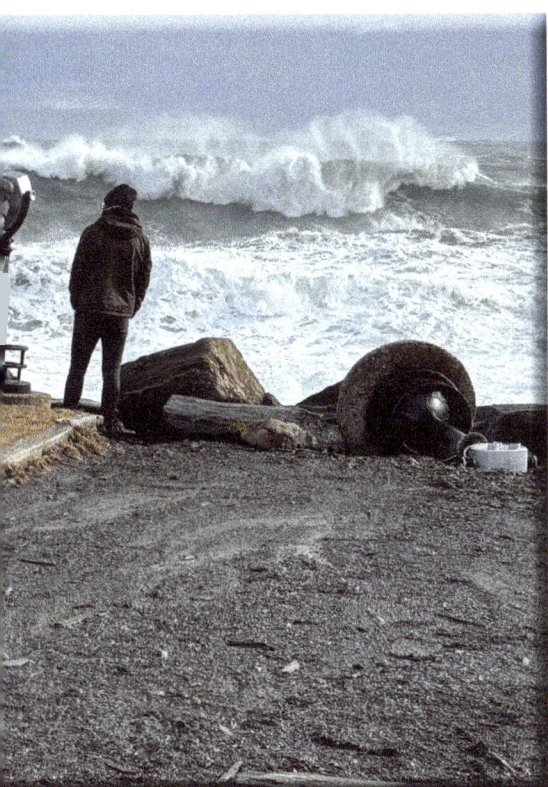
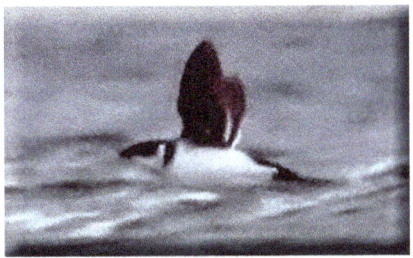
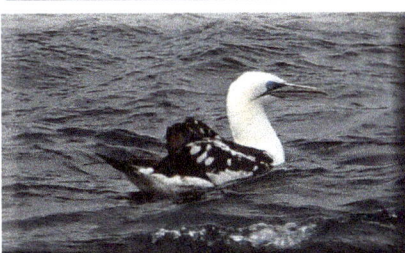
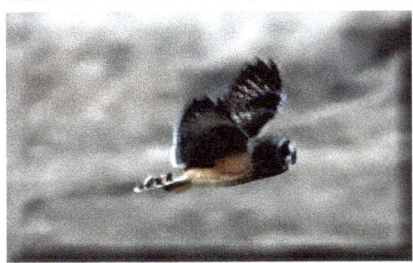

birding friends showed up within minutes. These Internet based birding message sites would be invaluable over the next 12 months. Every state, region and even county seemed to have their own tech sitting on GroupMe, Discord or WhatsApp. At times, finding these sites was more difficult than finding the birds.

The next day, a southern Maine GroupMe tipped us off to a beautiful male King Eider at Biddeford Pool—East Point Sanctuary. We spent 90 minutes staring out to sea looking for this most beautiful of ducks. We had numerous brief glimpses of the hard to find Thick-billed Murre, appearing and disappearing in the storm enhanced surf but never found the 'King'.

Later that day, we journeyed 30 minutes from our house hoping to see a pair of Short-eared Owls that had been observed late the previous afternoon. We joined a young birder who was already there and watched and waited, watched and waited.

Suddenly, Ethan spotted one flying in the distance, and then found where it landed on the ground. It took wing again and was joined by the second owl as they searched for and plunged at prey. For the next half hour as the sun sank slowly below the horizon, the three of us watched in awe as these breathtaking creatures floated moth-like over a rolling farm field. Truly magical.

We didn't necessarily have to travel to find our Maine winter birds, a casual walk through our neighborhood added us three new birds for the year – a group of Golden-Crowned Kinglets, foraging with a flock of Chickadees in the pines along our road – a Pine Warbler doing the same, and then a Carolina Wren a few trees over.

After 13 days birding primarily in Maine, our tally registered 107 birds for the year. We had stopped looking at the eBird standings which showed over 2,000 birders ahead of us. Our total species to date was very close to the plan we had drawn up ... but increasingly, our plan looked rather lame.

Sax-Zim Bog

This was a week we will always remember.... for breathtaking birds and incredible cold.

The Sax-Zim Bog is one of America's premier birding locations, where Canada's vast Boreal forests (think Spruce) reach down into the USA, providing access to species that are difficult to find in the Lower 48 States. The 'Bog' encompasses 300 square miles of Spruce, Alder and Tamarack forest ... wet, spongy, poorly drained areas, and neighboring farm fields with a few hardy homesteaders.

In the winter, temperatures regularly hover below zero, and we experienced wind chills far below that during our entire visit. Sax-Zim has recorded the Lower 48's record cold daily temperature many times over.

Our primary target was the charismatic Great Gray Owl - one of the few birds that Ingrid had seen but Ethan had not. We also hoped for a second chance at seeing a Northern Hawk Owl.

On Sunday, January 14, we boarded a United Airlines flight to Minneapolis with a layover in Chicago. From there we would rent a car and make the 3 hour drive to the Bog. A long day, but nothing too challenging. Or so we thought.

Upon landing in Chicago, things went bad quickly. The gate of our connecting flight was changed four times and the expected 8:30 pm departure time was changed to 9:00 PM.,

Then 9:45 PM.

Then 10:05 PM.

Then 11:00 PM.

Then at 11:30, the flight was canceled. Fortunately, Ingrid had the foresight, when things began to be delayed, to book us the only remaining hotel room left in the city of Chicago. So, after midnight we found ourselves walking through city streets in sub-zero weather, dragging our birding gear and luggage, looking for an over crowded shuttle bus.

Just what we imagined when we planned our Big Year.

The next morning, back at the airport, United Airlines began to delay our flight to Minnesota again, and we began to realize that if we were to get to the Sax-Zim Bog by Monday morning we would have to take matters into our own hands.

So we rented a car in Chicago and made the eight hour drive to the Bog.

On the trip home three days later, United canceled our connection out of Newark, and we ended up taking an Uber to LaGuardia, where we flew to Boston and then rented a car to get home to Maine.

Suffice it to say, we never flew on United Airlines again.

After our long journey, we finally arrived at our Sax-Zim lodge, Alesches' Accommodations. The common area, complete with a roaring fire, was shared by other birders and wildlife photographers. We enjoyed hearing their stories but were concerned that several were heading home in the morning having failed to find our much longed for Great Gray Owl.

Morning arrived, and the temperature was -14 with a 'feels like' temperature of -33. We walked the inn's grounds and soon observed a flock of Red Crossbills on a feeder, only about 20 feet away. These were our first Crossbills of the season, and we were thrilled to see them so close up.

We took this as a good omen. Later we learned that this was only the second time that Red Crossbills had ever been seen at the lodge.

As we traveled across the country for our Lower 48 State Big Year, we avoided hiring guides whenever possible. Using guides is, in the opinion of some, akin to 'corked bats and steroids'. But, we made an exception to this rule for the Sax-Zim Bog. It's too vast, too cold. The roads can be challenging, and the birds are very spread out.

After doing our research, we hired Judd Brink, a man with years of experience in the Bog. He was very excited to help us, and the three of us set off across the snow packed roads of the Bog in search of birds.

Our first sighting of the day was a Northern Hawk Owl, the bird we had missed a week earlier in Maine. Given its name because it looks like a hawk in flight, this bird seems to have a real attitude. It appears to glare at you with an angry look. Feeding on small rodents, which it hunts by sight and sound, it likes to perch on top of trees looking for prey.

Judd kept us busy until well after dark, scanning the roadside for the elusive Great Gray Owl while adding new bird after new bird to our year list.

One of the remarkable things about the Sax-Zim Bog is the elaborate private feeding stations that homeowners set up near the road. Visitors are invited to stop and

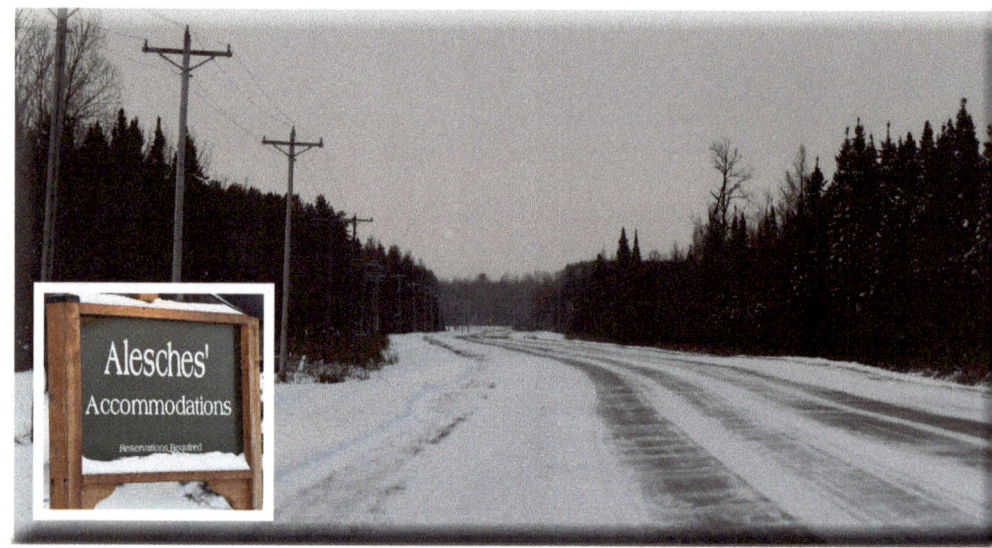
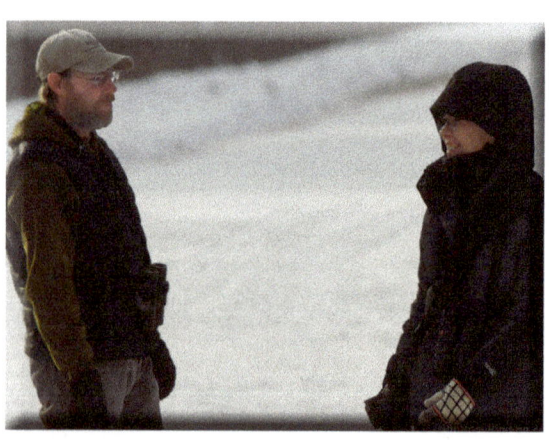
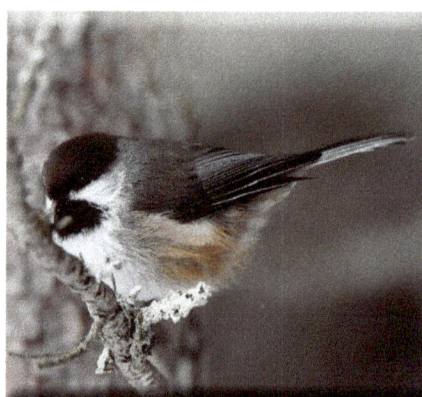

Sax-Zim Bog Jan 16-17
Counter Clockwise from Top-Left
- Icy Roads
- Judd Brink and Ingrid
- Boreal Chickadee
- Great Gray Owl
- Gray Watermelon (Great Gray Owl)
- Evening Grosbeak (Female)
- Pine Grosbeak
- Black-billed Magpie
- Northern Hawk Owl

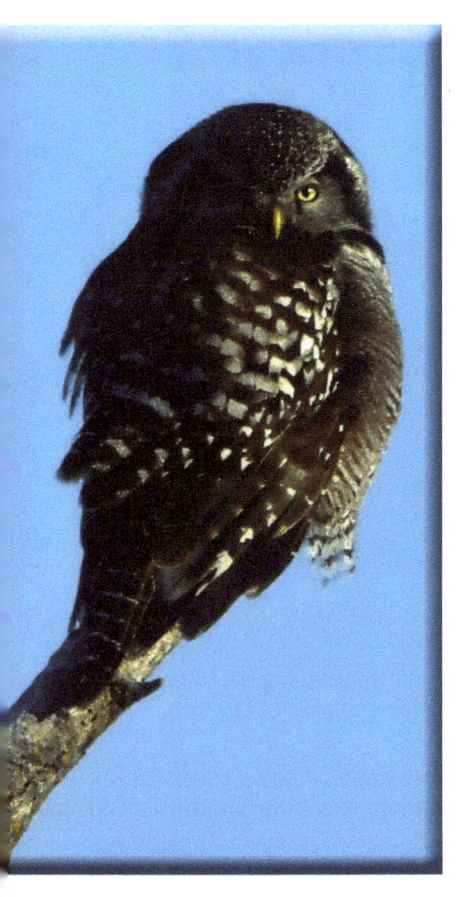
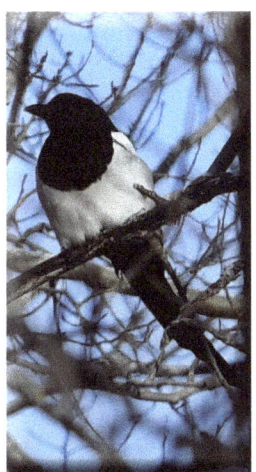
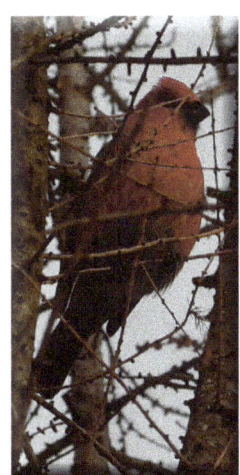
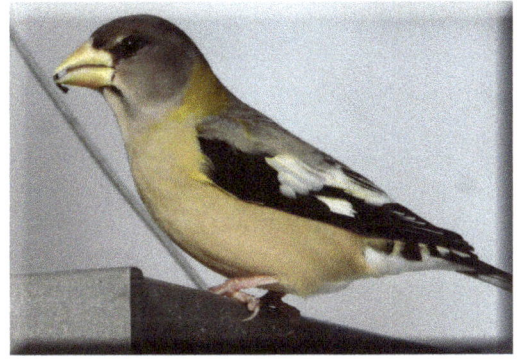

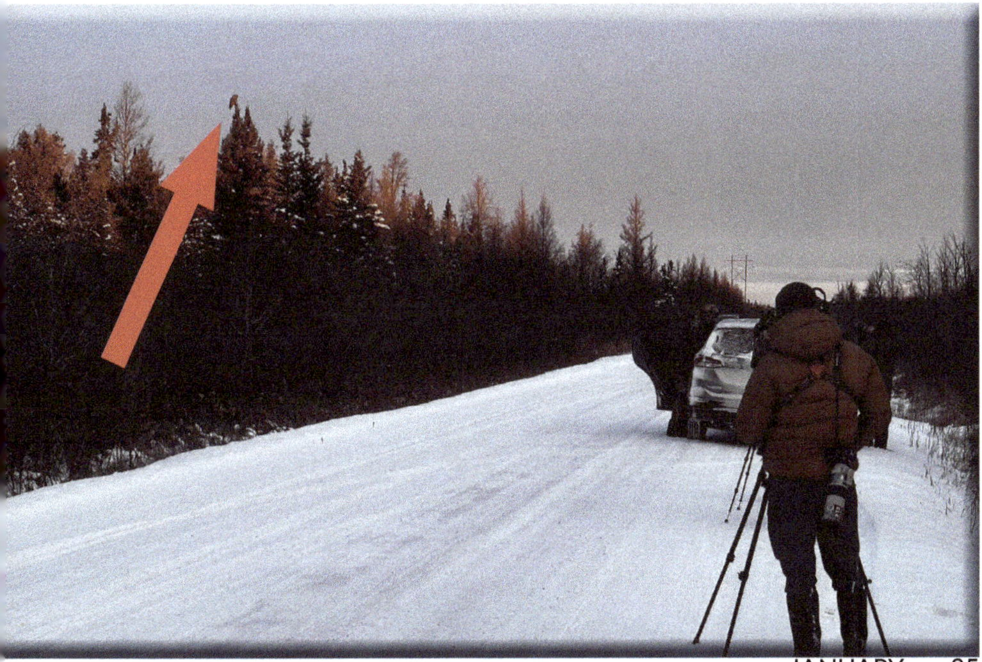

Lifer Pie

Eating a piece of pie after spotting a 'life bird' (a bird species seen for the first time) is a quirky and celebratory tradition among birders. It's a way to savor the excitement of adding a new species to one's life list—a collection of all the bird species one has identified over time. The pie tradition adds a fun ritual to birdwatching, symbolizing the 'sweetness' of achieving a new milestone.

During our Big Year we quickly realized that we had to limit our pie consumption to 'very special life birds' ... as we each added over 200 'lifers' during the year.

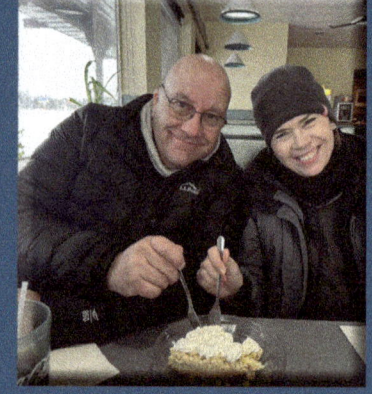

watch the feeders as birds come in.

Judd has his own, somewhat secretive, feeding station hidden in the woods where we stopped for over an hour and added 3 more birds to our year list.

As darkness began to fall, we drove up and down the road combing the trees for the Great Gray to no avail. However, we were treated to a dozen or so Ruffed Grouse feeding on the catkins of Birch trees, as the Grouse came in to roost for the night.

The next morning, we piled into Judd's Subaru Outback and once again began to scan the trees for a "gray watermelon with a white bow tie," as Judd aptly describes the Great Gray.

At exactly 7:41 AM, we received an alert on the Sax-Zim messaging site that there was a GGOW on Admiral Road.

Suddenly, we were moving down the Bog's icy, snow-packed roads at break-neck speed. Twenty minutes later, we observed the silhouette of a "gray watermelon" sitting at the top of a Spruce tree. We had at last sighted a Great Gray Owl! We crept as close as we dared to the bird and watched it for about 30 minutes until it flew off. Ethan stoically tried not to cry as the tears would have frozen to his face.

The rest of the day was spent trying to find long-shot Woodpeckers and getting better looks at some of our earlier sightings.

During our four day trip to Minnesota we added 15 new birds to our year list. Thanks to Judd's expert help, we went home having found more of our target birds than we had expected and had a lot of fun along the way.

We spent most of the next week preparing for our ten week road trip.

Part One would take us from Maine to Florida, across Alabama, Mississippi and Louisiana followed by two weeks of chasing birds along the Gulf Coast of Texas and the Rio Grande. From there we'd fly back to Maine for three weeks before returning for another week in Texas.

In Part Two, we'd move on to New Mexico and Arizona before embarking on the long drive home through Colorado, Kansas and the Midwest, hoping to catch migrating and breeding birds as we went.

All of this took place in our 2023 Subaru Outback Touring Edition, a vehicle that we bought specifically for this adventure. We had a lot of gear - binoculars, cameras, spotting scopes, field guides, food and clothing for all kinds of weather. We were going from New England winter conditions to the Arizona desert, and we needed a car that could hold all of our gear and handle any road conditions we might encounter.

We made lists, pages and pages of lists, of everything from mosquito netting to hand warmers. Packing was quite a challenge!

We did manage to squeeze in some birding amidst all of the packing, picking up both Bohemian Waxwings and Cedar Waxwings and a surprise Ruby-crowned Kinglet sitting on a wire … a real treat to see this bird in January.

Driving the Atlantic Coast

On January 28, we left the cold confines of the north and headed south to the Sunshine State, Florida. So far we had seen 131 birds in our Lower 48 State Big Year, and there were some 2,000 birder across the country that had seen more.

After loading up the car, we left our Maine Coon Cats and our home in the hands of our trusted house sitter. Our first stop was Newton, Massachusetts for a birthday party for Ingrid's dad. At 4:30 we made our apologies to the family and jumped on the Mass Turnpike with the intention of reaching New York State before bed.

Unfortunately, the actual weather forgot to check with the predicted weather and we watched the dashboard thermometer drop below 32 degrees. The expected rain turned into unexpected snow and rapid accumulation. Within 20 minutes we realized we would be in trouble if we kept driving, so we found a hotel in Sturbridge, Massachusetts, two hours short of our planned first night's destination. Not the start we had hoped for!

When morning arrived, the snowplows had cleared and treated the roads, and we were off to find a Pink-footed Goose.

The Pink-footed Goose is a winter resident of Europe. It spends the summer nesting in Greenland and Iceland. Every so often, one of these geese flies west instead of

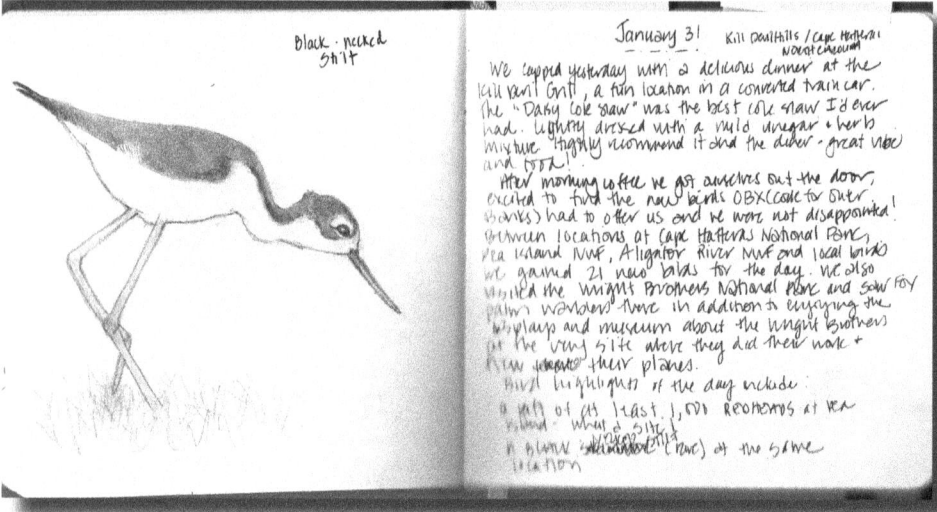

east in autumn and excites birders in the US. Our quarry had been hanging out with a large flock of Canada Geese in a community park in Lincroft, New Jersey.

Unfortunately, the Pink-footed Goose is brown, gray and black (like Canada Geese). The two species are about the same size, eat the same stuff and act just the same. To find a single bird, in a flock of three hundred birds, is a little bit like playing "Where's Waldo". But, we got lucky, and after about 5 minutes of scoping, we found it.

Two hours later, we found another rarity - a Barnacle Goose in Smyrna, Delaware.

This wayward bird from Greenland/Iceland is white and black and easy to separate from the Canada Geese. Except, it took us quite a while to find the flock. Our Big Year endeavor would have been so much easier if birds would just stay in one place!

Birds are coded by scarcity, with very common birds being Code 1 and extinct birds designated Code 6. The Pink-footed and Barnacle Geese are both designated Code 4. Thus, we were delighted to get two rare birds on day one of our road trip.

We spent the night in Ocean City, Maryland and picked up another five birds for the year before dark.

Kill Devil Hills, North Carolina, near Kitty-hawk where the Wright Brothers made their first flights, was our next stop. There we stayed 2 nights, spending the day seeing the birds that make the mid-Atlantic home each winter.

We saw hundreds of enormous Tundra Swans, thousands of beautiful Redhead Ducks, and lots of first of the year wading birds. These barrier islands yielded us 25 new birds for the year.

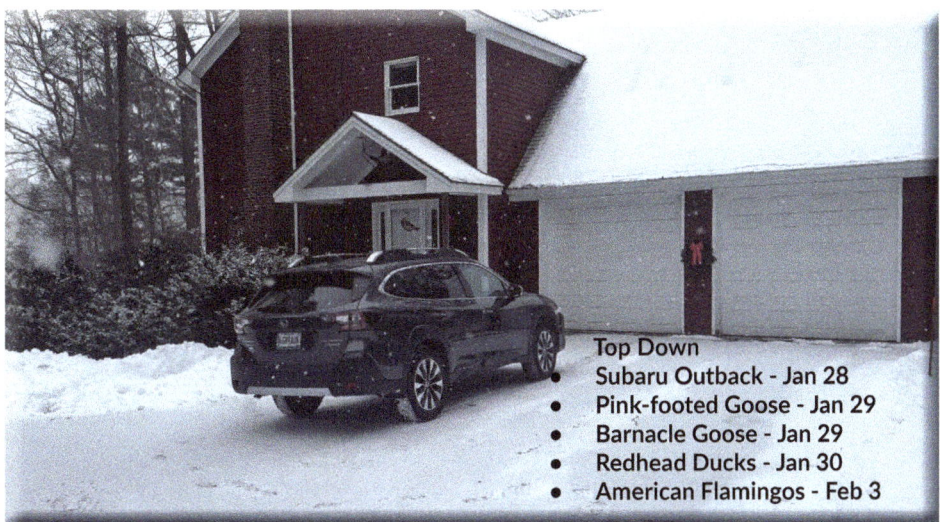

Top Down
- Subaru Outback - Jan 28
- Pink-footed Goose - Jan 29
- Barnacle Goose - Jan 29
- Redhead Ducks - Jan 30
- American Flamingos - Feb 3

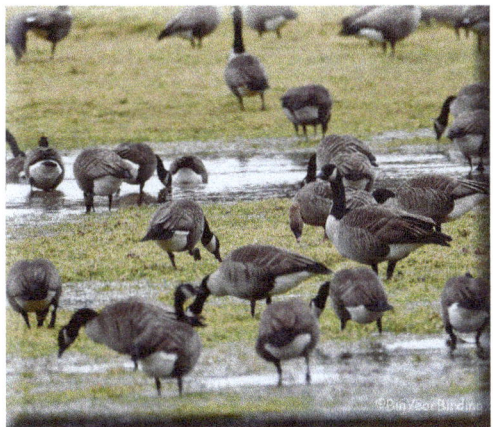

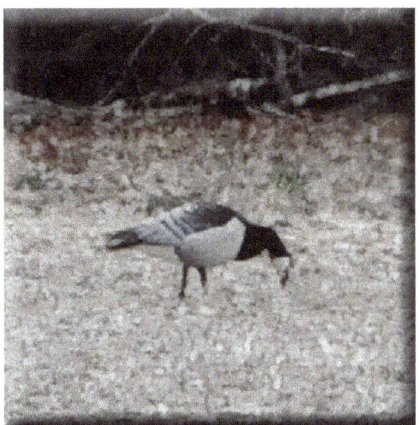

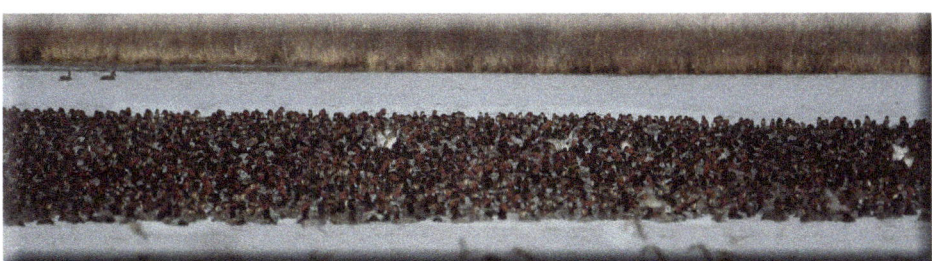

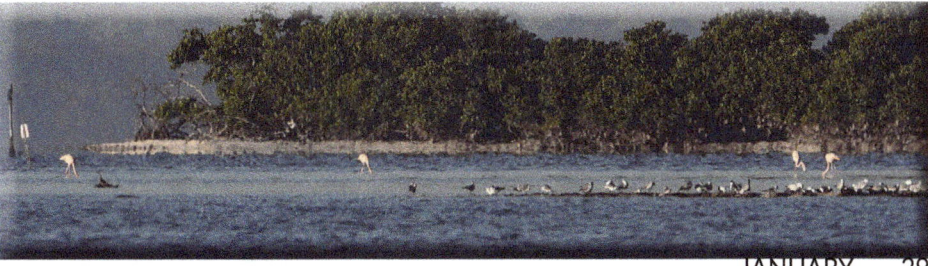

1st Bird of the Year

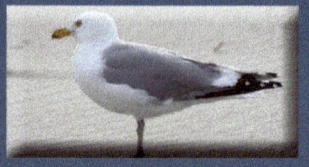

We observed our first bird of the Year in Salisbury, Massachusetts ... the ubiquitous **Herring Gull**. We have no idea how many Herring Gulls we saw over the course of the year, but no doubt, it was in the hundreds of thousands.

In October it was renamed the American Herring Gull (see splits on Page 103).

January 1, 7:10 AM

50th Bird of the Year

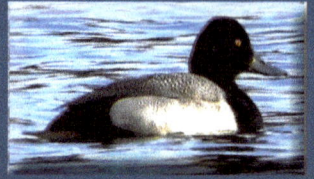

A male **Lesser Scaup** was seen on Grondin Pond in Scarborough, Maine, a large duck pond in a residential community. Each winter, Grondin Pond is host to a wide variety of waterfowl, until it freezes over.

January 2, 1:47 PM

100th Bird of the Year

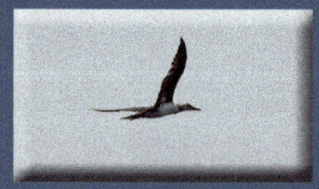

After a massive wind and rain storm that caused tremendous damage and closed many roads throughout the State of Maine, we observed this late in the season **Northern Gannet** flying south over the heavy surf in Cape Elizabeth, Maine.

January 10, 11:00 AM

150th Bird of the Year

While observing thousands of Redhead Ducks, hundreds of shorebirds and dozens of Tundra Swans on the Outer Banks of North Carolina, we were surprised to see the normally secretive **American Bittern** fly up out of the marsh and relocate to a distant location.

January 31, 8:34 AM

Our next goal awaited in Georgetown, South Carolina ... the endangered Red-cockaded Woodpecker.

Unlike other woodpeckers, the Red-cockaded nests only in living Long-leaf Pines, drilling chambers in the trees from 7 to 50 feet off the ground. They move about in family groups, called clans, made of mother, father and young males (or helpers). Each chamber can take the clan up to a year to carve out, with the males doing all the work.

The birds also drill small holes around the nesting cavity. This forces pitch and sap to flow down the tree, discouraging snakes and raccoons from attacking the nest.

Naturalists working to restore the Red-cockaded Woodpecker population mark nesting trees with two white bands near the trunk. A local naturalist gave us the location of a stand of Long-leaf Pines with four nesting trees in it. The birds had been active there that week.

We arrived at about 2:00 in the afternoon and began the wait. Four hours later it was dark, and we had not seen nor heard the birds.

The next morning, Friday, we rechecked the stand ... still no birds ... and headed south forty-five minutes to the Francis Marion National Forest to try again. Stop one produced nothing. Stop two, same result.

Just as we made the decision to cut our losses and head to Florida, a medium-sized black and white woodpecker flew right in front of us and into a nearby tree. It was a Red-cockaded Woodpecker! Evidently, the bird sensed our disappointment and took pity on us.

After this triumph of historic proportions, we pointed our once shiny black car toward Florida and Flamingos. Before we became serious birders, we assumed Flamingos were relatively common birds in Florida. On the contrary, they are quite rare ... in Florida and the rest of the country.

That all changed last year when Hurricane Idalia swept flocks of American Flamingos up from the Bahamas and deposited them all over the United States with verified reports in Wisconsin, Michigan, Kansas, Texas, Kentucky, Louisiana, Ohio, North Carolina, Virginia, South Carolina, Alabama and of course Florida. The wayward birds immediately started south and by January of our Big Year only two small flocks remained in the USA, one on Merritt Island near Cape Canaveral and the other near Ft. Meyers, both in Florida.

At about 4:00 PM we rolled onto Merritt Island. We stood right where dozens of other birders had observed the birds over the last week, stared at the same nearby island where dozens of other birders had seen the birds, and saw nothing. The sun was setting right behind the island, and we could see nothing but bright, iris frying, skin burning sun. Our quest for American Flamingos would have to wait till morning.

When morning came, the sun was at our backs, and there were the American Flamingos right where they were supposed to be, about a quarter mile away across the bay.

We were amazed at their size (up to six feet tall). They dwarf every other bird around them, and their feathers are a vibrant pink that no plastic lawn ornament could ever imitate.

Thus began one of the more wonderful days of birding we have ever experienced starting with a Painted Bunting at the Merritt Island Visitors' Center and followed by 6 miles of incredible Florida birds. Simply exhilarating!!!

Our final bird of the day was the Florida Scrub-Jay. This completed our Grand Slam of lifer Scrub-Jays (California, Woodhouse, Island and now Florida) which began over seven years ago. We hoped to see them all again in 2024.

Scrub-Jays

The Scrub-jays of North America are a fascinating example of how species can evolve and adapt to different environments, eventually becoming distinct from each other. Initially, the Scrub-jay was considered a single species, simply called the Western Scrub-Jay, but further research revealed substantial genetic, behavioral, and ecological differences. Today, birders recognize four separate species: the California Scrub-Jay, Woodhouse's Scrub-Jay, Island Scrub-Jay, and Florida Scrub-Jay. Each species occupies a distinct range and has unique adaptations suited to its environment, illustrating the dynamic process of specialization.

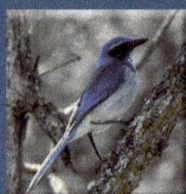

The California Scrub-Jay is found primarily along the Pacific Coast, from Oregon through California and into Baja California, Mexico. It inhabits Oak woodlands, chaparral, and urban areas, and is known for its bold and curious nature. California Scrub-Jays have a striking blue-and-gray coloration, with more intense blue hues compared to their relatives.

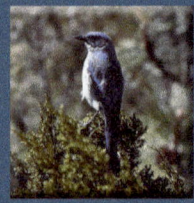

Woodhouse's Scrub-Jay ranges across the interior West, from Nevada and Utah to Texas and central Mexico. It prefers arid, open habitats with Pinyon Pine and Juniper woodlands and is generally more shy and more subdued in appearance than the California Scrub-Jay. It has a slightly grayer plumage with a more slender bill.

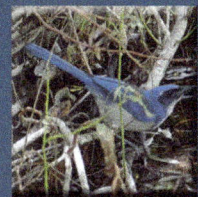
The Island Scrub-Jay is the rarest of the group, living only on Santa Cruz Island off the coast of southern California. This isolation has led to unique evolutionary traits: Island Scrub-Jays are larger and more vibrant in color than their mainland relatives, with deeper blue plumage and a stout, powerful bill.

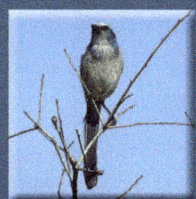
The Florida Scrub-Jay is the only Scrub-jay species found in the southeastern United States, specifically in Florida's rare and endangered scrub habitats. This species is entirely dependent on Florida scrub lands, a habitat characterized by sandy soil and sparse vegetation, which is frequently maintained by wildfires.

The split of the Western Scrub-Jay into four species arose from studies in the early 2000s, which identified distinct genetic lineages, behavioral differences, and environmental adaptations among the birds. Researchers found that each group had developed unique calls, social behaviors, and physical traits that corresponded with the demands of their specific habitats. As more sophisticated genetic analysis became available, scientists were able to confirm these differences at a molecular level, solidifying the case for recognizing separate species. This split from a single species into four showcases how geographic isolation and ecological niches can drive specialization over time.

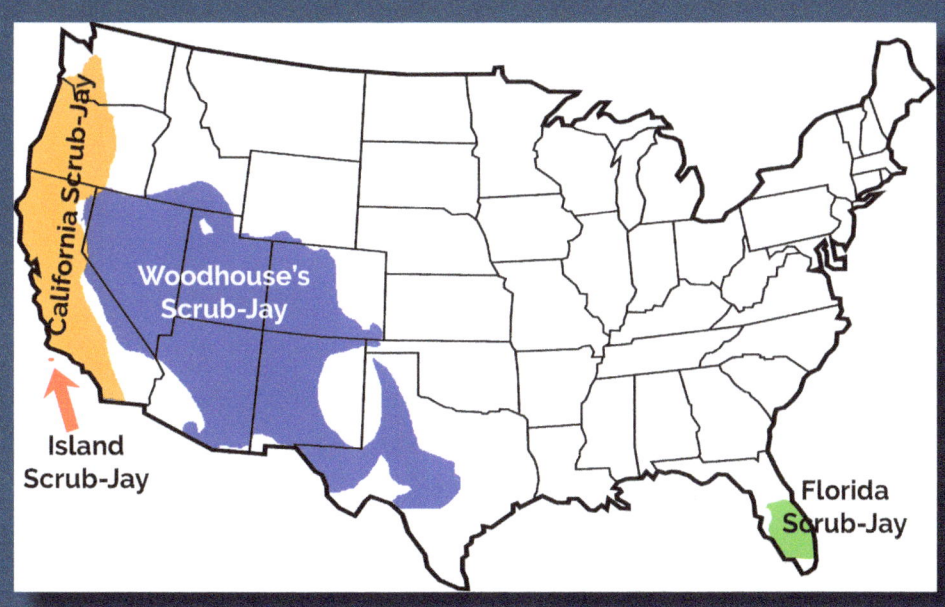

February

Travel	#
Plane Flights	8
Rental Cars	0
Nights Away	29
Boat Trips	1

State	Year Birds
Florida	90
Louisiana	4
South Carolina	8
Texas	105
Total	207

Florida

As expected, after our booming first day in Florida, the pace of new birds slowed, but we did not! Despite two days of steady rain and wind, both of which make songbirds hunker down much like us humans, we were determined to find what we could. The variety of shorebirds and wading birds in Florida were a help here, as they are less bothered by bad weather.

The first days of the week were spent in the vicinity of Cape Canaveral. Unfortunately, several of our destinations turned out to be gated or otherwise private

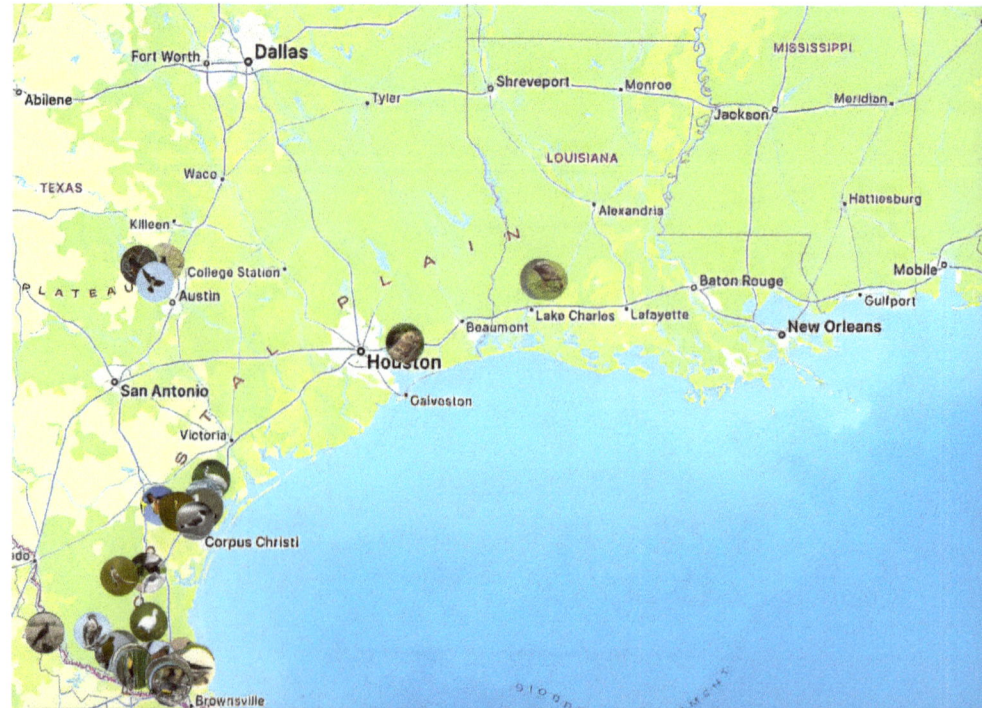

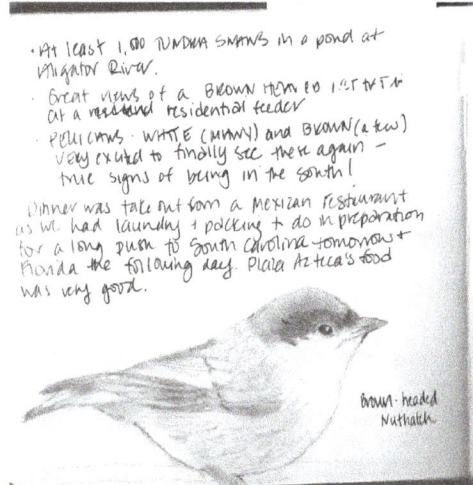

communities. Ahhh, to know that the bird you are seeking may be waiting just on the other side of a wall. That Egyptian Goose feeding on a pond-side lawn in Melbourne? Forget it! Despite these obstacles, we managed to tick off an average of 8-12 new birds each day.

On February 6 we packed up Great Auk (that's right, we named our Subaru Outback after an extinct bird) and headed for Homestead, Florida, just north of the Everglades. On the way we found a flock of Gray-headed Swamphens, an awkward, yet beautiful, rail.

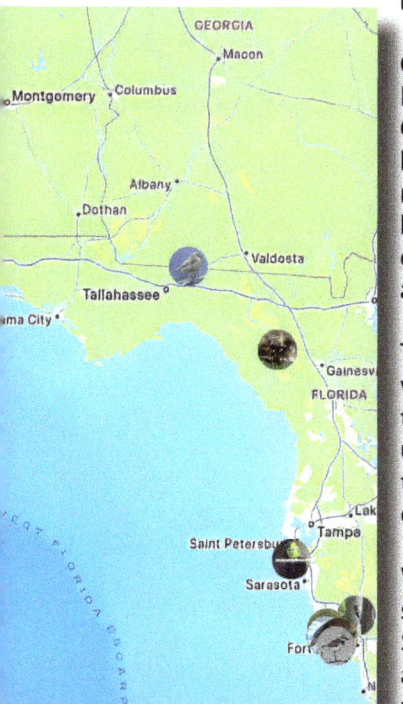

On Thursday, we ventured out to find a Common Myna, a species native to India and Southeast Asia. Common Mynas were brought to the USA as caged birds for their beauty and their mimicry. A few Mynas have escaped into the wild and established a breeding community around Miami, making them countable Big Year birds. We found two walking on a lawn in an urban area of Homestead.

The Everglades, while providing stunning vistas, were a bit disappointing from the birding perspective. Perhaps we were in the wrong places or just unlucky. The reptiles were cool, but birds were hard to find. We did see a Mangrove Cuckoo, however, one of our target birds.

We reached Fort Myers after a journey across the state and began the search for our next target bird. Some birds were almost handed to us. We'd see a report, go to the location and the bird was right there - almost too easy. But then we'd remember

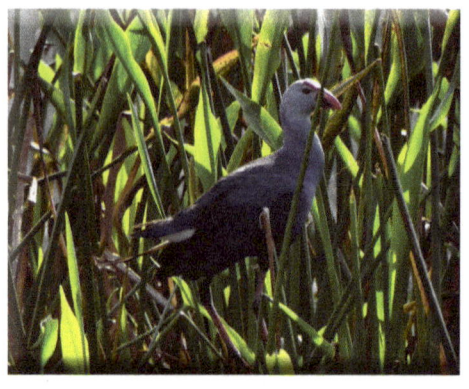
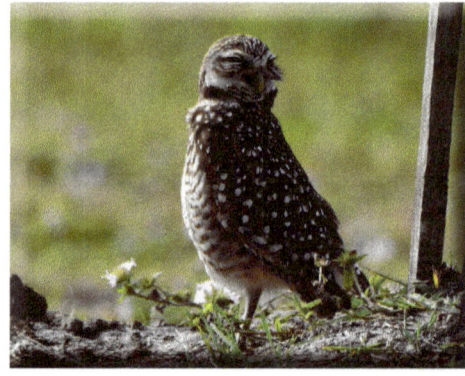
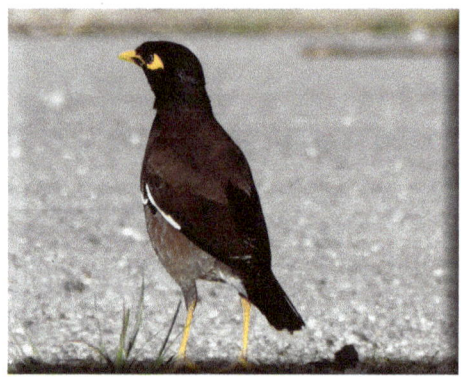
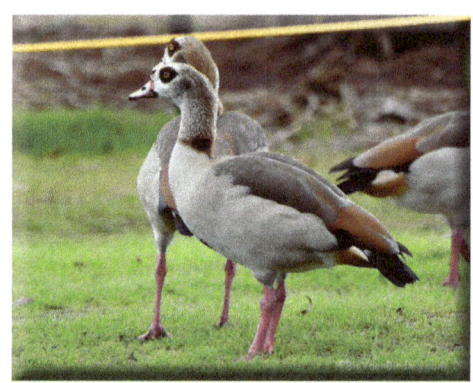

the birds that made us wonder why we continue this silly sport. Like the Wilson's Plover.

What we thought was going to be a pretty quick pick-up turned into a two mile hike across a beach full of sunbathers, partiers and dogs. We felt out of place and looked it - so much so that one beach-goer asked us if we worked for National Geographic!

There were a few birds about, but not the Wilson's. We kept walking and scanning, walking and scanning and finally found the bird across a mudflat at the extent of our binoculars. Not the most satisfying view, but one more tick.

Being in Fort Myers, we of course had to go see our beloved Boston Red Sox Spring Training facility. On the way, we stopped at a Little League field in Fort Myers hoping to find Burrowing Owls that nest near the playing fields. We pulled into the parking lot and immediately saw four Burrowing Owls staring at us.

A minute later, we heard some cackling and looked up to see several Monk Parakeets building a nest. They are noisy, social birds. No wonder a group of parakeets is called a 'chatter'!

A tourist pontoon boat took us out into the bay at sunset to view the other colony of Flamingos in the state, at Black Skimmer Island. The 11 birds, mostly juveniles, were so close we could almost touch them.

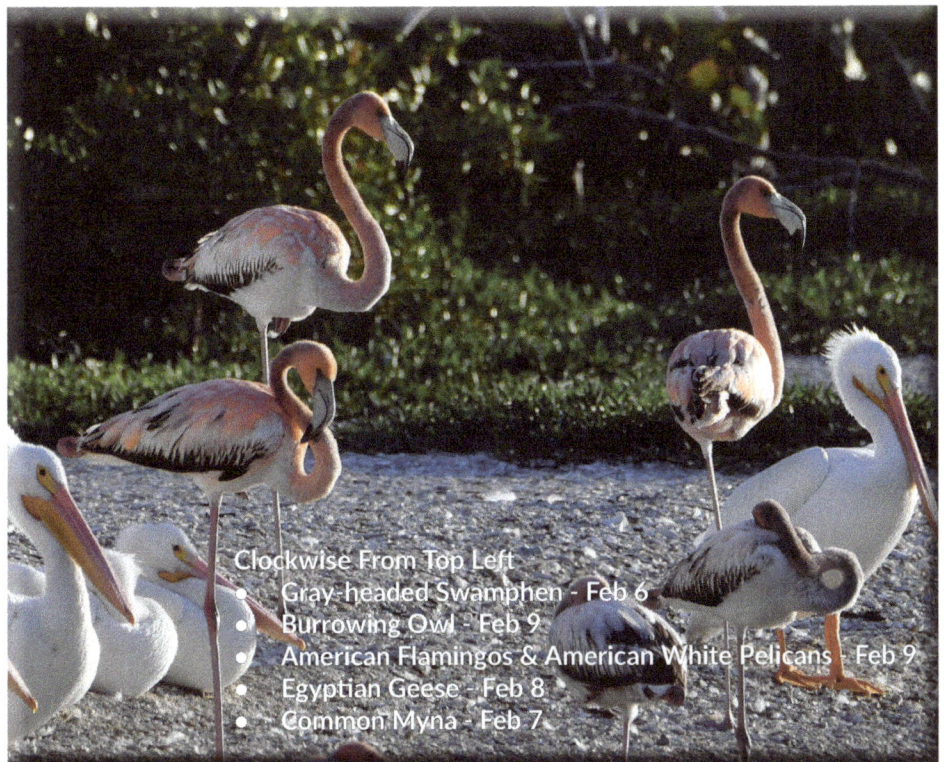

Clockwise From Top Left
- Gray-headed Swamphen - Feb 6
- Burrowing Owl - Feb 9
- American Flamingos & American White Pelicans - Feb 9
- Egyptian Geese - Feb 8
- Common Myna - Feb 7

As we returned to the harbor, we were treated to two more first of the year birds coming in to roost for the night - a Yellow-crowned Night-Heron and a Black-crowned Night-Heron.

Those elusive Egyptian Geese hiding from us in gated communities? We finally found a flock of seven at a PUBLIC golf course!

Exotics

Species from Asia and South America brought into southern Florida as pets make up many of South Florida's 'exotics'. Escaped and released birds over time have established breeding colonies. Now that these colonies have existed for a number of generations, they are countable in a Big Year.

Moving around one of America's largest cities finding unfamiliar birds was a bit overwhelming to us. So, we hired David Simpson, a well-known Florida birder and naturalist, as our guide. For nine hours we moved from neighborhood to neighborhood, finding Parakeets at one stop, Macaws at another. It was an incredible day!

February 14 was notable, not only because it was Valentine's Day, but also because it yielded zero new birds for us. As we made our way through Alabama, Mississippi and Eastern Louisiana, there were no birds to chase along our route. Ethan tried

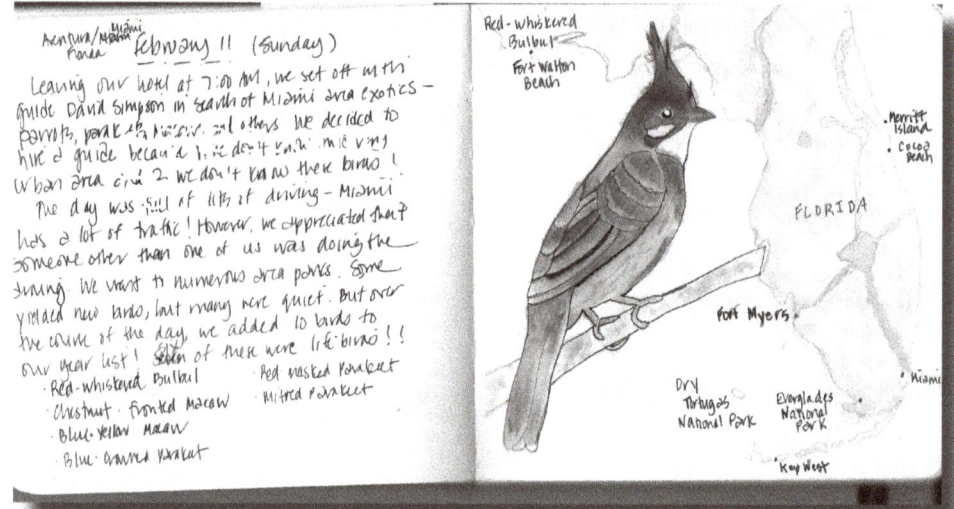

very hard to turn every rest area bird into a new one, but those ubiquitous Yellow-Rumped Warblers we'd seen in high numbers in every state we'd been in simply refused to cooperate!

Determined to change this situation, we found a hotspot along the next day's route at a landfill area in Louisiana. Here we picked up four new birds for the year. You might be surprised to know how many birds can be found at landfills and water treatment plants!

Checking the nearby sightings, we noticed several from Anahuac National Wildlife Refuge. We first visited this wonderfully birdy wildlife drive in April, 2017. It was a bit of a detour, but we couldn't pass it up. Here, the birds helped us pump up our year count by 3 - the most exciting of which came at the end, a majestic and very

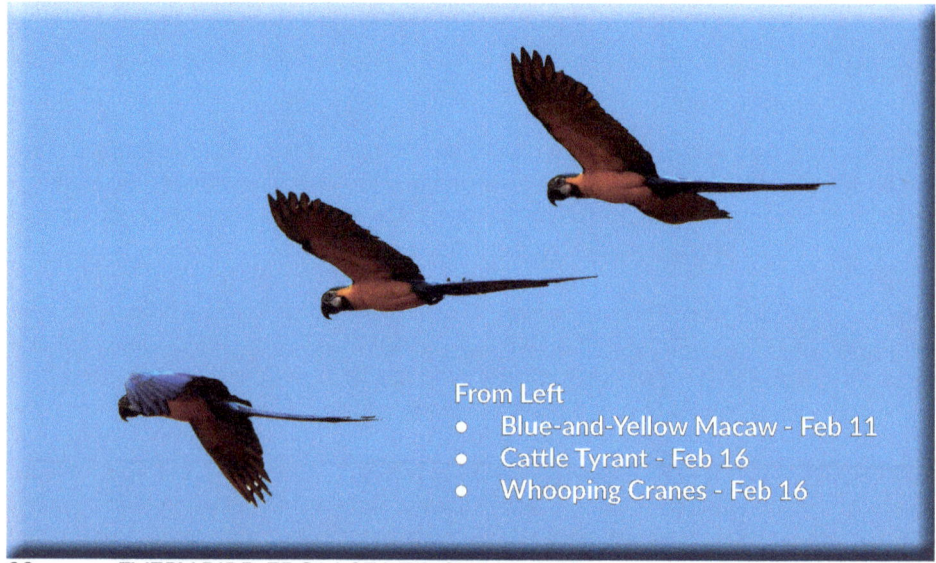

From Left
- Blue-and-Yellow Macaw - Feb 11
- Cattle Tyrant - Feb 16
- Whooping Cranes - Feb 16

accommodating White-tailed Kite.

Leaving Victoria, Texas on Thursday morning, we were excited to try our luck on a tip we got from good birding friend Eddy Edwards. Eddy had observed 20 Whooping Cranes the day before in a field just north of Corpus Christi. They were there, just as Eddy had promised. We also enjoyed views of Sandhill Cranes as there were several of them there as well.

Corpus Christi, the home of an off-course Cattle Tyrant, was our next stop. The Cattle Tyrant should have been in South America following cattle around, in a flock of its kind. But this particular bird missed that memo and had been hanging around a busy intersection since November, enjoying the insects provided by dumpsters in the parking lots of nearby restaurants. We had had our fingers crossed for weeks that this bird would still be present when we finally arrived in Texas, and we were thrilled that he stuck around for us.

Our birding luck took a turn for the worse on Saturday, as Mother Nature decided to send the Lower Rio Grande River Valley a nasty front of rain and wind. We were out chasing birds anyway, especially the many rarities to be found in Brownsville. But, despite our best efforts, we could not find these birds. They were likely hunkering down to ride out the storm. Cold and soaked to the skin, we decided to call it quits for the day, warm up with hot cocoa and start again tomorrow. All was not lost though - we did pick up eight new birds for the year.

Texas

Birding is often a lot of excruciating, mind-numbing waiting. Such was our quest for the Fan-tailed Warbler. Normally a resident of Mexico and Central America, a single bird strayed north and had been observed near "the styrofoam" in Brownsville.

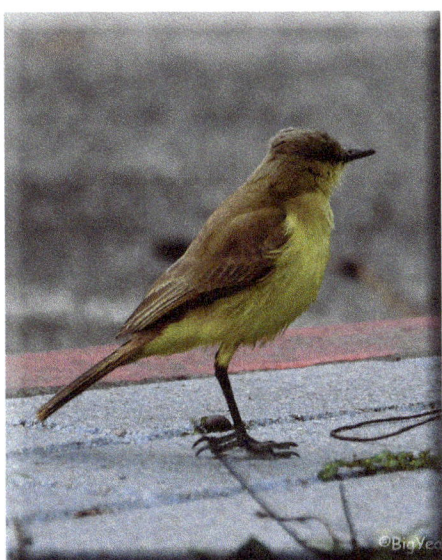
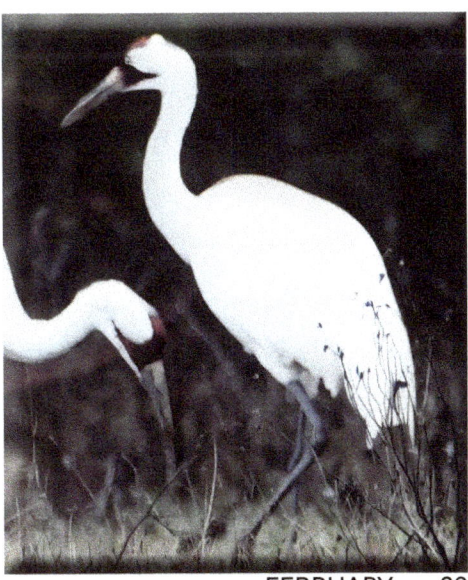

Since we'd left Maine, we'd been reading reports of this 'magic' styrofoam and imagined a huge block of foam insulation at a construction site. Instead, the styrofoam was a tiny piece of rubbish at the bottom of a dry stream in a claustrophobic hole in the woods. There we joined fifteen other birders silently staring at the filthy trash. Some had been there for 7 hours at a clip.

Now that's entertainment!

We visited the styrofoam on two different days, striking out on the first visit and getting lucky on the second. On the latter, the bird showed for a brief glimpse after only 20 minutes of waiting and then again 15 minutes later when it put on quite a show, including walking across one birder's feet.

Earlier in the morning, we broke a couple speed limits getting to a Gray-Collared Becard. The Gray-Collared Becard is another Mexican expatriate. El Niño had changed weather patterns over the last few months, perhaps driving some of these rare birds into Texas. On this, our third trip to see the bird, it disappeared a minute after we arrived. Our visit was unsatisfying, and the photo was poor, but the bird counted toward our Big Year.

Another rarity we 'saw' was a Golden-crowned Warbler who played hide and seek with us for 20 minutes in Harlingen, Texas. A professional birding guide, Cameron Cox, was helping his client find the bird, and he graciously helped us 'get on it' too. A lover of thick underbrush, the Golden-crowned Warbler was just a few feet from us.

Parrots are noisy, entertaining birds. Oliveira Park in Brownsville, Texas is a beautiful residential park full of soccer fields, skateboard pipes, tennis and basketball courts. We visited the park in December 2018 to watch the Parrots come into roost and were there again to add them to our Big Year list.

Just before sunset, as the lights for the athletic facilities went on, the Parrots began to arrive. In the hundreds. The squawking was deafening.

The funny thing, the kids playing soccer and the parents and grandparents watching the kids playing soccer never looked up at the swarming mass of green and red birds. Nor did they seem to notice the dozen birders and photographers standing on the sidewalks. An everyday occurrence for them, but thrilling for us!

The Brownsville Landfill is a legendary birding spot, one that Ethan insisted we visit. Over the years the dump has been a place to find Tamaulipas Crow, Chihuahuan Ravens and rare gulls. There were so many birds - mainly Vultures and Laughing Gulls - it was impossible to get an ID on anything else. Due to the usual less pleasant characteristics of dumps, we did not stay long!

One of the most iconic birds of the US southwest is the Greater Roadrunner. This bird is so elusive that despite his best efforts, even Wiley E. Coyote can't capture

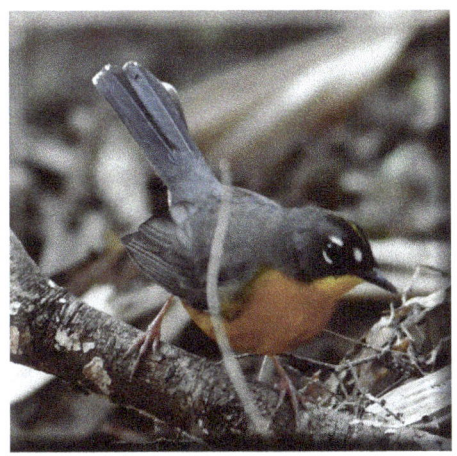 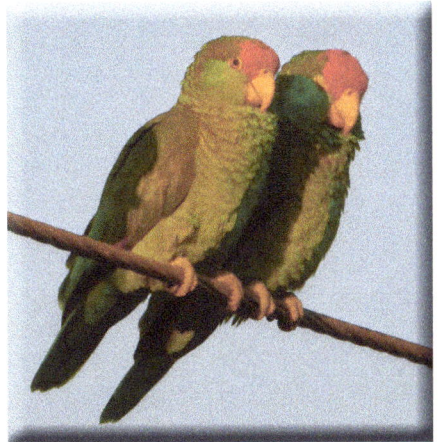

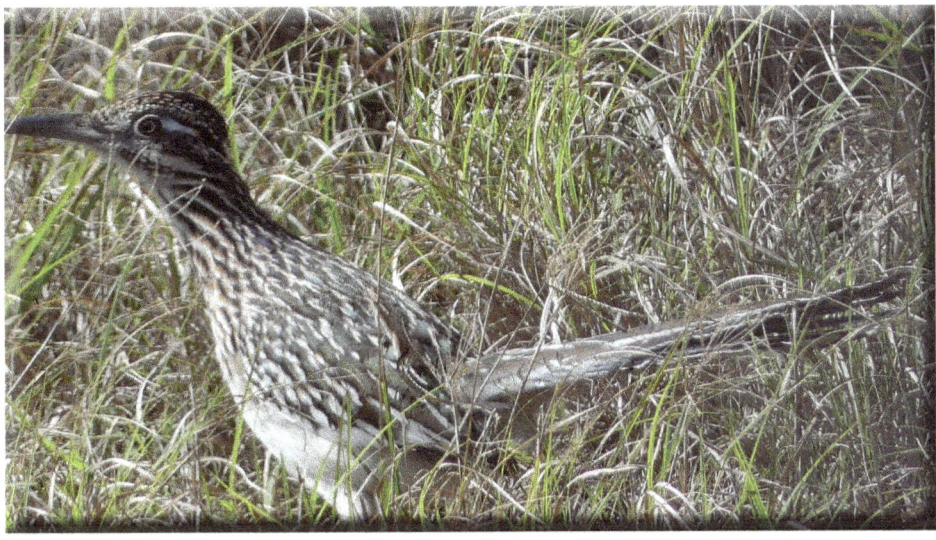

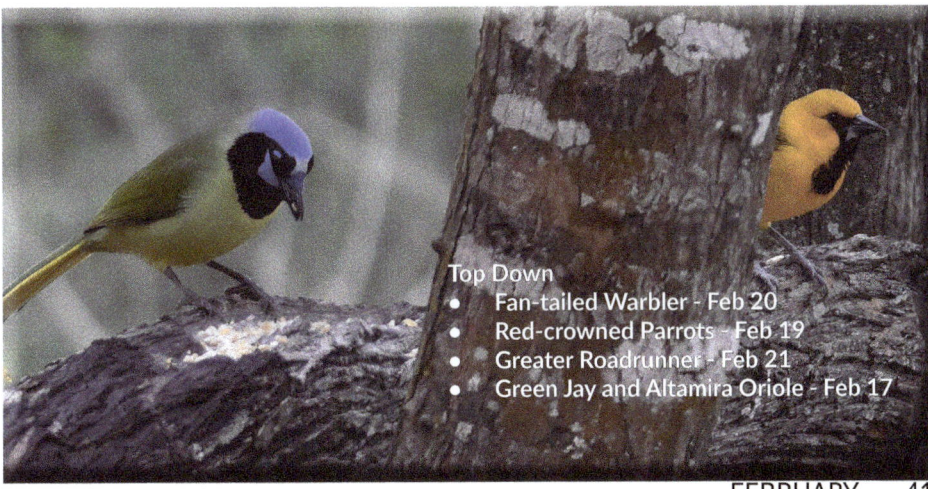

Top Down
- Fan-tailed Warbler - Feb 20
- Red-crowned Parrots - Feb 19
- Greater Roadrunner - Feb 21
- Green Jay and Altamira Oriole - Feb 17

him! And we haven't had much luck over the years either. Before this week, the only time we had seen one was when one ran across the road, living up to its name, in Patagonia, Arizona a few years ago.

Thanks again to our friend Eddy we were given a tip about one of their favorite spots, near the entrance to a nature preserve in the Rio Grande River Valley. We drove the road carefully, scanning for this rascally bird and came up empty.

After walking around the preserve, we also came up short on a rare Blue Bunting reported there and headed out. As we drove the road again, Ethan spotted a hooked beak poking out of tall reeds at the edge of the road. We stopped and waited. Lo and behold, a Roadrunner came into view. We quickly grabbed our cameras and barely got photos before he darted out of sight once again.

Leaving the Rio Grande Valley behind, we drove north to Port Aransas. On the way, we came upon an enormous flock of Snow Geese and the smaller and cuter Ross's Goose. As we watched the birds from the highway, the ranch owner pulled up and invited us to enter the ranch and get a better view. It is amazing how many times during our Big Year we benefited from the kindness of strangers.

Two of the most beautiful birds of the week were the Altamira Oriole and Green Jay.

While our detour north to Port Aransas gave us quite a few new birds, the main reason we were there was to take a boat out into the intracoastal waterways to get better views of Whooping Cranes. This violated every competitive rule of Big Year Birding ... making a detour to see a bird that you have already seen. But we didn't care. Whooping Cranes are amazing, and we saw about 20 of these endangered birds. This included 4 juveniles. Only 16% of Whooping Crane nests are successful, so every juvenile is a small victory.

Santa Margarita Ranch

Santa Margarita Ranch became Birding's 2024 equivalent to Fenway Park. The ranch sits quite literally on the border of the US and Mexico, and like Fenway it has a giant wall! Also, due to its unique location on the Rio Grande, it fields a roster of heavy hitting birds much like the Red Sox of the good 'ole days.

Thanks to this year's El Niño weather pattern and droughts in Central America, several rare species moved north into the USA. Santa Margarita Ranch, with its diverse riparian and desert habitat, it is an appealing landing spot for the birds.

For the past several months we had drooled over the rare bird reports from Texas and chewed our nails worrying that they would be gone when we got there.

Access to the ranch is restricted and one must go with a guide. We joined one on Saturday evening to see the rare Mottled Owl. While some owls can be seen during the day, the Mottled Owl, a resident of Mexico and Central and South America, is

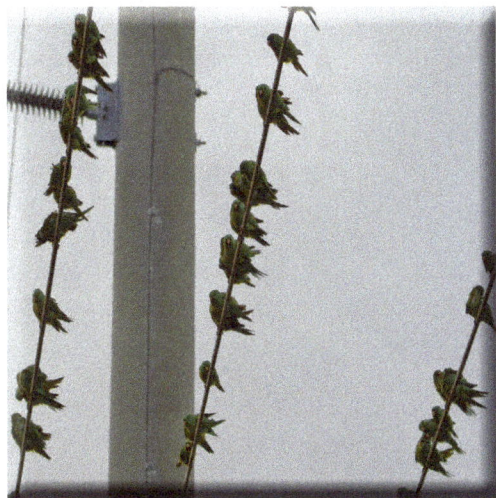
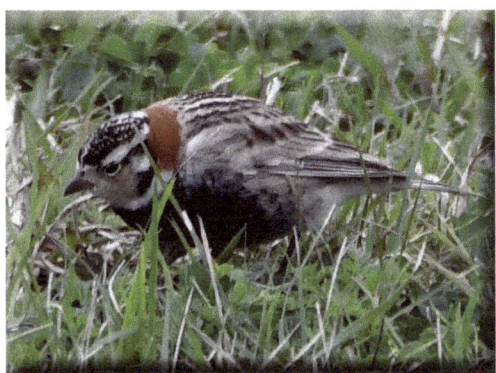
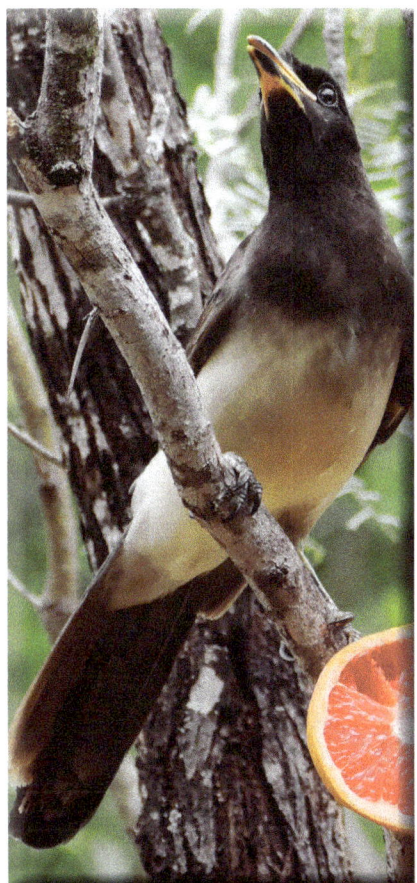
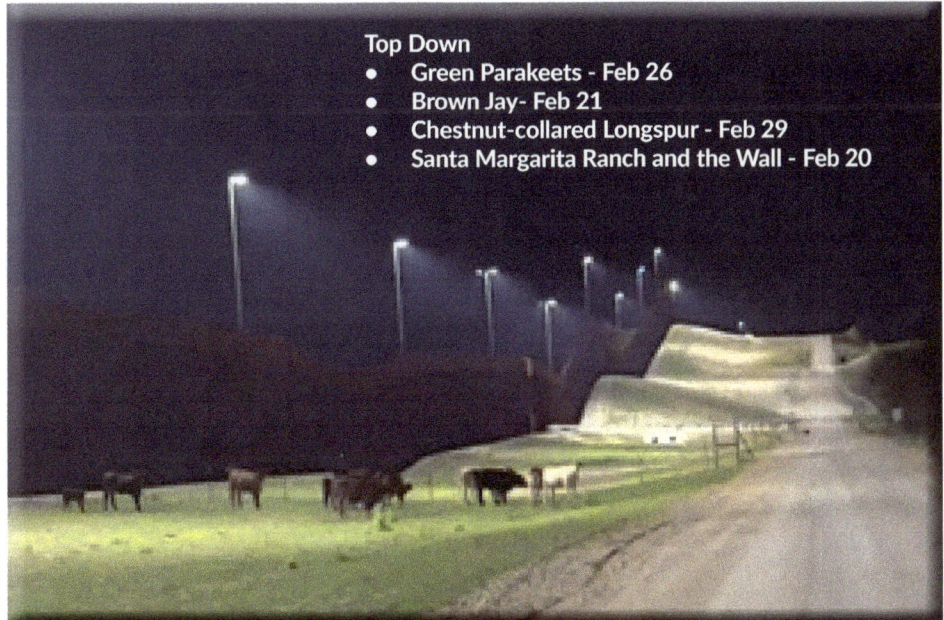

Top Down
- Green Parakeets - Feb 26
- Brown Jay - Feb 21
- Chestnut-collared Longspur - Feb 29
- Santa Margarita Ranch and the Wall - Feb 20

FEBRUARY 43

200th Bird of the Year

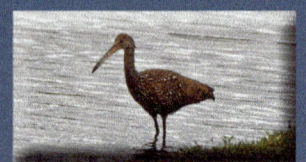

A Florida Bird, in recent years individual Limpkins have been seen all over the eastern USA and even in Canada. We saw this odd looking wading bird in a small pond near a convenience store parking lot in Melbourne, Florida.

February 4, 8:44 AM

250th Bird of the Year

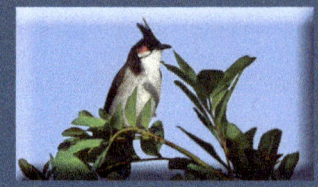

The Red-whiskered Bulbul is a stunning cage bird, native to Africa. Escapees in Florida have established a small breeding community and thus are countable in a Big Year. We saw our first Red-whiskered Bulbul singing at the top of a bush in Miami, Florida.

February 11, 8:03 AM

300th Bird of the Year

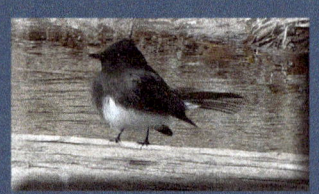

While in a Brownsville, Texas cemetery looking for a rare Warbler, we saw our first Black Phoebe of the year. A beautiful bird known for its bobbing tail, we would see hundreds more over the course of the year.

February 18, 1:35 PM

350th Bird of the Year

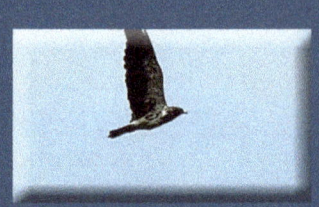

We spotted our first Swainson's Hawk of the year from the bluff at Santa Margarita Ranch, along the Rio Grande River in Roma, Texas.

February 25, 9:05 AM

strictly nocturnal.

We set off under a full moon, assisted by headlamps and flashlights, through a door in the border wall and down a trail on the ranch. About a mile and a quarter in, the guides played the call of the Eastern Screech Owl. The Mottled Owl immediately responded with his own call, which sounds like an old man telling kids to get off his lawn. The Owl then made a couple of passes over our heads, giving us stunning views.

We returned to the ranch before dawn the next morning for a full day of birding. We began on a bluff overlooking the Rio Grande where we could see across into Mexico. This presented a unique problem. We had to be careful because only birds on the US side count in a Big Year. Fortunately, over the next two and a half hours, all of the birds were on the US side or obligingly flew into US territory, if only briefly in a few cases.

Further down the same trail we had been on the night before, we searched the river's edge for the Bare-throated Tiger Heron, a primal looking heron of mangroves and marshes. While we combed up and down the river throughout the day for him, it appeared he took that day off. Several other fantastic birds were out and about though, and we ended the day with a whopping 102 species. Sweaty and exhausted from miles of hiking in 90 degree weather, we were thrilled to add 22 new species to our Big Year list and 12 to our life lists!

Over the next two days, we picked up birds at state parks and nature preserves in the Lower Rio Grande River Valley as well at urban Parrot and Parakeet roosts in McAllen and Weslaco.

The Green Parakeets of McAllen are well organized and predictable in their habits of returning to the same shopping center every night. Not so the Parrots of Weslaco. They frequent the same residential neighborhood each evening, but they don't always return to the same place. The result is a frenzied contingent of birders racing through the streets in pursuit of the flock. We imagine parents telling their children to be sure to be home well before dark for fear of one of these crazy birders running them over in their cars!

We were in search of rare Lilac-crowned Parrots that had been reported in the flock. They did not make it easy with their constant movement from tree to tree and street to street, but we managed to find two and are happy to also report that we did not hit any children or wandering dogs!

Another adventure was a return trip to the fallow farm fields of Edinburg for the elusive Mountain Plover. Here we drove slowly over dusty dirt roads among windmills and farm equipment scanning and occasionally stopping to scope the fields.

Despite our best efforts over a couple of hours, we emerged from the fields with our car a new shade of dusty gray but no bird. We reminded ourselves that we'd have another chance at the Mountain Plover in the Pacific Northwest over the summer.

A move from the Lower Rio Grande Valley to Hill Country outside of Austin, Texas was next. There we found an exciting new lifer, the Chestnut-collared Longspur. It was feeding in the company of a large flock of American Pipits in grass near a lake outside of Austin. It took quite a lot of searching, and just as we were about to give up, he flew up from the grass as we walked by him on an adjacent path. Thrilled to see him, we shared the joy with three other equally happy birders who had joined the search.

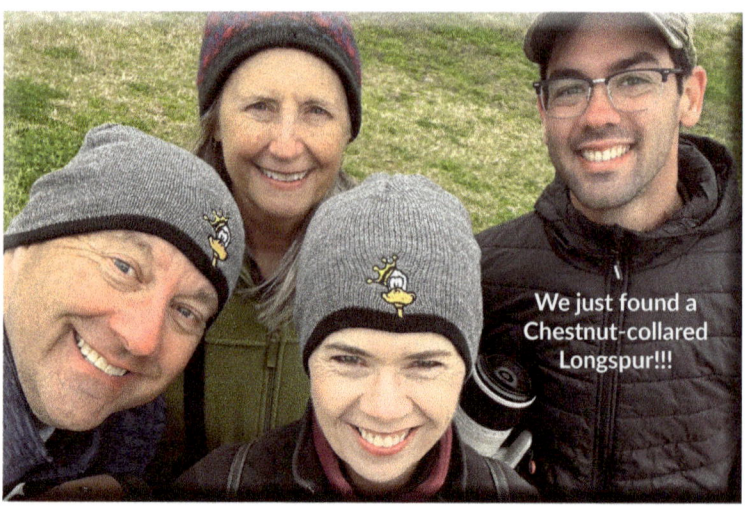

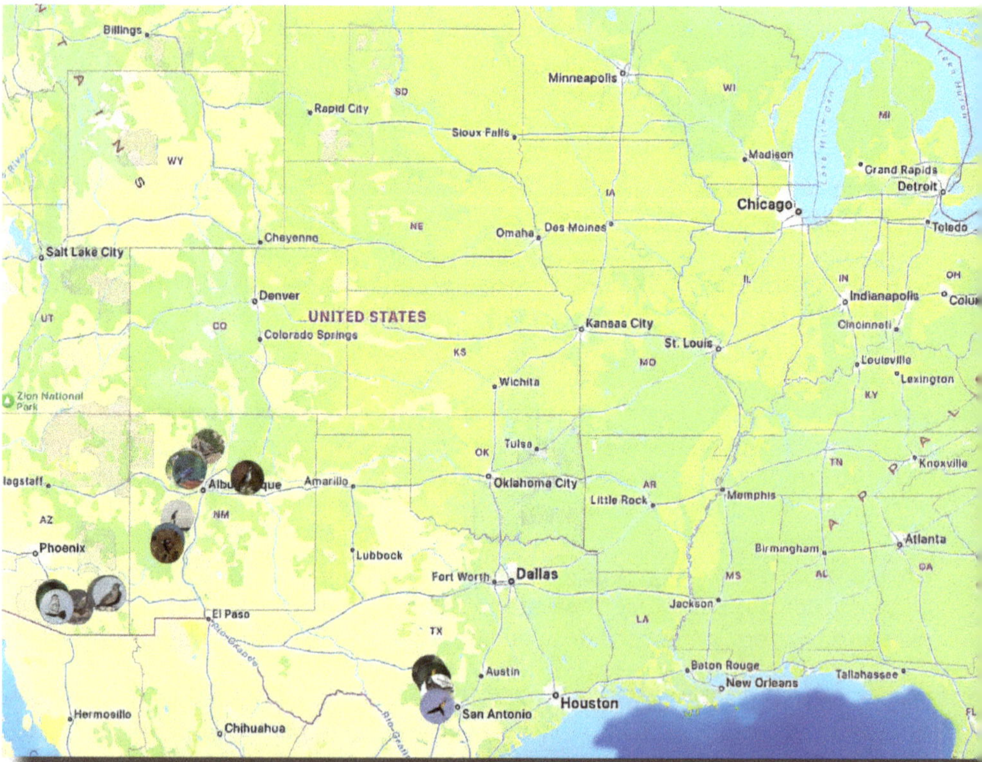

We just found a Chestnut-collared Longspur!!!

EVERY BIRD FROM SEA TO SHINING SEA

March

Travel	#
Plane Flights	4
Rental Cars	2
Nights Away	13
Boat Trips	0

State	Year Birds
Arizona	29
Maine	4
New Hampshire	1
New Mexico	17
Texas	7
Total	58

Back in Maine

Sometimes our bliss at finding a new bird is sharply brought to a halt.

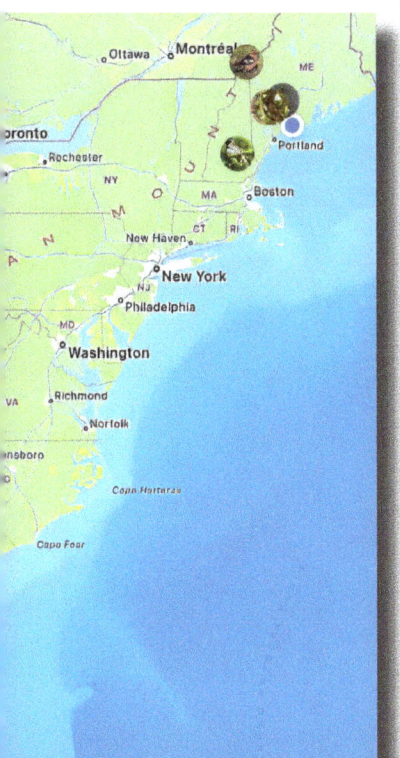

Such was the case with the Ferruginous Hawk, a large uncommon raptor of arid grass and farmland. Incredibly, after only 20 minutes of searching, we found this magnificent bird perched on a power pole. We took multiple photos and were thrilled to add a Ferruginous Hawk to our year list.

During a lovely dinner with our son and daughter-in-law, Brad and Tanner, in San Antonio that evening, we learned from an eBird reviewer that it wasn't a Ferruginous Hawk but a very pale and very common Red-tailed Hawk.

Red-tailed Hawks do not look like this in New England, but there are regional differences in species, and the mostly brown birds we are used to seeing can be almost white in the south. So, with tears in our eyes, we removed the Ferruginous Hawk from our list and continued our search for one.

On March 4 we left our car at Brad and Tanner's house near San Antonio and flew home to Maine for two and a half weeks. We had just completed the longest trip of the year, 36 days on the road. During this road trip we added 243 birds to our year list, bringing us to 374 species. We also climbed in the standings from 2,000 something place to being in the top ten.

Back in Maine, we worked on getting a few outstanding Maine birds before our return to Texas. Target bird one was the Purple Finch. Some years this is an extremely common bird and comes to our feeders, singing loudly in the morning. This year, however, due to a bonus Spruce cone crop in Canada, very few dropped down. A friend a few towns over had three Purple Finches visiting her feeders, but they were uncooperative on a visit to her house.

The second target bird was the White-winged Crossbill, again a bird that lives on Spruce cones, and was, for the most part, still in Canada. We visited Reid State Park, near our home and one of our favorite places to find this bird. But we struck out, despite walking the roads for a couple of hours.

The final bird we really wanted to get in Maine before hitting the road again was the secretive Northern Saw-whet Owl. One night we visited a number of spots near our house and listened for this bird's bizarre tooting call. We heard none.

Winter Birds

On March 9 we took another shot at the Northern Saw-whet Owl. We decided to try Eaton Farm, a nearby wildlife preserve run by a local youth camp. With meadows

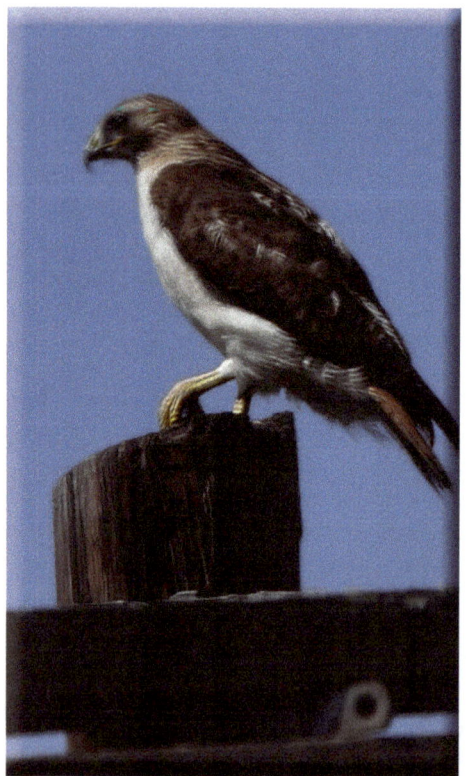
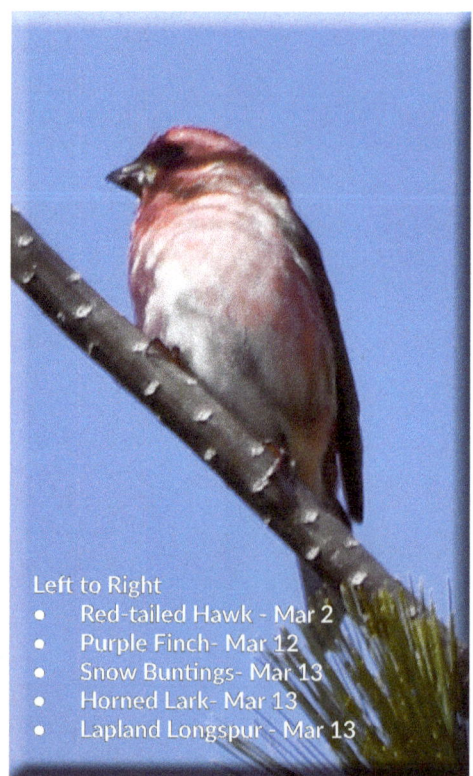

Left to Right
- Red-tailed Hawk - Mar 2
- Purple Finch- Mar 12
- Snow Buntings- Mar 13
- Horned Lark- Mar 13
- Lapland Longspur - Mar 13

surrounded by forest, Eaton Farm appeared perfect for an owl looking to hunt for mice and voles.

Arriving right about dusk, we didn't hear the 'toot toot toot' song of the Saw-whet. But, we did hear the 'peent peent peent' call of the American Woodcock all around us. In mid-March each year, the male Woodcock will emerge from the woods as the sun sets and sing his 'peent' song in an effort to attract a female. The male will then leap into the air, flying up hundreds of feet, before spiraling back to the ground. This spiraling creates a twittering sound as air hits the Woodcock's wings.

We stood in the parking lot surrounded by American Woodcock display 'peents' and 'twitters' and glimpsed the occasional shadow of a bird soaring into the air. Then, suddenly, we heard an almost metallic 'toot toot toot'. We had our Northern Saw-whet Owl for the year!

And, we found our first Purple Finch of the year as well this week.

Having ticked off virtually all species in Maine, we traveled south to Hampton Beach, New Hampshire to find a grassland bird of the Great Plains, the Lapland Longspur. In the Northeast they can often be found with flocks of Snow Buntings and Horned Larks.

We found the flock of Snow Buntings and Horned Larks within a minute of arriving.

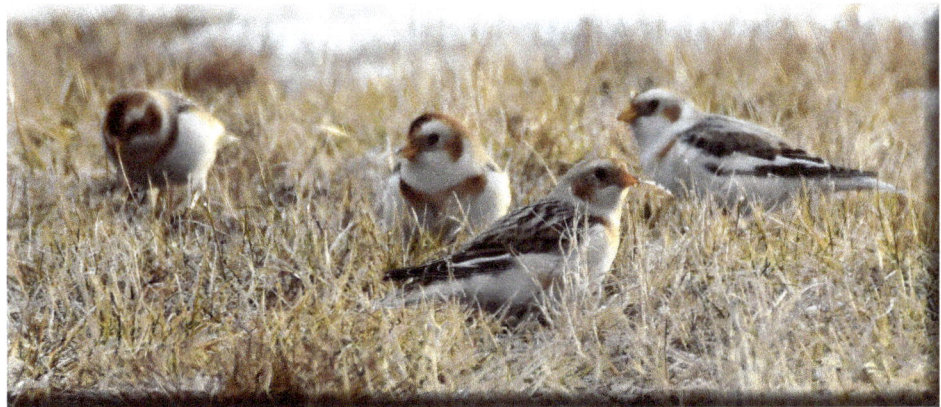

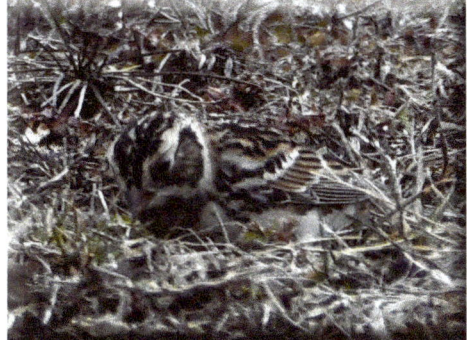
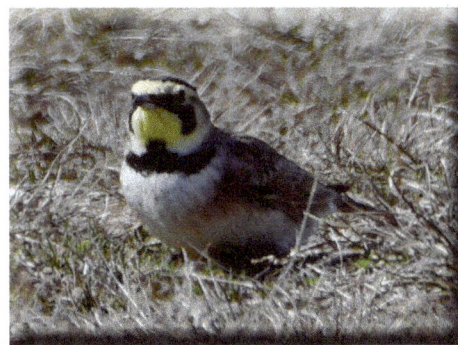

So finding the Lapland Longspur should have been easy, right? Wrong! Imagine 50 constantly-moving brown and white birds, all with slightly different plumage. Every couple of minutes they leap into the air, fly around in circles, and then land 50 yards away.

It took us an hour to find the one bird that was not like the others and only confirmed it was a Lapland Longspur via a fuzzy photo when we got home.

We have a saying, "The camera giveth, and the camera taketh away." Sometimes we leave the field certain that we have seen our target bird only to get home and learn from our photos that we were wrong. This happens more than we would like. But every once in a while, the camera rewards us with confirmation that we really did see a bird we weren't 100% sure of. This was the happy case with the Lapland Longspur.

Our final target bird before we headed back to Texas was the White-winged Crossbill, a stocky finch with a curious adaptation ... a crisscrossed bill that allows it to easily extract seeds from the cones of conifers. Some winters we see lots of Crossbills when they drop down out of Canada to feed on Pine and Spruce. But other years, when the Canadian cone crop is plentiful, White-winged Crossbills are really hard to find.

With no report of this bird anywhere in the Northeast, we decided to drive a couple hours north to the Saddleback Ski Resort where we had seen White-winged Crossbills in the past. It was a bit of a long shot, but certainly not the dumbest thing we tried during the Big Year.

Shortly after passing the ski lodge and heading into the condo area, Ingrid noticed some birds eating salt in the middle of the road. We lifted our binoculars, and, incredibly, there were four White-winged Crossbills.

Sandia Crest

After 19 days in Maine, we picked up our car outside of San Antonio and began the two day drive to Albuquerque, New Mexico, with a few stops for a bird or two along the way, of course.

Our first stop was in Texas Hill Country, north of San Antonio, for an elusive Golden-cheeked Warbler. This bird is very picky. It winters in a tiny area of Central America before migrating to an equally small area of Texas in the early spring. When we returned to Maine from Texas on March 4, there were no Golden-cheeked Warblers in the state. When we came back on the 23rd, they were all back, singing from the tops of Oak and Juniper trees.

We were delighted to come upon five Golden-cheeked Warblers in our initial one hour stop. To be more accurate, we heard five birds and got fleeting glances of three. Its reputation of being easily heard but a challenge to see proved true. The

Golden-cheeked was a new life bird for us.

As we progressed toward New Mexico, we were a little surprised to hit snow on the Texas panhandle. But, it was nothing that could stop a pair of Mainers driving an AWD Subaru, so we continued on.

The landscape was fascinating as we moved across the Prairie, passing mile long trains, cattle ranches and small towns.

Our birding destination for the day was Sandia Crest, the highest point in the Sandia-Manzano Mountains of New Mexico. We made the thirteen mile drive up to 10,679 feet on snow covered switchback roads to reach a single bird feeder maintained by a local Audubon group. It's the best place in the United States to see Rosy-Finches. Living above the tree line, feeding on seeds exposed by wind-driven snow, Rosy-Finches are not exactly the easiest birds to find.

Ethan does most of the driving on our expeditions, and while he is confident and relaxed in his driving, all of that goes out the window when navigating up or down mountains. But we made it, despite the falling snow and bitter winds. We soon found the bird feeder and saw dozens of Black Rosy-Finches, Brown-capped Rosy-Finches and a couple of Gray-crowned Rosy-Finches, in addition to a few Mountain Chickadees. All lifers and a real thrill!

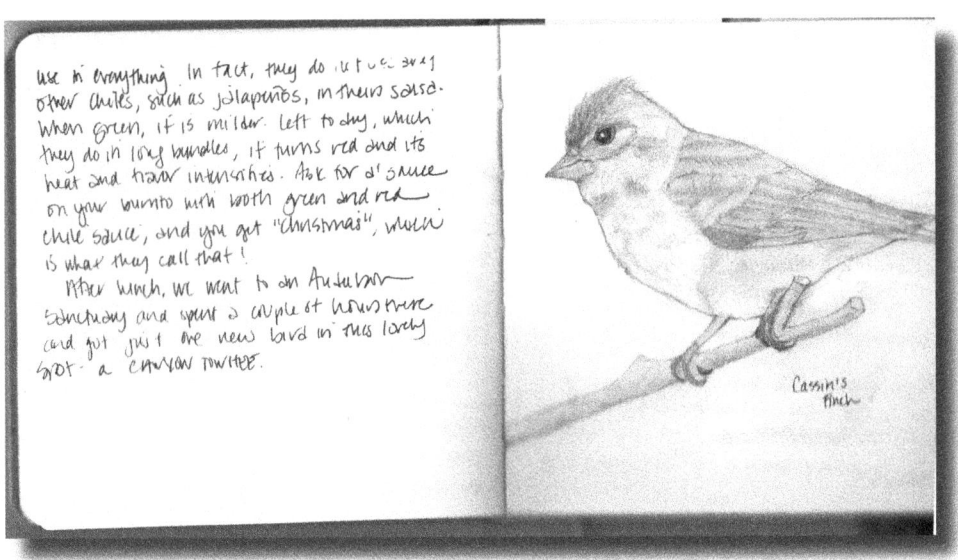

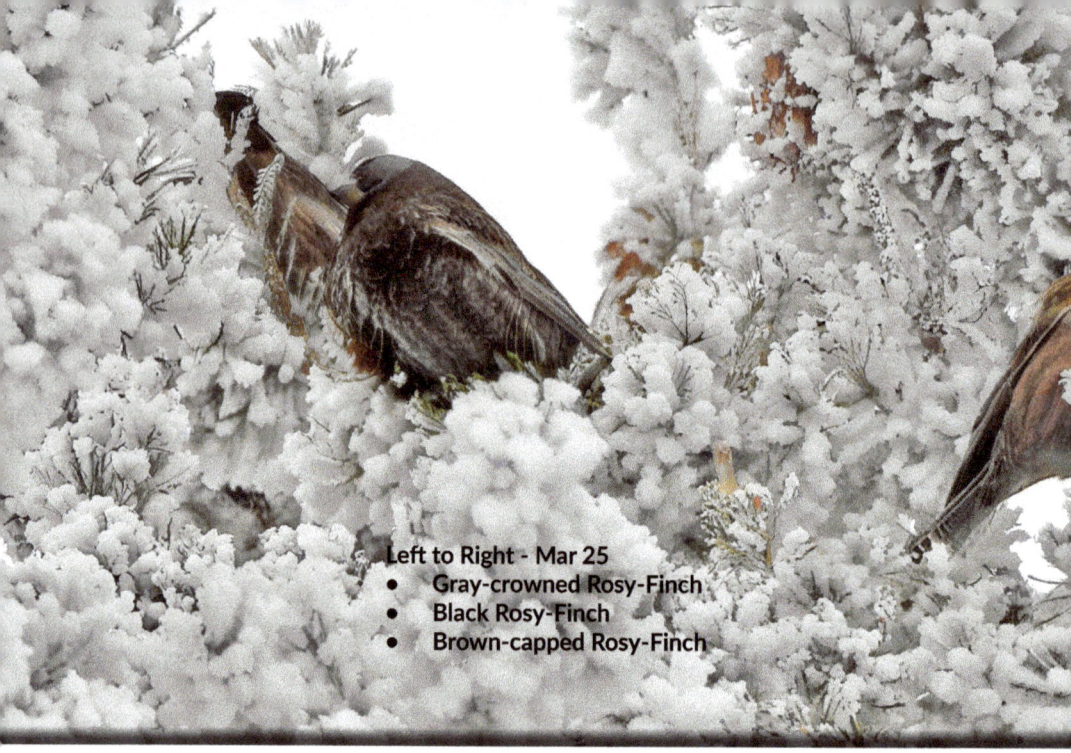

Left to Right - Mar 25
- Gray-crowned Rosy-Finch
- Black Rosy-Finch
- Brown-capped Rosy-Finch

Drive to Arizona

After leaving the Rosy-Finches of Sandia Crest, we took a break from birding and spent the morning exploring old Santa Fe. After our tour, we headed to the Randall Davey Audubon Center outside of Santa Fe. This lovely sanctuary is built into a hillside and is surrounded by bird feeders, and thus, birds. While we enjoyed great views of many species during our time there, we added just one new bird to our list for the year, the Canyon Towhee.

New Mexico's nickname is "The Land of Enchantment", and it is easy to see why. Stunning red rock mountains border the horizon throughout the state. Depending on the time of day, angle of the sun, and weather, the rock color changes from bright reds and oranges to soft golds and browns. Truly mesmerizing. And while the habitat is primarily desert, there is an unexpected lushness to the landscape that we did not see in Texas.

As we made our way from Albuquerque to Portal, Arizona, we were thrilled by the scenery but also the new birds we were able to see. Our first stop was the famed Bosque del Apache National Wildlife Refuge in San Antonio, New Mexico. On the road to the reserve, Ethan spotted an interesting looking meadowlark perched on a fence wire. We stopped, listened to it, studied it, checked our field guide and confirmed we were looking at a Chihuahuan Meadowlark. This is a relatively new species that the ornithologists split from the Eastern Meadowlark, and thus a new lifer for us!

While we did not get the Wilson's Phalarope that had been reported at Bosque, we met many friendly birders, a few of whom were from our home state of Maine. And, we learned why this location, with its attractiveness to migrating waterfowl, is so beloved among birders.

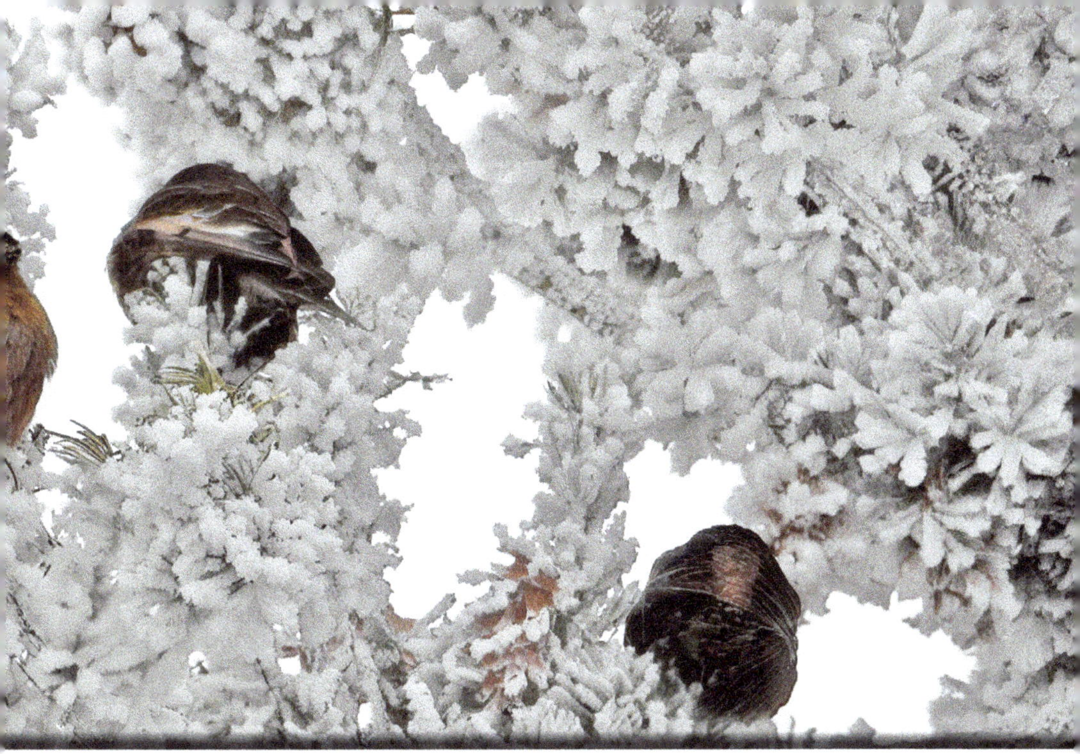

A stop at the interestingly named Elephant Butte Lake State Park in Sierra, New Mexico was next. At this remote, almost other-worldly location we observed a large flotilla of waterfowl. Among them were both Western Grebes and Clark's Grebes.

Believe it or not, a town called Truth or Consequences, New Mexico was our next stop. The town was literally named after the game show in an effort to win a 1950's contest.

Arriving late in the afternoon at our AirBnB in Portal, Arizona we were treated to yet another gorgeous Southwestern landscape. The area is much like New Mexico, just five minutes away. Edward Abbey's *Desert Solitaire* evokes images of the landscape that are second only to the experience of seeing it in person.

As there were bird feeders right out our door, we quickly settled in and added new

400th Bird of the Year

Almost identical to the Western Grebe, our 400th Bird, the Clark's Grebe, has white all around the eye. The slightly larger Western's black cap descends below the eye.

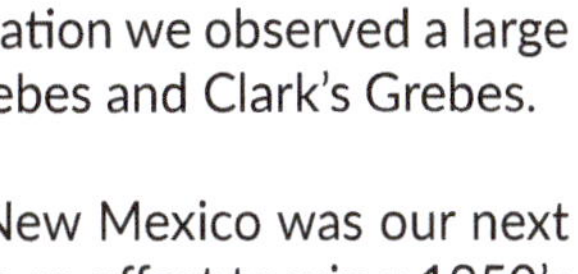

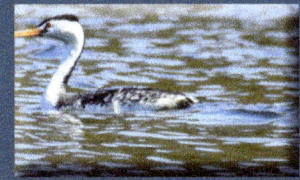

March 28, 1:13 PM

birds to our year list - Black-Throated Sparrow, Lucy's Warbler, and the delightfully entertaining Gambel's Quail.

The next morning, we were visited by a beautiful Phainopepla, a bird we do not often see. It sat atop a bush for a while, giving us extended views - not something we always get with constantly moving birds.

Portal is a mecca for birders. One reason is Cave Creek Ranch. The ranch caters to birders and has feeders throughout the property. Fortunately for those not staying there, the ranch allows day visitors for a $5 fee. Well worth the investment. Especially when a truly remarkable bird makes an appearance.

The Elegant Trogon is a stunning but very secretive bird that appears in southern Arizona each summer before moving back below the border in the fall. When we first birded Arizona in 2018 we failed to find an Elegant Trogon, perhaps because it was mid-April and most of the Trogons had yet to arrive. Now we were searching the Cave Creek Ranch for one in late March, even earlier!

Fortunately, the ranch had a single, early male Trogon, and after 3 plus hours of searching and waiting, it appeared. Ethan had wandered off when Ingrid spotted it. She quietly called Ethan back by whispering, "Trogon, Trogon, Trogon" until she got his attention.

This was Ingrid's most hoped-for bird of the year. As it flew off, she hugged Ethan and declared, "Okay, now I can die happy."

Little did we know how close that trite cliche came to being realized.

One of the things we enjoyed most about this year was the people we met while birding. People of all ages, from all over, who share our passion for birds. And, they often pass on tips about where to find birds. Such was the case at the ranch where

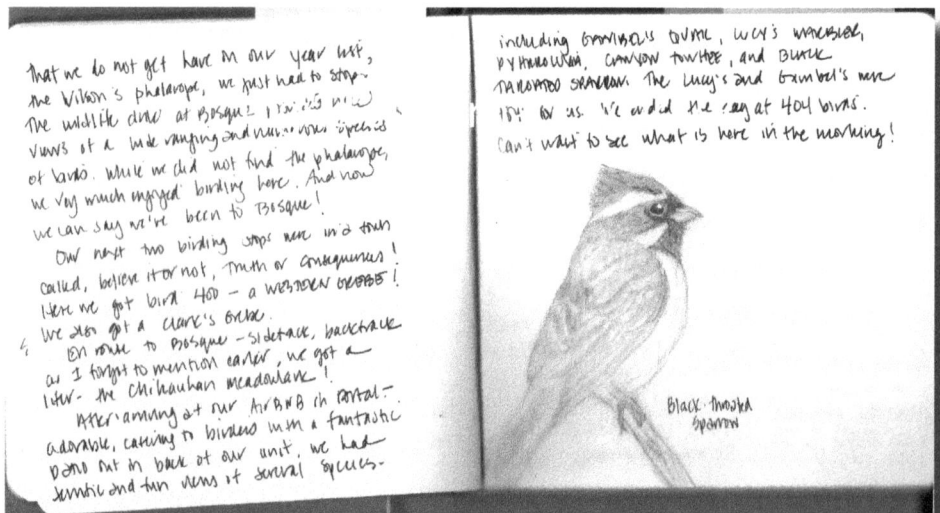

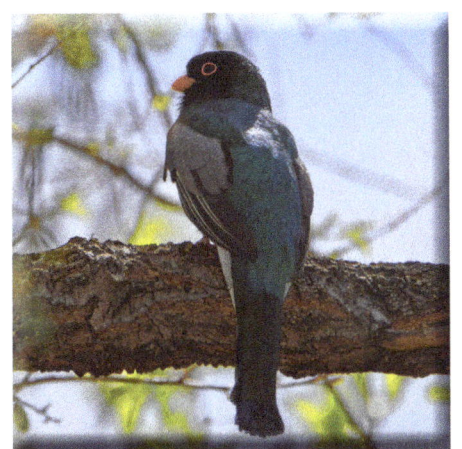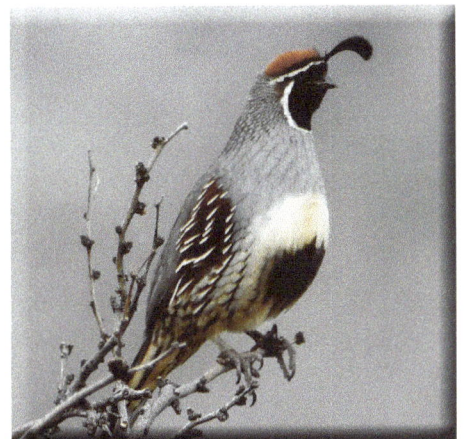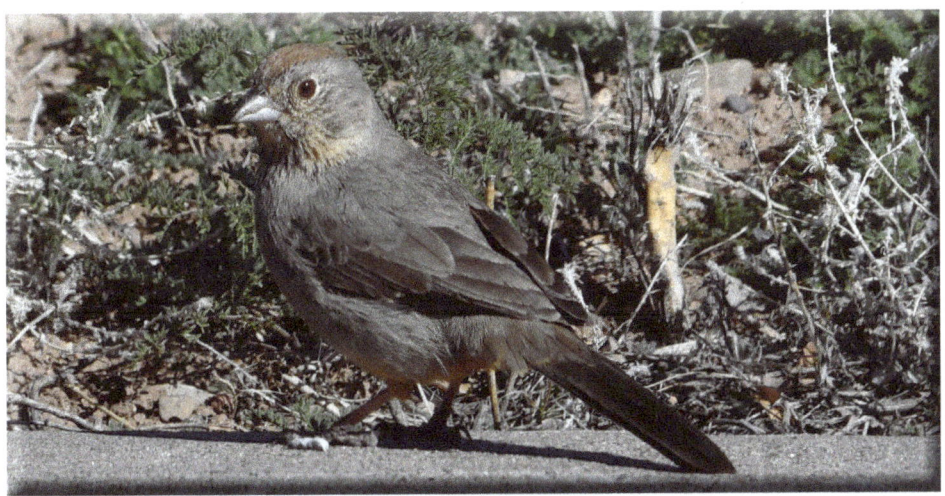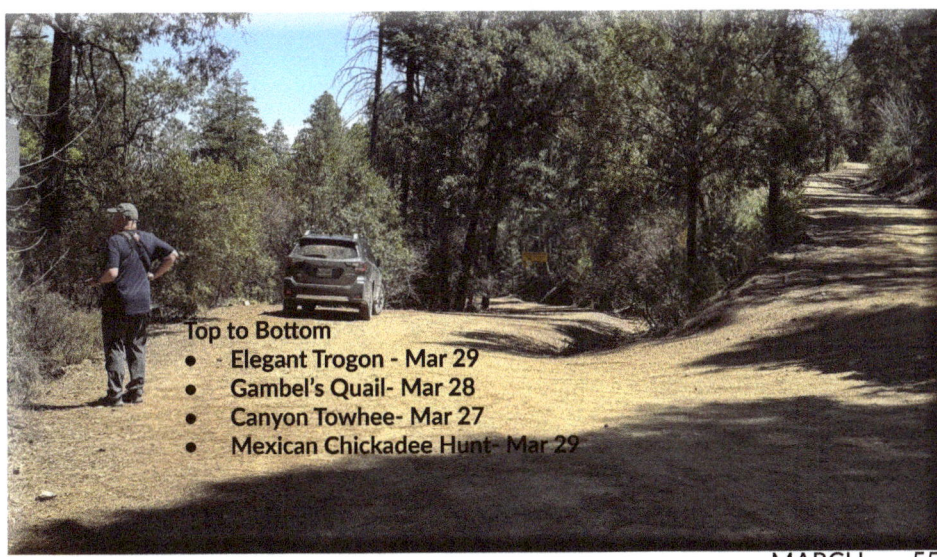

Top to Bottom
- Elegant Trogon - Mar 29
- Gambel's Quail - Mar 28
- Canyon Towhee - Mar 27
- Mexican Chickadee Hunt - Mar 29

we heard about some Mexican Chickadees further up the road. We set off determined to find these exotic birds.

Remember our white-knuckle-drive up the mountain to see the Rosy-Finches? That was a walk in the park compared to the Mexican Chickadee chase. With great appreciation to Subaru, we traveled up a mountain road that was rocky, narrow, steep, and rivaled anything we had thus far encountered. Of course, there were numerous road signs warning us how bad the road was, but we had Mexican Chickadees to find!

After 15 minutes at the Chickadee spot and a chance to recover from the drive, a flock mercifully landed in a tree overhead.

On the trip down the mountain road to Paradise, we drove through three streams, traversed large rocks, and oh so carefully inched past another SUV on a curve with a steep cliff drop-off into the valley below. This day could easily have had a very unfortunate ending.

In the evening, we had owls to chase at the Portal Library and Post Office. Our birding friend Kathie Brown had told us an Elf Owl could be found there. After about 45 minutes of waiting, a Western Screech-Owl called, followed shortly after by the Elf Owl.

On the way west to our next destination, Patagonia, we stopped at the San Pedro House in Sierra Vista and added a Green-Tailed Towhee and an Abert's Towhee to our year list, as well as a Gila Woodpecker.

Once in Patagonia we hurried to the Paton Center for Hummingbirds as late afternoon fell. The Paton Center's array of feeders is to hummingbirds what a 'Make Your Own Sundae Bar' is to a class of fourth graders. The feeding frenzy is so intense that you'd think these birds were starving. Not a chance! Here we added the Anna's and Violet-crowned Hummingbirds to our year list.

This week was very lucky for us. We added 38 new birds, and 13 lifers!

eBird

eBird is an innovative platform created by the Cornell Lab of Ornithology that allows birders to record, organize, and share their sightings. Launched in 2002, it has become a cornerstone for birders of all levels, offering tools for logging sightings and tracking personal bird lists while simultaneously contributing to a vast global database of bird observations. By using the eBird website or mobile app, birders can report real-time sightings, upload photos and audio, and view checklists tailored to specific locations. This ease of access has encouraged millions of birders to contribute, creating one of the largest and most comprehensive citizen science databases in the world.

The data collected on eBird is invaluable for researchers and conservationists, providing insights into bird population trends, migration routes, and habitat preferences. Scientists use eBird data to monitor species at risk, track changes due to climate shifts, and identify critical areas that need protection. For instance, distribution maps generated from eBird data have been instrumental in identifying essential stopover points for migrating birds. Conservation organizations rely on this data to make informed decisions about preserving habitats and guiding species conservation efforts. The platform thus serves a dual purpose, both enriching the birding experience for users and contributing significantly to scientific research and conservation.

Beyond its scientific contributions, eBird has created a global community for bird enthusiasts. Users can explore birding hotspots, share their lists with others, and participate in challenges like Big Days and Big Years, where they try to observe as many bird species as possible within a set time. The community aspect of eBird has made it more than just a data-gathering tool—it's also a social space that connects people who share a love for birds and the natural world. In this way, eBird has expanded the scope of birding from a solitary activity to a collective effort, empowering individuals to contribute to something greater while fostering a global network dedicated to understanding and protecting bird species.

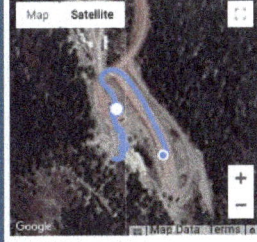

April

Travel	#
Plane Flights	0
Rental Cars	0
Nights Away	16
Boat Trips	0

State	Year Birds
Arizona	24
Colorado	5
Illinois	3
Kansas	4
Massachusetts	13
Maine	1
Missouri	3
New Hampshire	2
Utah	5
Vermont	1
Total	61

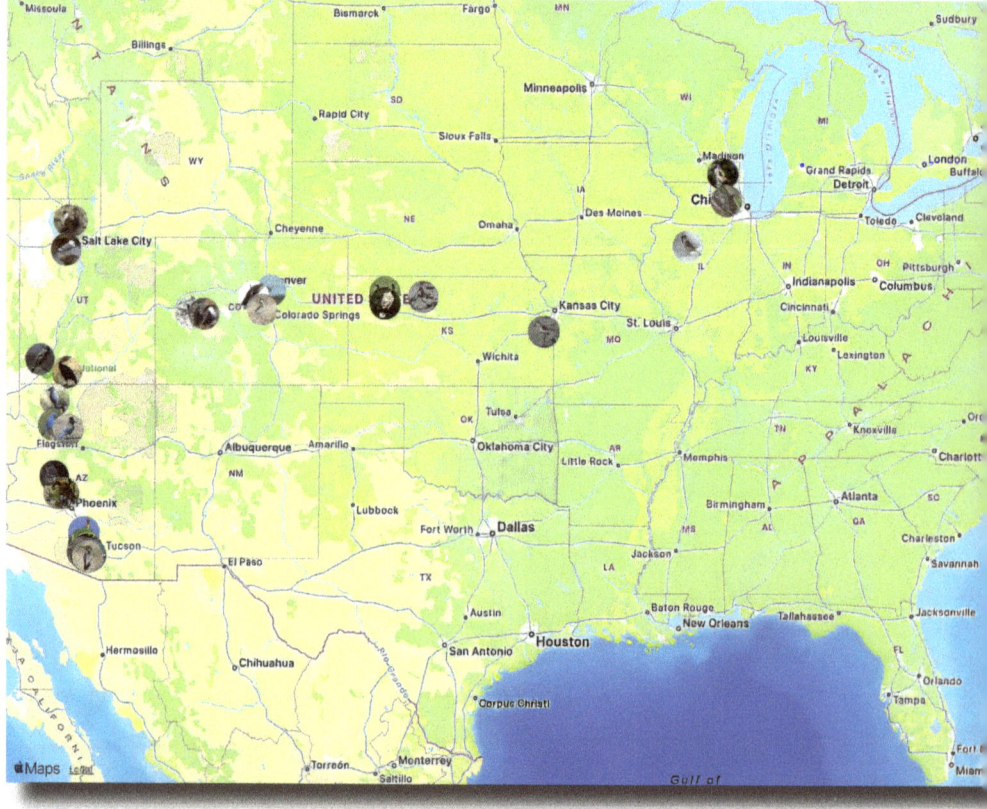

EVERY BIRD FROM SEA TO SHINING SEA

Hummingbirds and Owls

The Berylline Hummingbird is endemic to Mexico, but every once in a while one crosses into the U.S. and ignites a chase among birders. Such was the case with recent sightings of one in Madera Canyon, Arizona.

Situated twenty-five miles southeast of Tucson, Madera Canyon sits in the Santa Rita Mountains and is part of the Coronado National Forest. In addition to pristine hiking trails and incredible views, the canyon hosts a large diversity of birds and thus, many birders. In fact, there are lodges and cabins that cater to birders. They place seed and nectar feeders on the property and strategically locate chairs for comfortable viewing.

On our first visit to Kubo Cabins, there were several birders assembled, all bemoaning the fact that the Berylline's preferred feeder was empty. The wind did not help either as birds, like people, tend to hunker down in those conditions. After an hour, we headed back to Patagonia.

The next evening we had planned to go owling at night, but the wind remained high, it was raining, and we even saw some hail. So we bagged the owls and tried again for the Berylline Hummingbird.

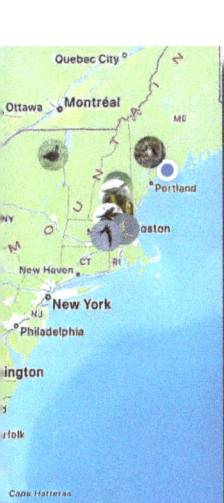

This was when bullies arrived.

Parked within a few feet of each feeder was a single Rivoli's Hummingbird, each determined to prevent the Berylline (and anyone else) from getting near THEIR nectar.

Once known as the Magnificent Hummingbird, the Rivoli's is large, beautiful, and very aggressive. It will try to impale any other hummingbird that enters his or her empire. While standing for two hours in the rain, we watched the poor Berylline attempt to get to the feeder and fail each time.

The next evening was calm and cold, ideal for owls. We donned our finest LL Bean winter gear and headed out to meet our guide, Jake Thompson.

On the way, we stopped one last time at the Berylline feeders. Only one Rivoli's sentry remained. The Berylline was able to slip in unnoticed by him over and over, allowing us to finally get a photo.

At the top of the Canyon, we met Jake, strapped on our headlights and set off up Old Baldy Trail. As we climbed, the night grew darker. We began to stumble over rocks and sticks as we looked up into the trees and listened for owls. The altitude didn't help.

Occasionally we would stop and listen while Jake made repeated whistles, spot-on imitations of the Spotted Owls and Northern-Pygmy Owls, hoping to call the birds in. All we heard, however, was a Great-Horned Owl, a Gray Fox and a rushing stream swollen by the recent rains. As we approached the stream it became clear that there was no easy way of crossing. We agreed that we would not proceed down the trail any further.

Before long, we heard the two-note call of a Northern Pygmy-Owl. Next, the Whiskered Screech-Owl showed up - in the parking lot, of course. Getting a Spotted Owl had been a long shot, but we knew we had a good chance of trying for this later in the year.

We spent five nights in Patagonia, Arizona, using it as a base to head out in numerous directions for birds - including Patagonia State Park, the Paton Center for Hummingbirds, Box Canyon and Canoa Ranch.

Most nights we would return 'home' to Patagonia and run headlong into a comical band of Javelina carousing and browsing among neighborhood gardens and trash cans. Javelinas are cute (but stinky) wild pigs that roam the streets of Patagonia at night.

Onward to Tucson and Phoenix, we were impressed by how quickly the scenery changed. Ocotillo cactus were more prolific - the suddenly abundant and majestic Saguaro cactus even more so. Spring in the desert is stunning. Both Tucson and Phoenix are lovely cities with gorgeous parks and open space and a warm, dry April climate that we reveled in.

One of our primary goals in Phoenix was to see the Rosy-faced Lovebird. When we arrived on Thursday afternoon, we searched areas where they had been recently seen. We thought this was going to be an easy one. But no Lovebirds revealed themselves to us.

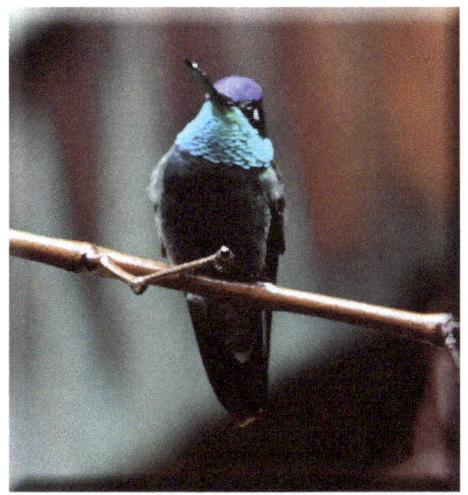
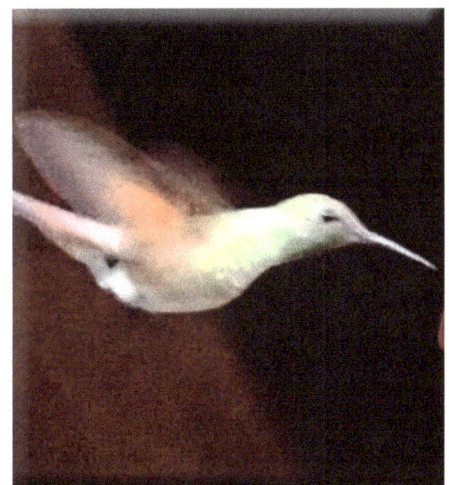
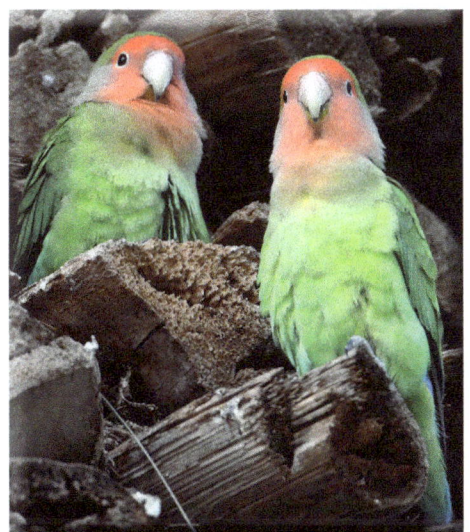
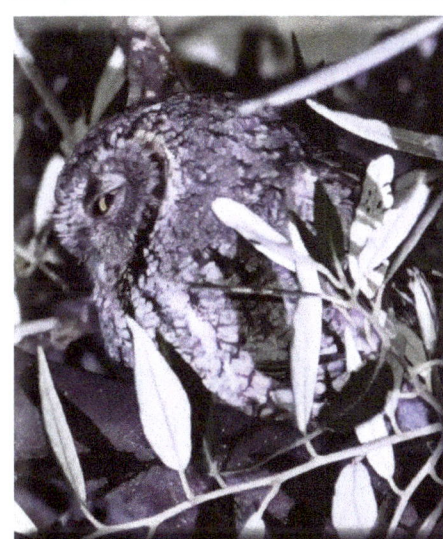
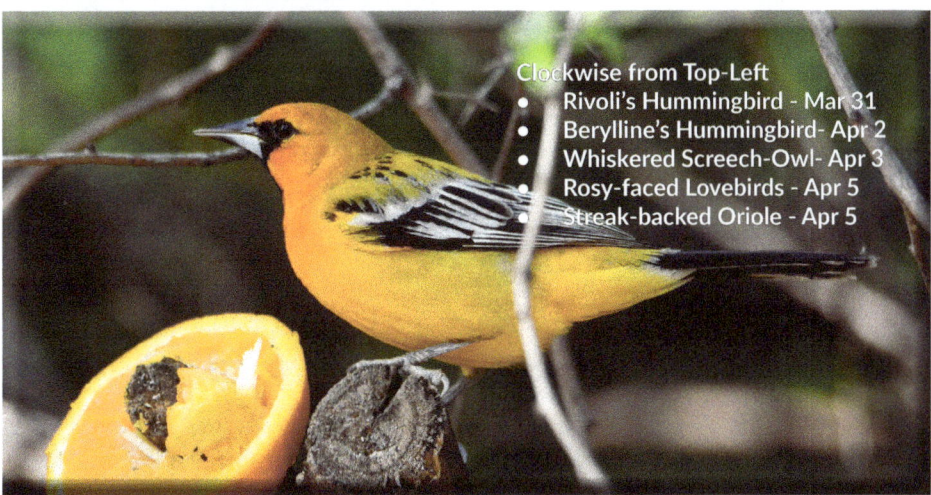

Clockwise from Top-Left
- Rivoli's Hummingbird - Mar 31
- Berylline's Hummingbird - Apr 2
- Whiskered Screech-Owl - Apr 3
- Rosy-faced Lovebirds - Apr 5
- Streak-backed Oriole - Apr 5

What to do about this turn of events? Why, turn to social media of course! Back at our hotel we checked a Facebook group, "Phoenix is for Lovebirds" and sure enough, buried in the comments of a post, were specific instructions about where to find some. Although a motorcycle gang kept us awake most of the night, we set off at dawn and found four of them exactly at the spot described!

Next, we were off to find a very special pair of rare birds that had been visiting a riparian park in Phoenix the previous couple of weeks, Streak-backed Orioles.

We arrived at the park and struggled a bit to find the correct location. Just as we turned the corner onto the Tiger-Moth Trail, we heard and then saw them, feeding on oranges left by other birders. While this pickup was almost too easy, it was luxurious, as it gave us more time to look for other birds.

Making our way from Phoenix to Flagstaff, we stopped along the way, happily adding a Gray Flycatcher and Steller's Jay to our year list. And, as fascinating as the birds we saw was the quick change in landscape.

Flagstaff, just two hours north of Phoenix, sits at 7,000' in elevation and is a whole other world. Surrounded by mountains and Ponderosa Pines, Flagstaff looks an awful lot like Northern Maine. It was 85 degrees in Phoenix the day prior, with brilliant sun. When we arrived in Flagstaff, it was 29 degrees and snowing!

Grand Canyon and Prairie Chickens

450th Bird of the Year

In a sloppy rain/snow storm in Flagstaff, AZ we were bringing our bags into the hotel when we heard and then saw our first Steller's Jay of the year ... #450.

April 5, 4:17 PM

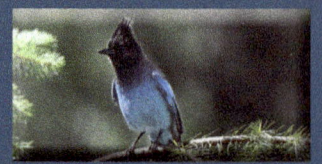

Neither of us had been to the Grand Canyon before, and we both had it on our bucket lists. Since it fit in perfectly with our birding plan, this was the time to make it happen.

The day got off to a great start with sightings of a Steller's Jay outside of our hotel and a Mountain Bluebird along the highway. We hoped our luck would hold for the California Condors near the North Rim of the Canyon later in the day.

After a lengthy wait at the entrance to the South Rim, we made our way to the visitor's center. This stop was important in order to make sure what we thought

From Top
- California Condor - Apr 6
- Greater Sage-Grouse - Apr 8

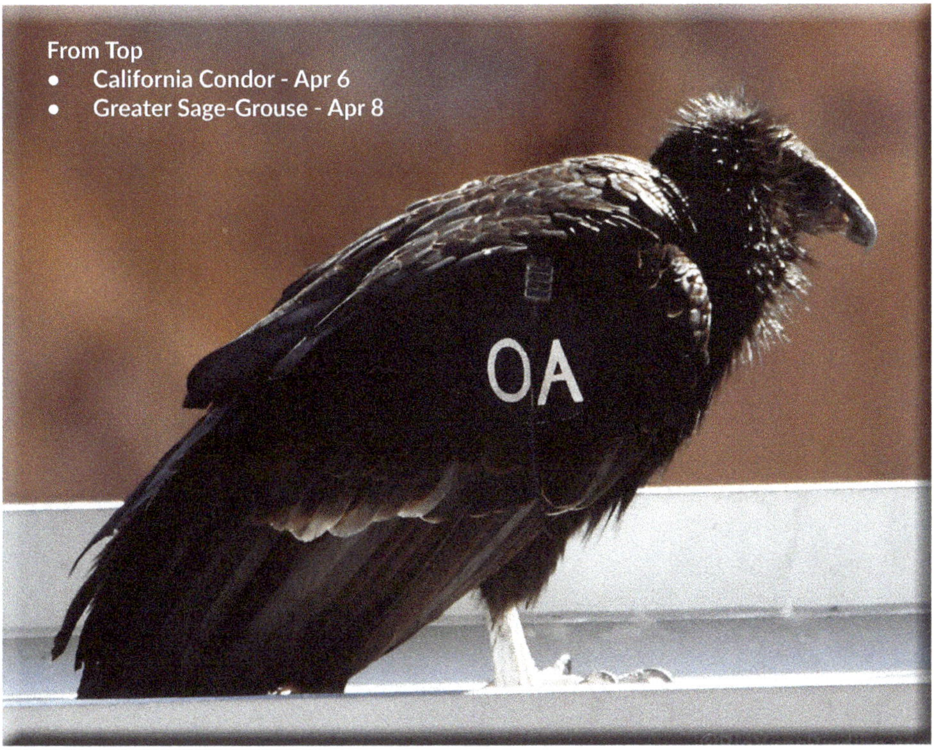

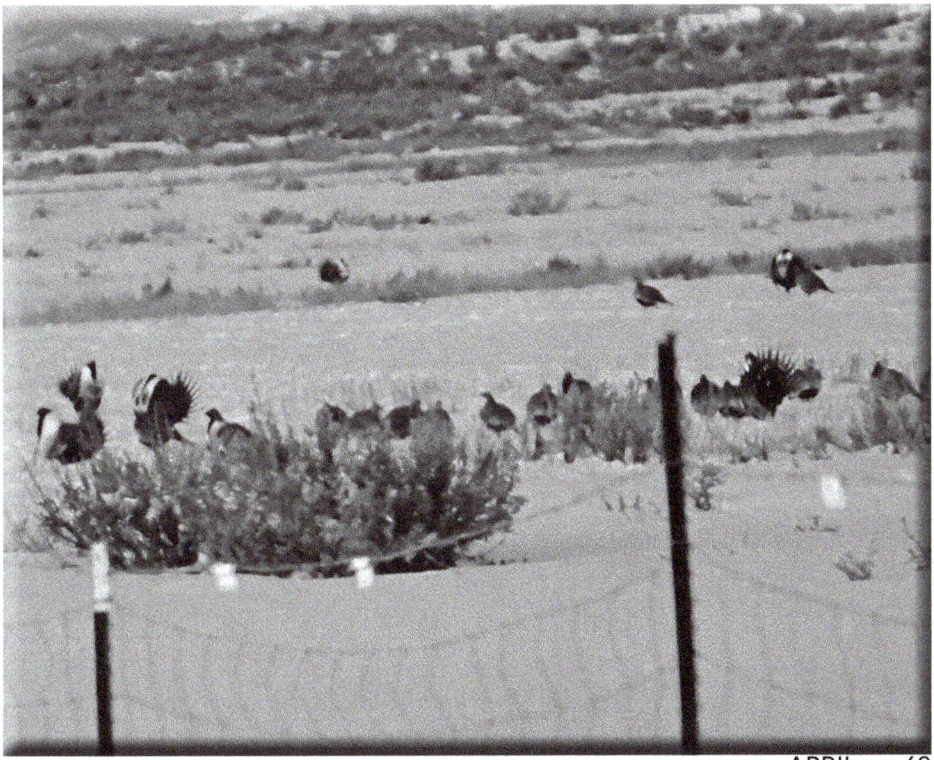

APRIL 63

was a doable route to the condors, truly was. Many thanks to the park ranger who confirmed that we had correctly figured out the directions!

As we walked the path from the visitor's center to the South Rim, we found ourselves looking for birds in the trees and bushes while others were focused on getting to the Canyon view. We stopped in our tracks and asked ourselves what we were doing. The Grand Canyon was just a few steps away, and we were looking for birds! We put the birds aside for the moment and made our way to the rim.

What we had seen in photographs of the Canyon over the years was surpassed only by what we beheld with our own eyes. The sheer size and depth of the Grand Canyon takes one's breath away. The colors, shapes and shadows scream out to be painted. We were both struck speechless.

After drinking in the view, we continued on to the North Rim and Page, Arizona, two and a half hours away. Page is home to the historic Navajo Bridge and the endangered California Condor.

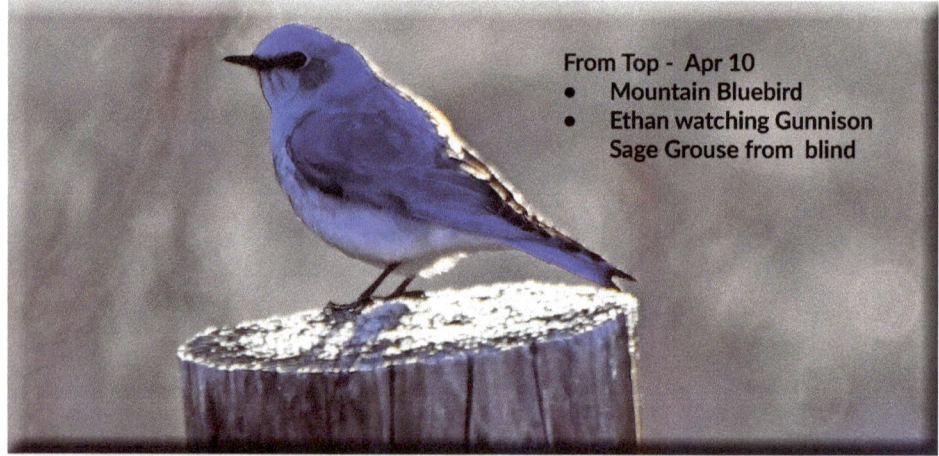

From Top - Apr 10
- Mountain Bluebird
- Ethan watching Gunnison Sage Grouse from blind

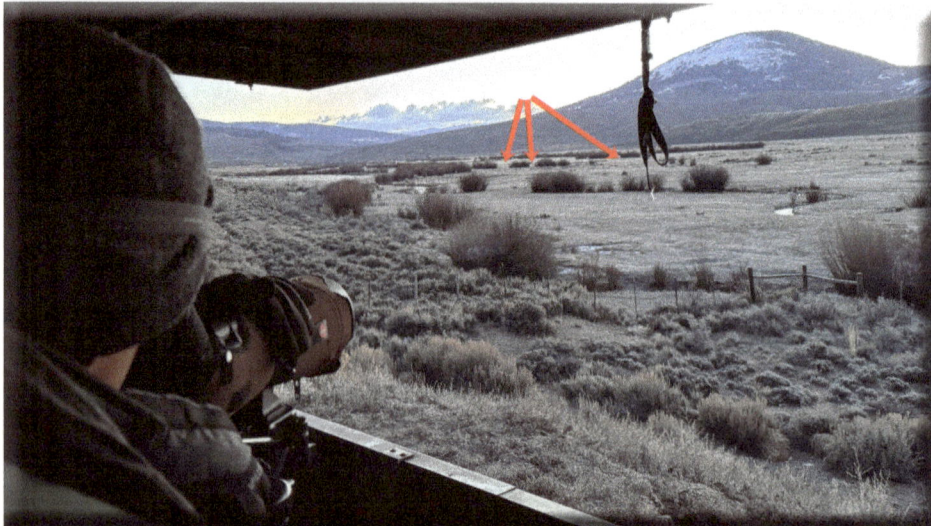

More Canyon views awaited us along our route as did extensive views of the Painted Desert. We cannot adequately describe either of these, but suggest that to really appreciate the impact of their presence, you must experience them in person if you can. The American West is a whole other kind of beauty, another world.

Navajo Bridge was a triumph of engineering built to replace a ferry route across the Colorado River. This was essential as the country expanded west. A safe, reliable route from Arizona to Utah was critical. The bridge opened to great fanfare in 1928.

Another scientific feat occurred in 1987 when wildlife biologists captured the country's 22 remaining California Condors and took them into a captive breeding program, later reintroducing them to the wild in California and Arizona. Navajo Bridge has become the nesting site for the Arizona population.

We were thrilled to observe two Condors from the bridge and see one, a juvenile, fly briefly from the rock cliffs to the bridge.

Our next stop was Kanab, Utah, a cute, little western town that was quite busy on this Friday night, especially at a local restaurant. We had climbed over 9,000 feet across more narrow, winding, switchback roads through northern Arizona with the sun setting in our eyes to get there and were ready for a good meal!

The next day was Sunday, and things were very quiet when we arrived in the tiny town of Coalville, Utah, as pretty much everything was closed. Coalville is just 20 minutes from the Henefer Greater Sage-Grouse lek, the reason for our stop-over.

Surprisingly, when we arrived at the lek just before dawn the following morning, a few grouse had already assembled. Soon after, more joined them, eventually bringing the number to 86, and these were just what we could see from our car.

The courtship display that the males perform is fascinating to watch, and the response from the ladies was pretty much what one might expect. When the guys weren't trying to impress the girls, they held chest pumping competitions among themselves. We couldn't help but find the humor in how this mirrored the behavior of humans!

Arches National Park was our next sightseeing destination today. Our daughter, Marita, who has visited many national parks, considers Arches her favorite, and it was easy to see why. The park sits atop an underground salt bed deposited when a sea flowed through the Colorado Plateau. It later evaporated. The salt bed is responsible for the arches, spires, balanced rocks, and eroded monoliths. The effects of weathering and erosion continue to shape the rock, as they have for millions of years.

The rock formations and monoliths are enormous and totally dominate the landscape. As we made our way up the scenic drive, we marveled at the sheer scale of the rocks, the intense red-orange color and the varied shapes, many cleverly named.

Balanced Rock, Delicate Arch, Fiery Furnace, Sheep Rock and Three Gossips aptly match the formations they refer to.

Utah has tremendous natural beauty. Expansive woodland and sagebrush landscapes sit in the shadows of majestic, snow-covered mountains. It has a vastness and otherworldy feeling that is truly wondrous to experience.

We finished the day in our 24th state of our Big Year, Colorado.

After some time to rest and recharge in Grand Junction, Colorado, we moved on to Gunnison, Colorado. Outside of town we found two Sage Thrashers at one of the many National Recreation Areas along the beautiful Blue Mesa Reservoir.

Gunnison is a lovely small college town, home to Western Colorado University and a nearby lek of Gunnison Sage-Grouse. On Tuesday evening we attended an informative lecture about the biology and conservation of this endangered Grouse. In addition to learning a lot, we enjoyed meeting other fanatical birders who would be joining us on the lek before dawn in the morning. One was 12 year old Killian Sullivan, a very impressive young birder from Ohio whose knowledge and passion rivals our own. He and his dad, Brandon, were on their own grand adventure. They referred to it as their "Crazy Chicken Tour"!

Bundled in as many layers as we could find, we left our hotel at 4:40 AM the next morning. When we arrived at the lek, we entered a shipping container refitted as a birding blind. One side had wooden shutters that can be lifted to allow for a view out to the lek. Before they were raised, we arranged ourselves on benches, set up our scopes, and then sat in total darkness after the light was turned off.

Total darkness, 20 degrees, sitting on cold benches inside an even colder metal container. After we chatted among ourselves for a bit, the cold really set in and many, maybe all of us, began to wonder aloud - what kind of crazy person does this?!

Fortunately, dawn finally arrived, the window shutters were raised and our attention shifted to scouring the lek for the Grouse. Numb fingers and toes were ignored...at least for the moment.

"I see them," announced our trip leader. "See that clump of willows way off at the base of the mountain? Go three willow stands to the left. See the one all by itself? Look back behind that. Beyond the fence. To the right of the thickest post. There are some Gunnison Sage Grouse, and one of them is displaying!"

With help from the younger eyes of Killian, we finally found four moving blobs about a mile from us. Not quite the view we had of the Greater Sage Grouse the day before, but it was a thrilling experience nonetheless. As unique as unique can be.

In addition to the Gunnison's, we enjoyed stunning sunrise views of Mountain Bluebirds and Black-billed Magpies. After two hours in cold storage, however, we were secretly relieved when the Grouse took wing - marking the time when we too could depart the lek.

After returning to our hotel to thaw ourselves out with a hot breakfast and hot showers, we packed up for our journey to Colorado Springs. We drove once again up and down steep, twisting mountain roads as we crossed the Rockies and the Continental Divide, continuing our trip east toward home where, thankfully, we have smaller mountains and wider roads.

Along the way we picked up a Townsend's Solitaire and Mountain Plover, which had eluded us despite our many attempts while in Texas. One nemesis bird off our list.

In addition to the Ferruginous Hawk, we now had a new challenger for the title of most annoying bird, the American Dipper. This would not only be a new bird for the year for us, but a lifer. We 'dipped' on this one again today.

On Thursday, we resumed our journey and headed for Hays, Kansas, our 25th state.

Our reason for being in Hays was to see the Greater Prairie-Chickens and Lesser Prairie-Chickens. Like the Grouse we observed in Utah and Colorado, the Prairie

Big Year Assistant

What does a retired software developer do before he and his wife begin a Big Year? He writes a mobile app to help!

Cornell Lab of Ornithology's eBird is a public platform that allows birders to record, organize, and share their sightings. eBird has an easy to use interface on the web and mobile devices ... and most serious birders use it on a daily basis.

eBird also has a free and documented API, which stands for Application Programming Interface, code that programmers can use in their own applications.

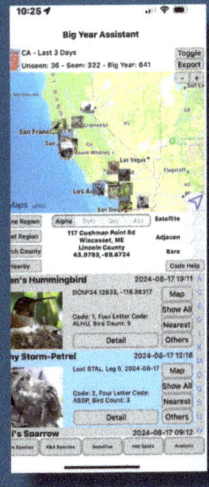

Ethan designed an App that he called The Big Year Assistant. It would give a real time view of birds in the Lower 48 States that the Whitakers had not picked up yet.

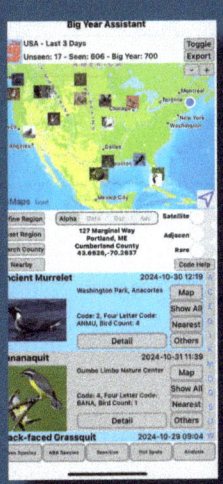

The Big Year Assistant was an indispensable tool through the year.
• What birds are in this county in Florida?
• In the last 2 weeks what birds are available in Colorado?
• Give me directions to the Ross's Goose.
• What Code Two Birds haven't we seen?
• Where were Snowy Owls seen yesterday?

There is no way to know how our Big Year would have gone without this App ... but it was of considerable help.

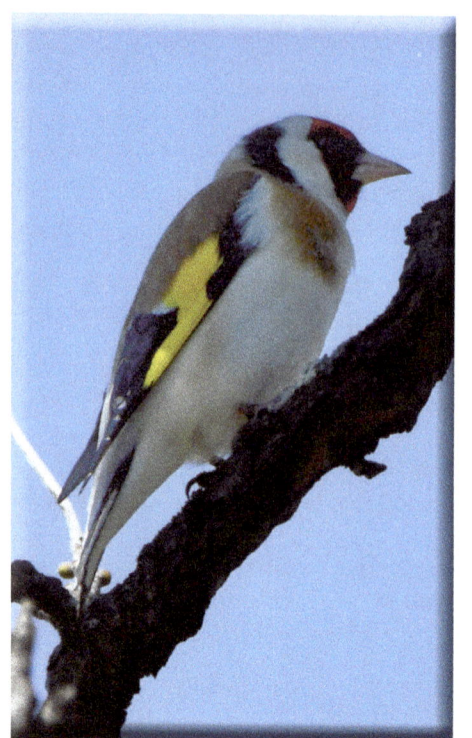
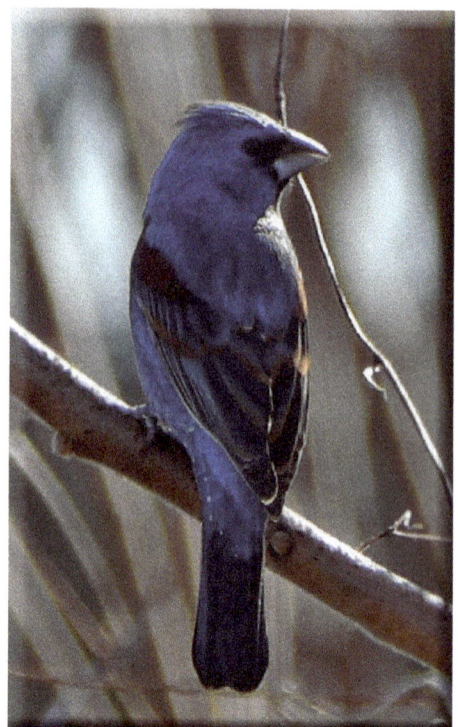

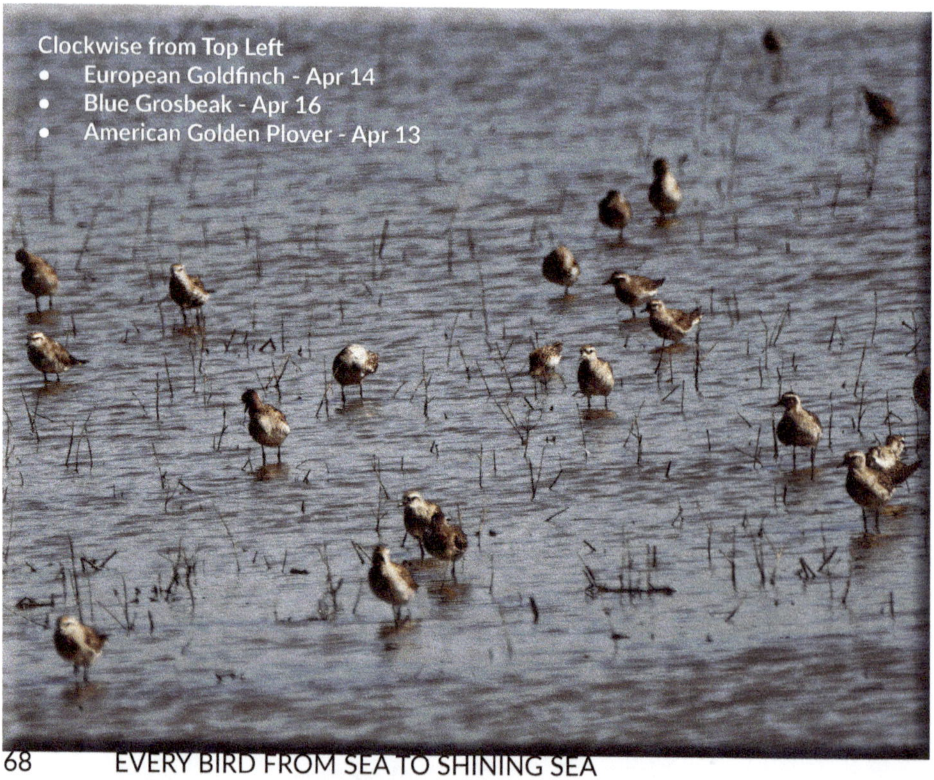

Clockwise from Top Left
- European Goldfinch - Apr 14
- Blue Grosbeak - Apr 16
- American Golden Plover - Apr 13

Chickens undertake an elaborate courtship ritual beginning at dawn.

While we still set out in the dark of night, this time we piled into a heated van, a definite upgrade from the ice box we endured at the Gunnison lek. Our driver had the distinct pleasure of chauffeuring 8 very sleepy, caffeine-deprived birders to the Prairie Chicken leks over mostly dirt roads for over an hour.

When we arrived at the first Lesser Prairie Chicken lek, dawn had just gotten underway. Our target birds weren't too hard to find thanks to our experienced guide, Jackie. But like the Gunnison's Sage Grouse, they were quite far out. Fortunately, they jumped into the air periodically, which helped us to spot them.

After visiting a second Lesser lek, we moved on to the Greater Prairie Chicken. Given that the sky was now lighter and that, as their name suggests, the Greater Prairie Chicken is bigger in size, they were much easier to see, and thus, a lot of fun to watch.

After several hours of birding, it was time to warm up with a hot breakfast. As we introduced ourselves to our table mates at the Hometown Bakery in Hays, we discovered to our great surprise that next to Ethan sat Andy Baker, who also lives in Maine! And just 30 minutes from us. What were the odds?!!

Driving from Missouri to Maine

While traveling from Hays to Kansas City, Missouri, we made an attempt along the way to find some American Golden Plovers reported at a rural airport. But, apparently they departed before we got there.

From Kansas City we moved to Springfield, Illinois. Our trip there got off to an unexpected start when Ethan, who rarely makes a mistake with directions, took us south for 90 minutes instead of east for 90 minutes in further search of American Golden Plovers.

As Bob Ross would say, however, this turned into a happy accident as we found over 400 American Golden Plovers as well as two other first of the year shorebirds - in what ended up being a terrific birding location.

What well-known person in US history lived in Springfield, Illinois? Abraham Lincoln, of course! As much as we wished we had the time to explore the Lincoln-related sites there, we could not stay long enough. Our time was getting short, and there were birds we needed to find in Chicago. This is one of the challenges of a Big Year. You go to so many interesting places, and there is so much you might want to see, but you just can't.

We were in Illinois to chase two European birds that have established breeding colonies in "the Land of Lincoln."

The first was the Eurasian Tree Sparrow.

We went to a lovely nature preserve, situated by a cemetery, where spring was well underway. As we were searching for the sparrow, we ran into Paula Aschim, a birder we had met in Texas. To our good fortune, she lived in the area and told us exactly where to find Eurasian Tree Sparrows at a different nearby nature preserve. We hurried over there, and bingo! Within minutes, we found two of these beautiful birds.

Chicago, one of very few places in the country where European Goldfinches can be found, was next. If we were going to add this bird to our 2024 list, we had to find it today as Chicago was not on any of our remaining itineraries for the year.

In the United States, European Goldfinches are kept as pets and have a propensity to escape from their cages. In Chicago and southeastern Wisconsin, so many of these beautiful birds have flown the coop that they have become 'countable' in this tiny geographical area.

We were prepared to spend several hours visiting a variety of locations in the city in search of them, but we found them at our first stop! It didn't hurt that these birds were at an office park, and this was a Sunday. No people noise or traffic noise. We knew that they sound like American Goldfinches, so when we heard a familiar sounding goldfinch-like song, it was clear we were getting warm. It took a bit of tracking, but we were able to photograph one as it rested.

Packing

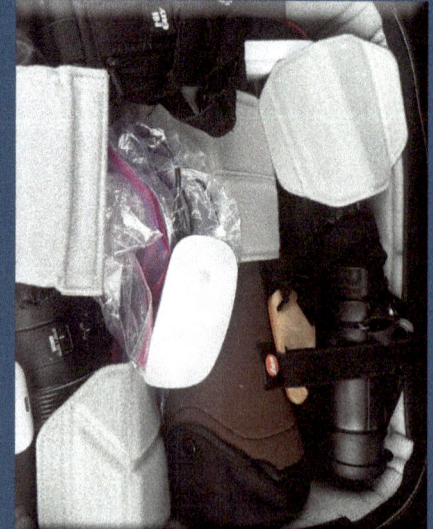

When we were traveling with our own car, a Subaru Outback, we tended to over pack. We hauled a box of books (birding, plant life and tourist guides). We brought a portable Keurig machine from hotel to hotel (we love our coffee). We had plastic bins with winter clothes, desert clothes and even dress clothes.

But when we had to fly, we had to make hard choices, because we rarely check bags.

Thus, each of use had a suitcases that fit in the overhead bin and a personal item that fit under the seat in front of us, we had to pack: two cameras, two computers, two sets of binoculars, a spotting scope, a tripod, clothes, toiletries, bug spray, suntan lotion, gloves, hat, etc. etc. etc.

Every trip was a challenge.

After many days of birding, Monday was a long-haul travel day for us. Thus, our binoculars and cameras got a rest while we made the nine hour push from South Bend, Indiana to Harrisburg, Pennsylvania. We did try to locate a Cerulean Warbler, conveniently reported near our hotel a few days ago, but we did not find him.

Thus began a relatively bad streak for us as we struck out on a number of birds the next day. Driving, searching and dipping, or missing out on a bird, can be oh-so frustrating.

Blue Grosbeaks appear occasionally in New England during migration but not in big numbers. For some reason, perhaps due to recent storms, there had been several reports across coastal New England over the previous few days.

One handsome male had been visiting a park in Boston, to much excitement from the birding community there. Several birders had even been so helpful as to post very specific instructions as to where to find him. Off we went, and within moments, there he was posing for us, ending our streak of bad luck!

On April 17th, we awoke in a Boston hotel, excited as this was the final day of our 81 day road trip. Our home in Maine was only 150 minutes away. First, however, we had to find a Blue-winged Warbler at an Audubon sanctuary in Marblehead, Massachusetts.

When we arrived, there were several birders present, but no one had seen the Warbler. We hoped that as it warmed up, the warbler would start stirring. In the meantime, Ingrid decided to check out some thrushes a little further down the trail. These Hermit Thrushes led her down another path where she soon spotted a bright yellow warbler scratching around in some leaf litter looking for his breakfast. Lo and behold, it was the Blue-winged Warbler!

Soon, Ethan got on the bird. As we told the other birders about it, they mentioned that a Scarlet Tanager was at the pond. We hurried over, and after a bit of searching, found this striking fellow high in a tree.

Our final stop was at a cemetery in Ipswich, Massachusetts where we had hoped to find a Prothonotary Warbler. While that was another dip, we did find a Baltimore Oriole. Spring really was underway in New England!

On January 28, we began our Big Year Road trip. Several weeks, fourteen thousand miles and 28 states later, we had identified 478 birds for the year. While we were very happy with our results, we looked forward to adding many more birds over the coming weeks and miles.

New England Birding

After weeks on the road, we were happy to return home, connect with family and watch for birds in our backyard while recharging our batteries a bit before our next planned journey to Florida. What is it they say about "the best laid plans of mice and men …"?

With laundry and unpacking completed, we scheduled a day trip to Boston so we could be there when Ingrid's dad met his new great grandson. Shortly before leaving the house, we learned that a Ruff, a European shorebird, had been spotted in Vermont. We quickly packed our bags and decided we would point our car there rather than back to Maine when leaving Boston.

We left Boston at 2:10, racing against sunset through mountain passes and over winding, narrow roads once again, this time through the Green Mountains of Vermont.

We arrived at the Ruff site hoping other birders would point us in the bird's direction.

Surprisingly, however, there were no other birders … just a cold brisk wind and darkening skies. We tried one spot after another and were becoming a bit discouraged when Ethan noticed a handful of Yellowlegs feeding a couple of hundred yards away in tall, flooded grass.

The two of us systematically worked our way through the birds … "That's a Greater Yellowlegs." "There's another Greater." "The smaller bird with the straight bill is a Lesser Yellowlegs." "Wait, that bird has orange legs and a down turned bill!" We had the Ruff.

Getting a confirmation photo was no easier than finding the bird, as the wind was blowing our tripods over and holding the camera steady was a pain, but we got one. A few seconds later the Ruff and his friends flew off to roost for the night.

It did not return the next day.

We returned home in the morning, once again looking forward to a respite from the road. Not so fast! We had not been home for more than half an hour when we learned that a Garganey had been reported - back in Massachusetts. We looked at each other, sighed, and made our plan for the morning. Out the door we would go before dawn…again.

Despite our best attempt, the Garganey was a one day wonder who did not wait for us. This is both the challenge and the thrill that makes birding such an addictive sport. Plan all you will, the birds may or may not oblige you.

Spring Migration

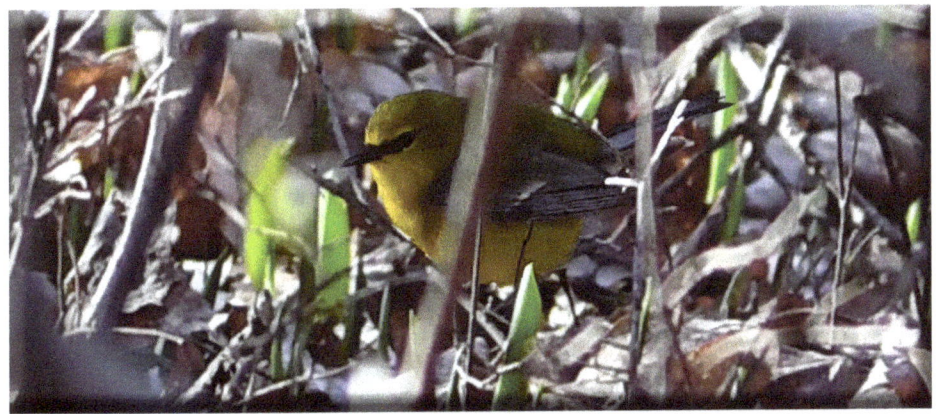

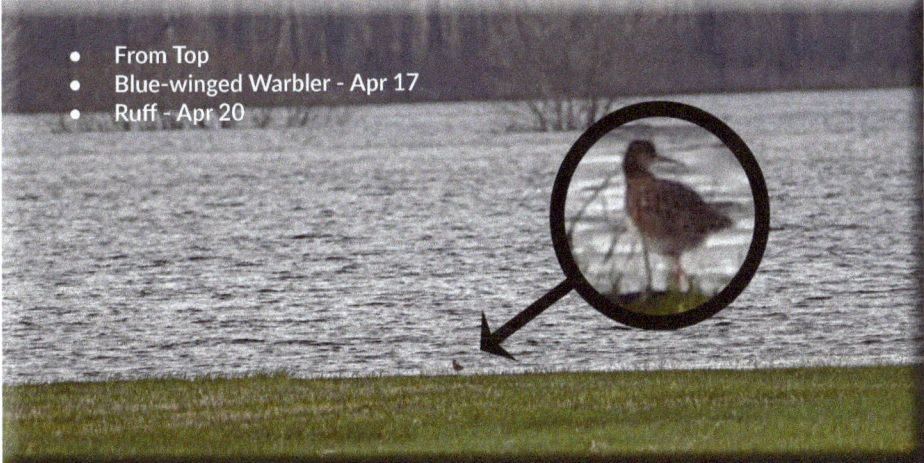

From Top
- Blue-winged Warbler - Apr 17
- Ruff - Apr 20

We had become rather impatient waiting for spring migration to arrive in full force in Maine, which generally occurs the second week in May.

Our upcoming trip to Florida was still several days away, and every time we searched locally for new birds, the gods threw roadblocks in our way. In one case, we ventured to a nearby wildlife management area in search of Kingbirds, Vireos and early Warblers and were met by dozens of hound dogs and their masters doing gun training. We were unable to access many of the prime birding areas there.

A road trip was in order, so we pointed our car toward Massachusetts once again.

Our first stop was the old Pease Air Force Base in New Hampshire. Here we were determined to find the Upland Sandpipers that had been reported. Using our spotting scopes, we found one grazing between the two runways as planes landed around him. We are never sure how wise it is to point high powered optical gear at commercial airplanes, but anything for a bird! The day was off to a great start!

Next, we returned to the Audubon sanctuary we visited the previous week in Marblehead. This time, we were in search of a reported Hooded Warbler. We dipped on this but picked up a few other first of the year birds - Ovenbird, Great Crested Flycatcher and Northern Waterthrush. We spent the night in Plymouth, Massachusetts, prepositioning ourselves within easy range of a couple of exciting birds in the morning.

Off and out of our hotel before dawn, we arrived at nearby Burrage Pond in Hamilton and made the long, but lovely trek into a bog, where we heard and eventually saw the King Rail exactly where he was supposed to be. Along the trail, we added several more species to our year list. We crossed our fingers that our luck would last.

After a quick pack-up and breakfast back at our hotel, we journeyed to Rehoboth, Massachusetts to search for Swallow-tailed Kites. These guys rarely appear north of South Carolina, but somehow 4 had found their way to Massachusetts and had remained.

We searched the skies at several reported sites throughout a half-mile area and then waited at a location with an expansive sky view. As we sat in our car with the skylight open and our eyes continually scanning, we negotiated how long we would remain. Ingrid suggested an hour. Ethan countered with two, so we settled on 90 minutes.

No sooner had that decision been made when Ethan, who had the foresight to tilt our side view mirrors skyward, spotted some raptors in one of them. We leapt from the car and saw...a couple of grackles. But then, there was one and then two majestic Swallow-tailed Kites swooping and gliding through the sky. A new life bird for both of us!

Time to make our way north toward home and a good cell spot where we could pull over and register for the Southeast Arizona Birding Festival taking place in August. Registration opened at 1:00 sharp, and we could not miss our chance to sign up for the trips that could get us the highest number of our target birds, without actually having to drive the nail biter canyon roads ourselves. As thorough prep work is to a good paint job, careful planning is to a successful Big Year.

A rainy day was on tap for Thursday, but we were eager to find a few more birds before we migrated to Florida on Sunday. There HAD to be some new migrants around. Soon, we learned about a pile of Warblers being seen at Laudholm Farm in Wells, Maine including a very early and secretive Mourning Warbler.

Off we went.

We drove through downpours with fingers crossed that the faucet would shut off by the time we arrived. We were in luck with the weather, but not with the Mourning Warbler, which we were unable to relocate. We did, however, find a Magnolia Warbler, one more new bird for the year.

As we were leaving Wells, our friend Richard Garrigus reported a rare Wilson's Phalarope at an old seafood canning plant, just 30 minutes away.

The Wilson's Phalarope is one of the few species in which the female is brighter and more boldly colored than the male. As a matter of fact, Phalaropes change traditional gender roles, with males sitting on the eggs and raising the chicks.

After the Phalarope tick, we stopped at a Portland birding hotspot that annually attracts a great variety of birds during spring migration. While we were still a week or so away from prime warbler movement, we were hopeful that we might find something at Capisic Pond. Sure enough, we did when birder friends Tova Mellen and Chuck Barnes quickly pointed us toward a Black-throated Blue Warbler and a Warbling Vireo in a marshy area of the park.

We enjoyed birding in Maine over our two week respite from the road, catching up with friends... and all of the birding gossip.

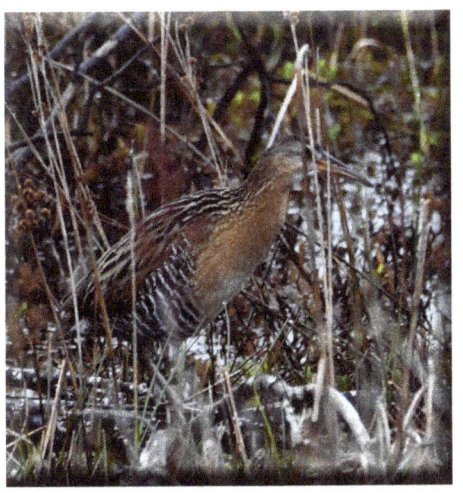
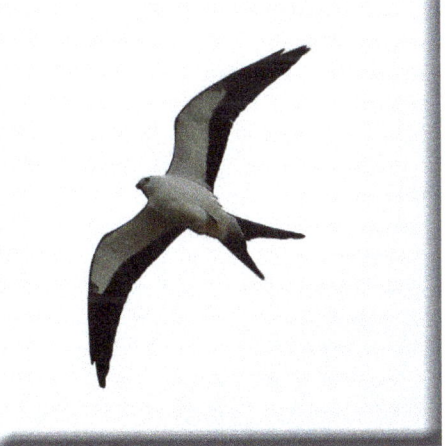
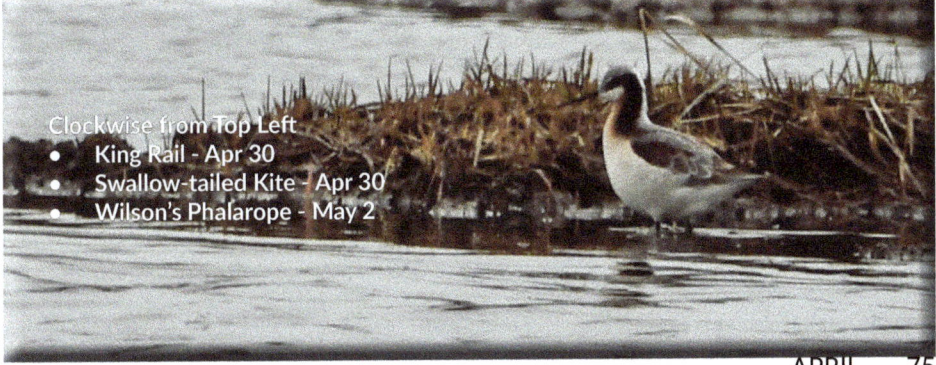

Clockwise from Top Left
- King Rail - Apr 30
- Swallow-tailed Kite - Apr 30
- Wilson's Phalarope - May 2

Chickadees

The Continental United States is home to six species of chickadees: the Black-capped, Carolina, Mountain, Boreal, Chestnut-backed, and Mexican Chickadees. These small, social songbirds are widely loved for their distinctive calls and curious behavior, though they vary greatly in range, appearance, and habitat preference. Each chickadee species occupies a unique geographic and environmental niche, with occasional overlap, particularly between Black-capped and Carolina Chickadees, whose ranges meet in the eastern United States. Chickadees are generally found in a range of woodland habitats, from deciduous forests to high-altitude Spruce-Fir zones, where they forage for insects, seeds, and berries.

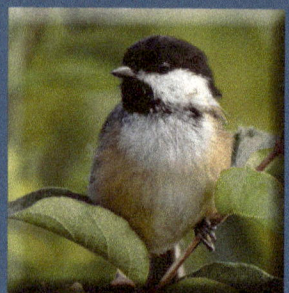

The Black-capped Chickadee is the most widespread, found throughout northern North America, from the northeastern United States to Alaska and down into some parts of the northern Midwest and the Rockies. This species favors deciduous and mixed forests, where it is easily recognized by its black cap, white cheeks, and fluffy, round body.

The Carolina Chickadee, similar in appearance but slightly smaller, occupies the southeastern United States and prefers lowland deciduous forests. Where the ranges of these two species meet, they often hybridize, creating offspring that display a mixture of characteristics, making identification challenging in these overlap zones.

Further west, the Mountain Chickadee inhabits high-altitude Pine and Fir forests in the mountainous regions of the western United States,

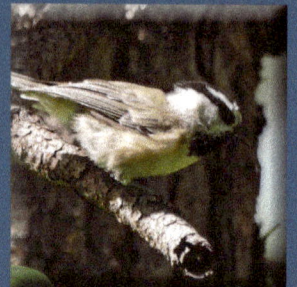

from the Rockies to the Sierra Nevada. This chickadee is easily identified by the distinctive white stripe above its eye, setting it apart from the Black-capped and Carolina Chickadees.

In boreal and subalpine forests of the northern United States, the Boreal Chickadee is common, distinguished by its brown cap and preference for coniferous forests. This chickadee tends to be quieter and less social than other species, adapting to the harsher climates of the far north. Despite their similar names, the Mountain and Boreal Chickadees do not

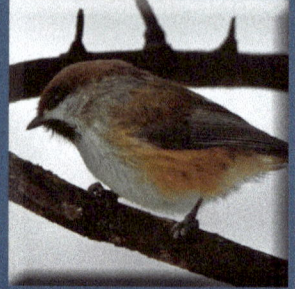

often cross paths due to their distinct habitat preferences.

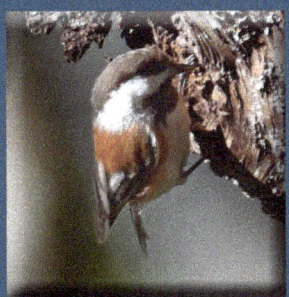

In the Pacific Northwest, the Chestnut-backed Chickadee is found primarily in coastal and wet coniferous forests from California to Alaska. Its unique chestnut-brown back and sides make it one of the most colorful chickadee species.

Finally, the Mexican Chickadee has the most restricted range of any U.S. chickadee species, occurring only in the high Pine-Oak forests of the Chiricahua Mountains in Arizona and parts of New Mexico. Mexican Chickadees have a distinctive, slightly larger appearance and a unique two-note call, adapted to their limited, high-elevation range.

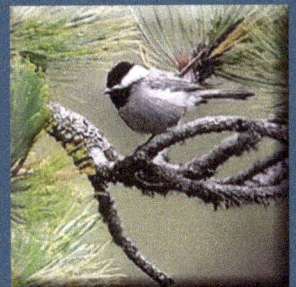

Together, these six chickadee species represent a diverse group, each adapted to specific habitats across the continent,

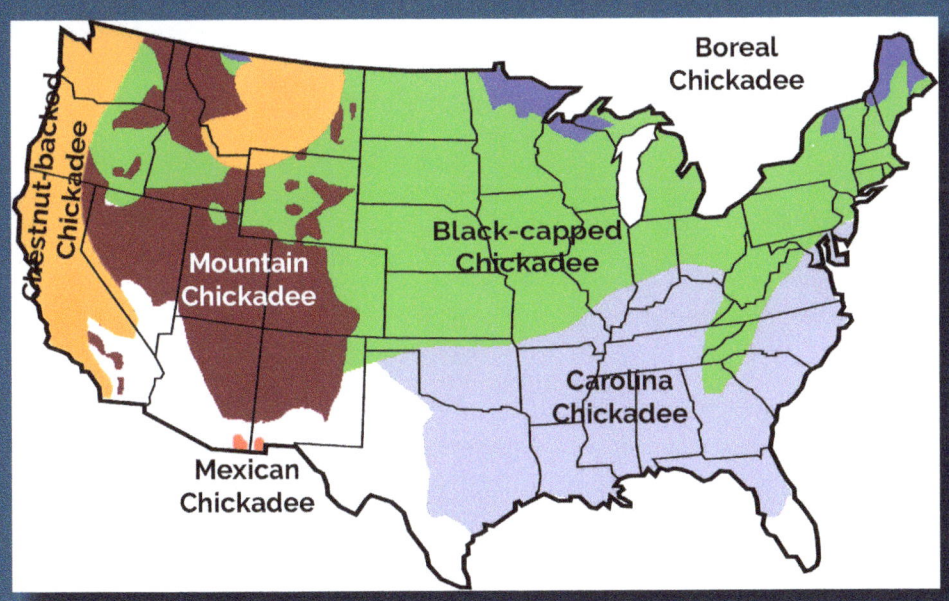

May

Travel	#
Plane Flights	4
Rental Cars	1
Nights Away	7
Boat Trips	2

State	Year Birds
Florida	27
Massachusetts	10
Maine	23
New Hampshire	2
New Jersey	1
Virginia	2
Total	65

The Dry Tortugas

The pre-dawn hours of May 5th found us with our car pointed toward the Portland Jetport. The silver lining in these inhumane middle of the night flights is that, weather and airline gods permitting, we arrive early enough in the day to get some birding in. In this case, the exotic birds that Miami is famous for.

Once in our rental car, we drove to Crandon Park in South Miami. Here, Indian Peafowl, aka Peacocks, are reliably seen. Crandon is a fairly large park, and it took us a bit of time and detective work to find the shady spot where they were resting to avoid the hot Miami sun.

Our next stop was a return trip to a park we visited in February, and our second attempt to find Yellow-chevroned Parakeets. We had learned that they like to eat the fruit of fig trees, but being from northern New England where pretty much the only fruit trees are apples, we had no idea what fig trees looked like. Google took care of that! Soon we found the birds high up, munching on figs

One of the best times to find Parrots and Parakeets is in the evening when they come to roost for the night. We were aware of a roost at Brewer Park and drove over there after dinner. As local tennis players hit balls across the net and families visited the playground, we watched and listened.

As dusk moved in and people moved out, the birds arrived. We were thrilled to find both Orange-winged Amazons (Parrots), White-eyed Parakeets and a first of the year Common Nighthawk. As we started the walk back to our car, we were treated to repeated tremolo calls from an Eastern Screech Owl. During our Big Year, we were fortunate to encounter several of these owls. But we never got tired of them.

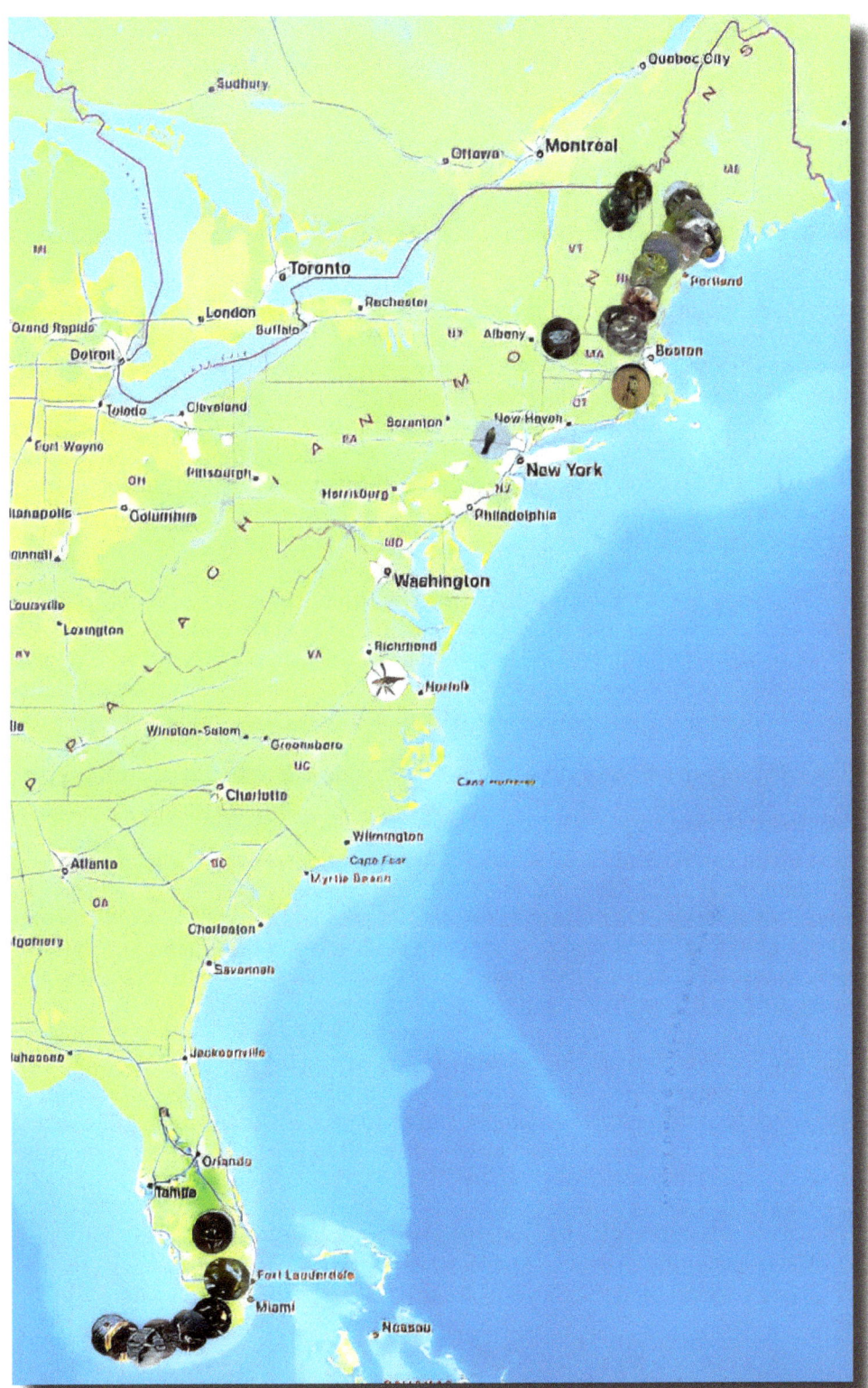

MAY

500th Bird of the Year

While hunting for Amazons (Parrots) at dusk in South Miami, a Common Nighthawk flew overhead.

May 5, 8:00 PM

The following morning we left the city heading north. Birding is not unlike placing a bet. We weigh the odds and cross our fingers. Then, we recalculate the odds as information comes in. Do we put our money on the finicky and unreliable Yellow-headed Caracara, a bird we had dipped on in February or the newly found rare White-cheeked Pintails at a location reported to be inaccessible on weekdays?

Choosing the Pintail for its proximity to another rare bird, the Shiny Cowbird, we headed in its direction. Following earlier reports and the helpful tips of another birder we encountered, we first found the Shiny Cowbird on the grounds of a rice mill - near a dumpster!

Unfortunately, we were not as lucky with the White-cheeked Pintails despite our best efforts at scoping the enormous flooded farm field for well over an hour. Or so we thought. While there, we believed we saw the pair, but they were far off and somewhat obscured by marsh grass. Months later, while reviewing photos, we discovered proof that we had indeed seen them. This time, the camera giveth!

Key West, where we stayed the night before taking the ferry to Dry Tortugas National Park, was our next destination.

Ethan had learned that Black-whiskered Vireos, White-crowned Pigeons and the Red Junglefowl could be found at a park in Islamadora on our route through the Keys. While early risers did laps in the pool, jogged and set out to fish, we looked through the trees for birds. We found both the Vireo and the Pigeon, but the Junglefowl was AWOL. No worries, we had several other places to check along the route. Fingers crossed, we would find it at one of those.

The day was very hot and humid and we had exhausted our supply of water, so a stop was required. No sooner had we pulled into a Publix parking lot when a Red Junglefowl walked by. We jumped out of the car with our cameras. Passersby chuckled in what appeared to be mocking disbelief as we photoed what turned out to be not one, but several Jungle Fowl.

It wasn't long before we discovered the reason for these peoples' mirth. These wild chickens wander the streets and parking lots of the Keys in equal numbers to gulls at a New England McDonald's plaza. That is to say, they are everywhere and are kind of a pest!

It wasn't long before we had all three of our priority birds for the day and could take our time a bit and enjoy the scenery. If you have ever been to the Florida Keys, you too no doubt have been in awe of the crystal clear, turquoise water, beautiful sand beaches and lush habitat.

Nightjars are a rather mysterious class of nocturnal birds that feed on insects caught in the air. They are generally medium-sized with short bills and legs and long wings. These include Eastern Whippoorwill, Common Paruque, and Common Nighthawk. They are sometimes referred to as goatsuckers due to an old myth that they drink the blood of goats.

The Antillean Nighthawk lives almost exclusively on the Florida Keys. Tuesday evening we found four of them near the Key West airport. We enjoyed watching them chase each other and snatch bugs out of the air, at least those that weren't biting us, that is.

Wednesday was a big day for us! Our trip to the Dry Tortugas was planned many months ago. This national park is legendary for its unique birds, and ferry tickets sell out far in advance. We bought ours the previous August.

As we waited to board the boat, we were surprised to see no other birders, and we

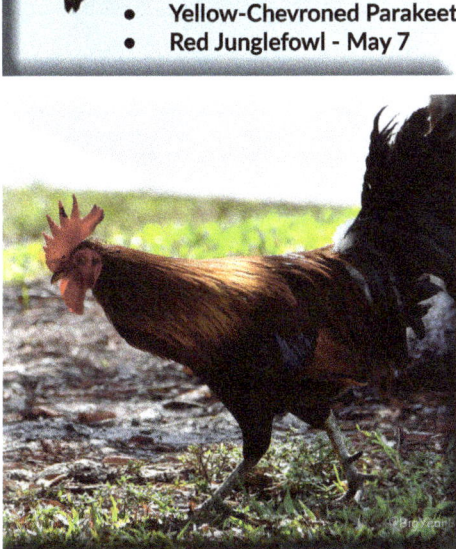
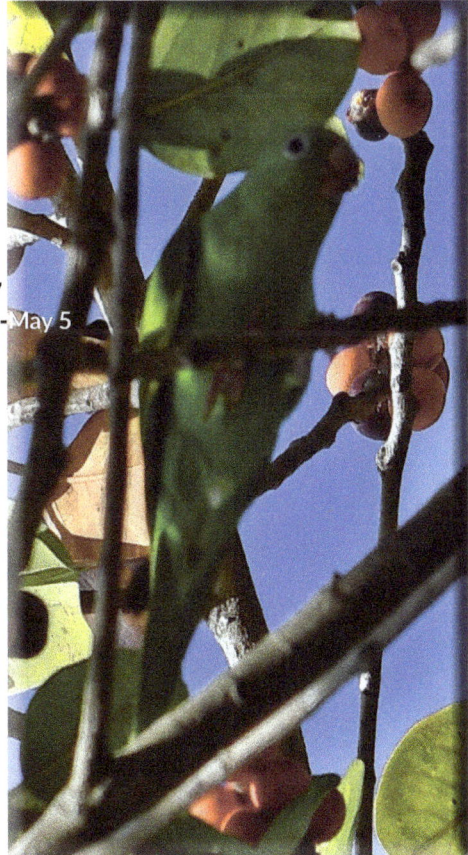

From Left
- Antillean Nighthawk - May 7
- Yellow-Chevroned Parakeet - May 5
- Red Junglefowl - May 7

found ourselves to be a bit of a curiosity to our fellow passengers who were dressed for a day of swimming, sunbathing and snorkeling. With our binoculars, cargo pants, cameras and spotting scopes we did stand out just a bit.

First used as a Civil War Era fort and later as a prison, mainly for Union deserters, Fort Jefferson on Garden Key in the Dry Tortugas, sits seventy miles west of Key West and requires a two and a half hour ferry ride each way or a seaplane trip to reach.

Whenever we take a pelagic trip, aka a boat trip to see birds that spend the vast majority of their lives at sea, we spend all of our time on deck so we can see as many birds as possible. This was the first time either of us can remember being on a pelagic trip in short sleeves. The Maine coast, even in August, is chilly when out on the water.

While we observed very few birds at sea, we did find two key species on our target list - Black-capped Petrel and Audubon's Shearwater, both life birds. The day was off to a good start.

After two hours on the water, Fort Jefferson came into view on the horizon. Our pass by Hospital Key, home to a colony of Boobies, was so near we could taste it. As we got closer, we could just make out the white and brown blobs on the shore. Yes, both the Brown Boobies and Masked Boobies were there! As we got closer, our excitement grew and others on the bow worked hard to help us - offering us their front row views and dashing after our hats when they blew off.

Shortly after arriving on Garden Key, we made our way up to the second level of the fort, and set up our scope to overlook the old coaling dock.

Garden Key is the nesting home of 4,000 Brown Noddies, a stunning life bird for us both. One would have to be blind and deaf not to see hundreds of them on any day in May at Garden Key. But we were in search of two smaller, darker birds - Black

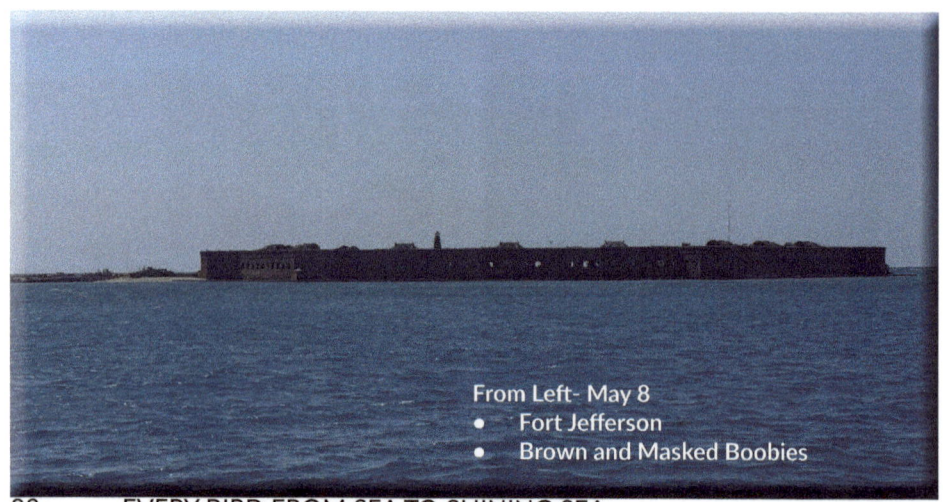

From Left- May 8
- Fort Jefferson
- Brown and Masked Boobies

Noddies. We were prepared to spend several hours scanning the Browns for the rare Black.

While Ethan set up the spotting scope, Ingrid began to scan with her binoculars. Almost immediately she announced, "I got one. I got the Black Noddy!" How adorable, Ethan thought. Ingrid believes she has scanned through 4,000 birds at a distance of 50 yards and found the one that was not like the other - not likely. He looked in the scope, and there indeed was the Black Noddy! After high fives and hugs we were off to find Bridled Terns.

As with the Black and Brown Noddies, there are thousands of Sooty Terns nesting by the fort, but only a few Bridled Terns. And of course the two species look almost exactly alike. The Sooty has a black back and wings while the Bridled has a dark gray back and wings.

In April, Andy, the Maine birder we met in Hays, Kansas, had described in detail how to find the Terns. Fortunately, we had written down every word, and we headed to the broken rocks below the old helicopter pad.

Here is where we began to have trouble. Every path to the helicopter pad was blocked by 'Area Closed' signs - a deliberate effort by the National Parks Department to prevent us from getting the tern! Ingrid had a brief view of one flying by, but it disappeared from sight before Ethan had a chance to see it.

Finally we came upon a cement pylon on the beach near the helicopter pad. We stood on it, holding onto a dead tree for balance. From there we were able to see two Bridled Terns on their nest, only 20 feet away! Miraculously, neither of us broke our necks.

We next made an attempt to find the Red-footed Booby that another Mainer, Alex Lamoreaux, had observed on Long Key a few days earlier.

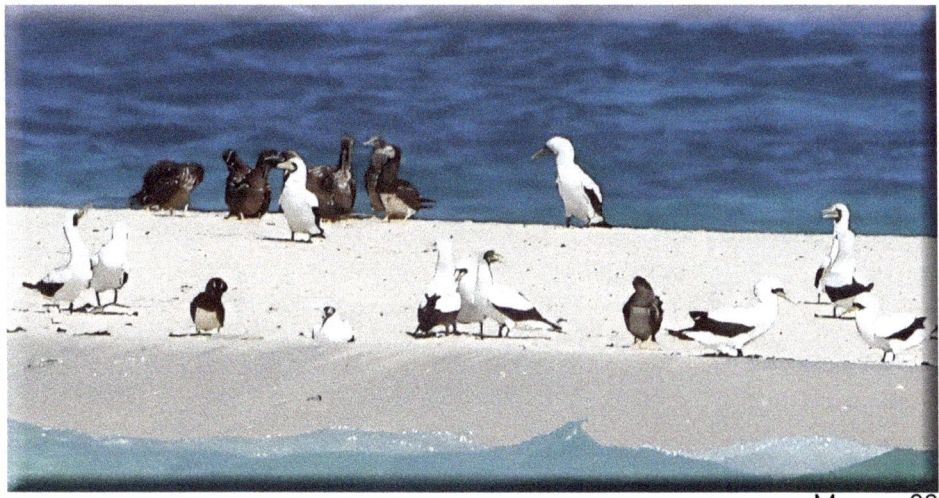

Long Key is about a half mile off of Garden Key and is inaccessible to foot traffic due to nesting birds. Needless to say, finding a bird in a tree at this distance, even with a powerful scope, is a shot in the dark, but we had to try. We searched for and found a candidate but did not see it clearly enough to make a confident ID. Very happily, we later found it in one of our photos.

The balance of our four hours on the island was spent combing the trees for warblers. We were thrilled to find a new species for the year for us, a Worm-eating Warbler, among numerous American Redstarts, Palm Warblers, and a Cape May Warbler.

Returning to Key West, we were both thrilled and exhausted from our day but enjoyed reliving every moment over dinner that evening.

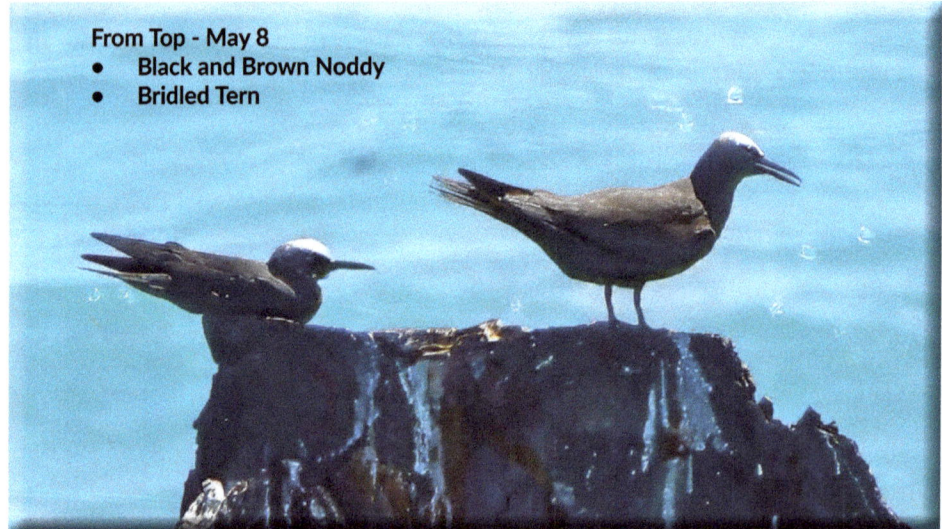

From Top - May 8
- Black and Brown Noddy
- Bridled Tern

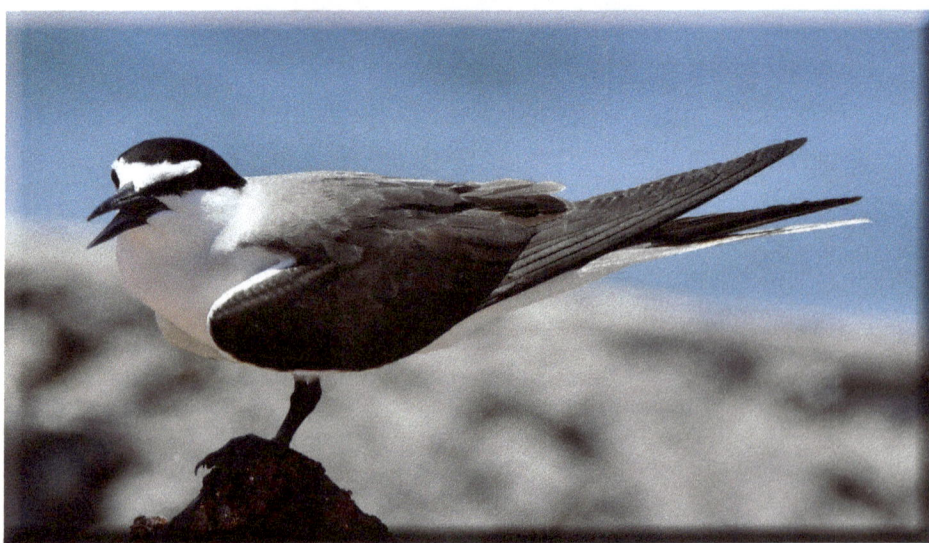

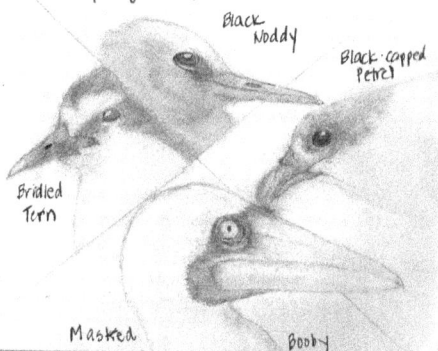

Massachusetts

Soon after we returned to Maine, we chased a rare bird on the Esplanade along the Charles River in Boston, just a few hundred feet from where Arthur Fiedler, John Williams and Keith Lockhart have conducted symphonies. Why this Chuck-will's-widow, a nocturnal bird of the American South, was sleeping next to an Outdoor Beer Garden at the Esplanade is anybody's guess.

Over the years we have had brief glimpses of Chuck-will's-widows darting through the sky chasing bugs at dusk. More often we have only heard their unmistakable "CHUCK will's WIDOW, CHUCK will's WIDOW" call well after dark. Seeing one this close was remarkable.

Ninety minutes later, we were in Concord, Massachusetts, not far from where the first shots of the American Revolution were fired. Here we found a Prothonotary Warbler, a bird of southern swamps.

We ended the day hiking up a mountain in Hadley, Massachusetts, the self-proclaimed asparagus capital of the world, to get two beautiful birds: the bright Yellow-throated Vireo and the Cerulean Warbler.

Earlier parts of the week found us on outings within a 50 mile radius of our home. Between Capisic Pond in Portland, Hinckley Park in South Portland, Hidden Valley Nature Center in Jefferson, Butler Head in Bath, and our own yard in Wiscasset we found several new Warblers and Flycatchers for the year.

Massachusetts, however, continued to beckon us. It is just far enough south of us to entice some of the more exotic warblers and other spring migrants in larger numbers than what we see in Maine.

Off we set to find a Kentucky Warbler in Dartmouth, Massachusetts close to the

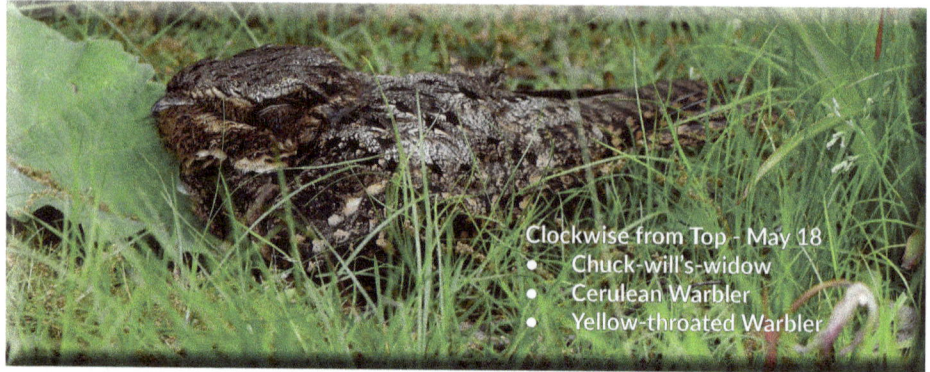

Clockwise from Top - May 18
- Chuck-will's-widow
- Cerulean Warbler
- Yellow-throated Warbler

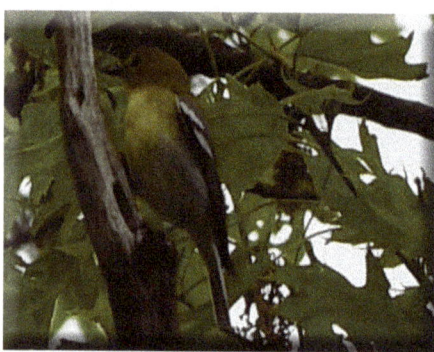
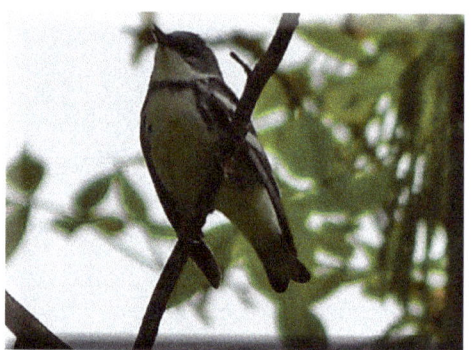

Rhode Island border. As this bird was very vocal and in the exact same spot it was reported to be the day before, it wasn't long before we found him!

Next we visited Allen's Pond in Westport and were thrilled to find both a Saltmarsh Sparrow and a Seaside Sparrow. While the former is not difficult for us to find in Maine, the Seaside is. Our final visit of the day was to Parker River National Wildlife Refuge on the north shore in Newburyport where Eastern Whippoorwills sing at dusk and dawn.

We arrived 45 minutes before dusk to learn that the gate to the refuge was about to close. Although we could have gotten out after the gate closed, according to one visitor, we decided not to chance it and waited and listened outside of the gate instead. Many birds were still singing, but as the sun set and dusk began to settle in, it grew quiet...too quiet.

Not having had much to eat and worried that we might miss a chance to find a place open late for dinner on a Monday night, we agreed that we would wait until 8:30 before packing it in and trying again another day.

Suddenly, just under the wire at 8:28, came the first 'whip' of the Eastern Whippoorwill's distinct call. It then completed its call, announcing its full name, exactly once! Since once was all we needed, off we went.

Unfortunately our luck for this trip ended there, as the next day we arrived at Marblehead Neck in search of a Hooded Warbler but found it oddly quiet. This was our second failed attempt to find a Hooded Warbler in this location. Perhaps it had joined the migration party and flown off the previous night.

Atlantic Puffins

Early in the week we traveled an hour north to Belgrade, Maine where each spring we stand on a rickety boat launch and peer out onto Messalonskee Lake and hope the Black Terns have returned.

Unlike the eleven other species of terns that we had seen in our Big Year, the Black Tern prefers freshwater to salt and, as its name suggests, is primarily black during breeding season. In the fall, the Black Tern's head and chest becomes white as it migrates south to its winter home along the coast of Central and South America. Fortunately, we found the Terns, sitting on buoys and swooping through the sky.

Wednesday was the first day of the season for Hardy Boat Puffin tours. We were there when the boat motored out of scenic New Harbor, Maine, headed for Eastern Egg Rock, North America's southernmost nesting island for Atlantic Puffins.

Like many birds with distinct or colorful plumage, Puffin feathers were once prized as ornaments for ladies' hats. In addition, their eggs and the birds themselves were collected for food. Due to Eastern Egg Rock's close proximity to the mainland (only 6 miles), Puffins on the island were over- hunted, and by 1885, there were no more Atlantic Puffins nesting anywhere on the island.

Fast-forward to 1973, when Stephen Kress of the National Audubon Society executed a plan to restore Atlantic Puffin breeding to Eastern Egg Rock. First, his team transplanted young Puffins from other breeding Islands, feeding and releasing them. By late summer, the birds would disappear into the North Atlantic where they lived

550th Bird of the Year

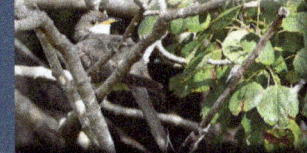

Yellow-billed Cuckoos are rare in mid-coast Maine and in parts north. But for the second year in a row we had one (or more) in our neighborhood. We heard it/them through out the spring and early summer ... and we had occasional sightings high in the tree tops.

May 25, 7:42 AM

at sea for 2 to 3 years before returning to the island to breed and nest.

Then through the use of Puffin decoys, Puffin recordings and even mirrors, the ma-

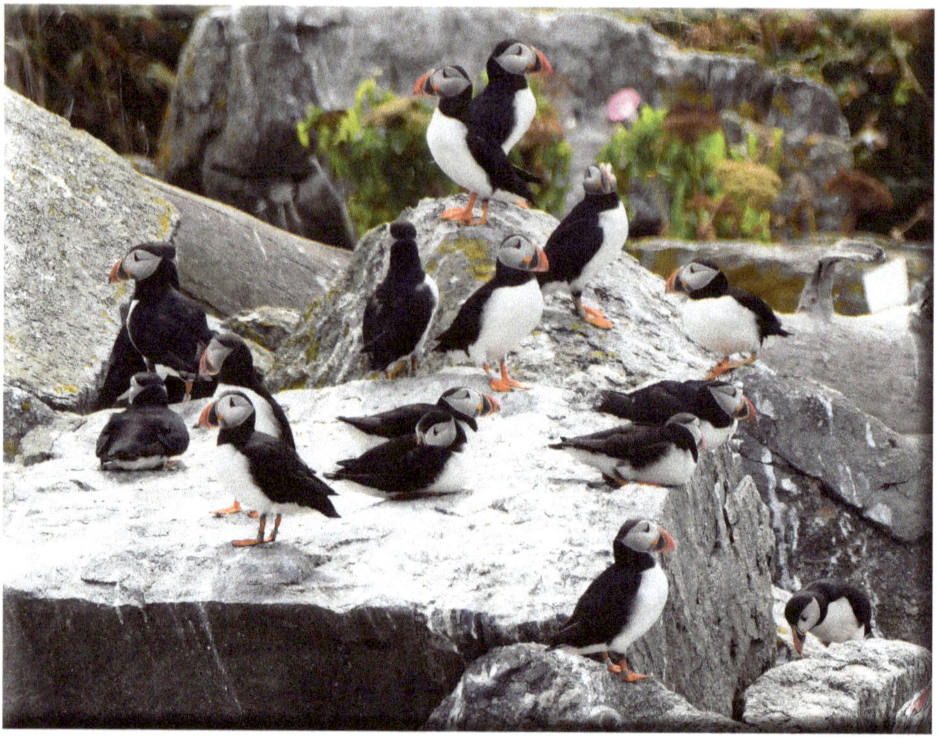

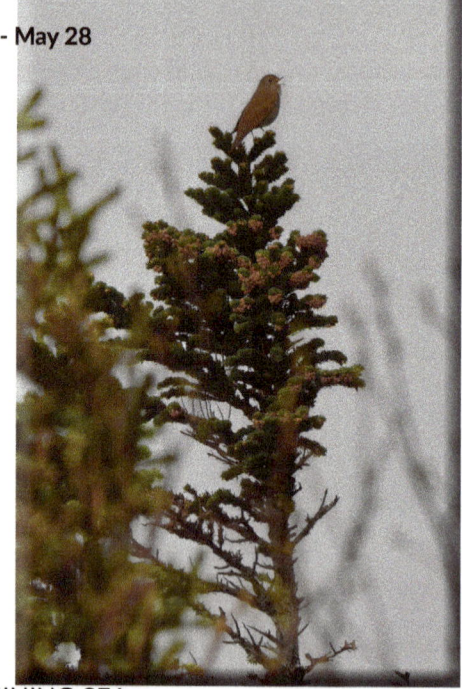

Clockwise from Top
- Atlantic Puffins - May 22
- Bicknell's Thrush - May 28
- Ethan and Ingrid on Mt. Washington - May 28

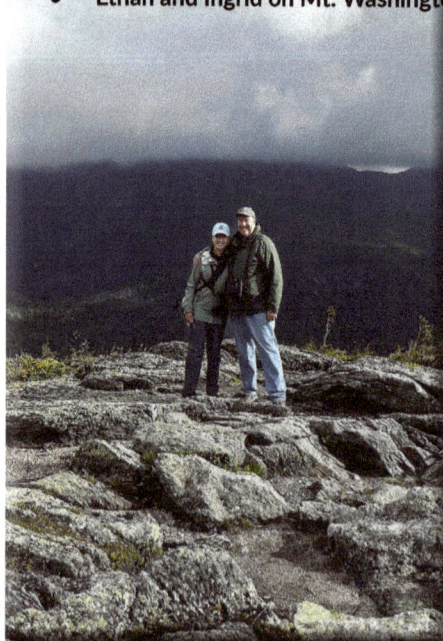

ture Puffins were coaxed back to Eastern Egg Rock. In 1981, the first pair returned to the island to nest. Thanks to the efforts of Steven Kress and the hundreds of interns who have worked on Project Puffin ever since, there are now approximately 3,000 puffins on Maine's seabird islands.

The day was unseasonably warm for May in Maine and a good one to be out on the water. As Eastern Egg Rock is only about 30 minutes from the harbor, it wasn't long before we spotted our first of approximately 30 Atlantic Puffins.

One cannot look at a Puffin and not smile. Its clown-like bill and tiny, football shaped body make it very entertaining to watch - whether darting through the air or bobbing atop the water.

We also saw our first Arctic Terns of the year. As well, a single Wilson's Storm-Petrel flew by the boat on our way back to the mainland.

The Bobolink is a ground nester, digging out a depression in the soil. This makes the Bobolink vulnerable to haying, human foot traffic and ground predators. As a result, its North American population has declined 56% since 1966.

We feel lucky to have a thriving Bobolink colony close to our home in Mid-coast Maine, at Salt Bay Farm in Nobleboro. We were delighted to find a first of the year Bobolink in our 'backyard'.

Mt. Washington

Mountain tops, cemeteries and swamps!

Our week began when we loaded into a van with eight other birders and headed up the Mt. Washington Auto Road in quest of a highly sought after bird, the Bicknell's Thrush, a tiny brownish bird that is very challenging to find.

The Bicknell's is a habitat specialist. It breeds only in alpine climates at 3,600 feet or more in elevation and only in Upstate New York, New England, Quebec and the Canadian Maritimes. Like many thrushes, it is a shy bird, often heard but not seen, preferring to feed on insects in dense stands of stunted Balsam Fir referred to as "krummholz".

The best way to find a Bicknell's Thrush is to listen for its singing, a raspy tangle of notes, or for its call, more or less a cough. They sing only from late May through mid-June.

As we twisted and turned our way up the narrow, but thankfully paved road, we marveled at the scenery on New England's tallest mountain - known for having some of the worst weather in the world. Fortunately for us, the winds weren't too bad. When we reached 5,000 feet and exited the van, it didn't take too long before we detected the first faint calls of the Bicknell's Thrush.

Due to the constant pounding of the elements, trees at this altitude only come up to one's waist, even though they may be a hundred years old. The wind also made it difficult to get a fix on the birds. Was the Bicknell's 25 yards to the left, to the right, or straight ahead? Ethan thought he saw one fly across a ledge and drop back into the krummholz. But, under these conditions, he couldn't be sure.

After an hour of futile searching, we moved about 400 yards down the mountain where the wind wasn't as strong. Here we could hear a Bicknell's quite well through the trees.

Just as we began to walk to our van and return to the base of the mountain, one obliging Bicknell's Thrush popped up to the top of the trees and put on a concert for us!

This bird would spend the summer nesting and raising its young in the krummholz before heading south in the fall to winter in the Dominican Republic.

Back on May 9th as we were finishing up our second trip to Florida, a photo of a Willow Ptarmigan on Cliff Island was circulating through the Maine birding community.

A Willow Ptarmigan is a rotund hen-like bird that lives year-round on the Arctic

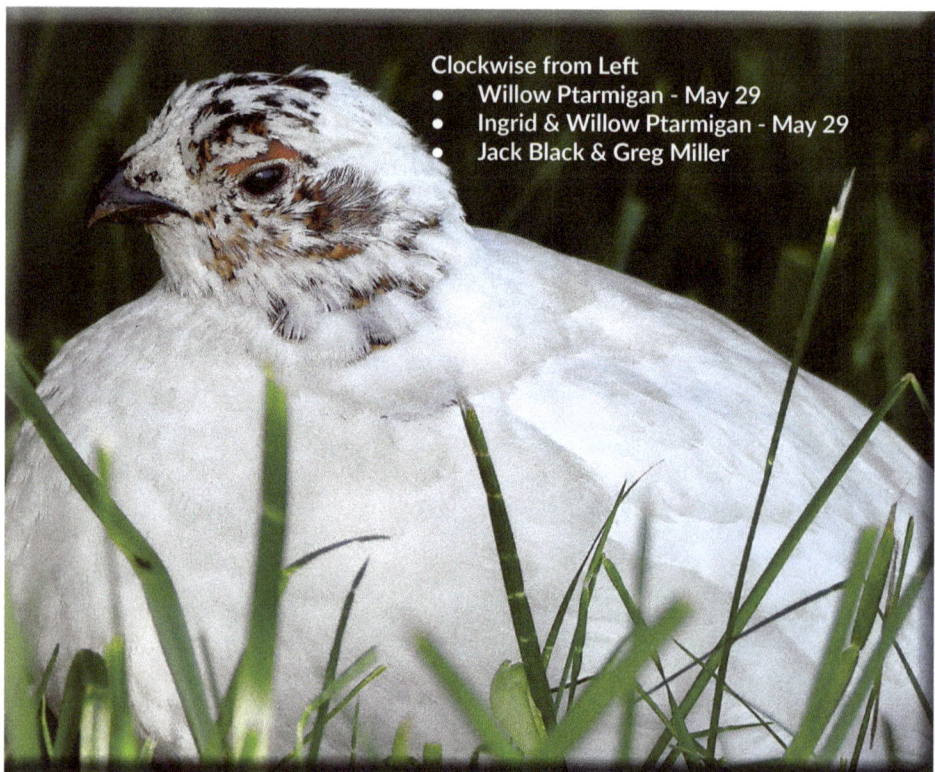

Clockwise from Left
- Willow Ptarmigan - May 29
- Ingrid & Willow Ptarmigan - May 29
- Jack Black & Greg Miller

tundra. While many of the birds that migrate through the US also nest in the Arctic, they generally return to warmer climates in the fall. The Willow Ptarmigan is ideally suited to brutal cold and snow, turning all white in the winter and reddish brown in the warmer months. They have heavily feathered feet that allow them to walk on top of deep snow and to excavate burrows for shelter. Due to their remote habitat, they have little fear of humans, often appearing tame and approachable.

The Willow Ptarmigan on Cliff Island spurred numerous birders to ferry to the Casco Bay island hoping to relocate the bird. By the time our flight got us back into Portland, most had given up; the bird was nowhere to be found.

A couple of weeks later, we received a heads-up from a birding friend that another Willow Ptarmigan, likely the same one, had been seen on a rural road in Waldoboro, Maine. This was about thirty miles from Cliff Island, which seemed a long way for a bird that spends most of its time foraging on the ground. But after a bit of research we found that Ptarmigans often migrate over water, with numerous reports of flocks landing on oil platforms and ships at sea. We searched the Waldoboro area where the bird had been reported but dipped.

Then on May 28, the bird was videoed sitting on the hood of a car at Small Point, a rustic private waterfront community a half hour south of our home.

With narrow dirt roads, home lots carved out of thick forest, limited parking and residents who guard their privacy, Small Point is absolutely the worst place for a rare bird to hang out ... at least from the perspective of birders who want to see it.

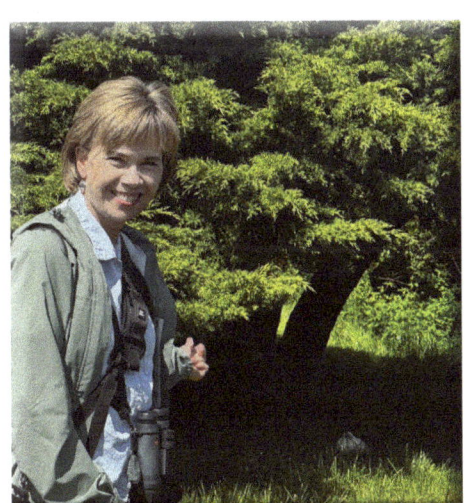

Doug Hitchcox, staff naturalist for Maine Audubon, was up for the challenge. He arranged with the homeowner for limited visitation, sent out a few initial invitations and created a private GroupMe discussion site for birders to coordinate their visits.

By the time it was our turn to visit Small Point, the bird had disappeared. We rode in with our friends Glenn Hodgkins and Anna Hodgkins and the four of us searched the area for over an hour but came up empty. While searching, we met legendary birder Greg Miller who was also looking for the Ptarmigan. In the movie "The Big Year", actor Jack Black's character was loosely based upon Miller and his 1998 Big Year.

As our allotted search time expired, we left Small Point figuring the Willow Ptarmigan had moved on. However, about ten minutes after arriving home, the GroupMe beeped...the Ptarmigan had returned to the homeowner's yard. Back into the car and back to Small Point we rushed and sure enough, this adorable white bowling ball with legs was resting under a shrubbery before emerging to forage on the grass.

The Ptarmigan had no fear of the paparazzi that had arrived, and we were able to observe the summer red and brown feathers beginning to replace the white, especially on the bird's head. After twenty minutes, we left to give others use of the parking space and lawn.

The next morning, another set of invitees arrived on Small Point only to learn that the Willow Ptarmigan had been killed during the night, probably by a Great Horned Owl, a predator that is known for decapitating its victims and only eating the head. Sadly, that is how the Ptarmigan was found.

So many birds look alike and identifying them can be challenging, even for birders who have been in the field for decades. Our friend the Bicknell's Thrush and its cousin, the Gray-Cheeked Thrush, are the proverbial twins separated at birth, virtually identical. They were considered a single species until 1995.

The best way to tell the species apart is by song (they sound different); by habitat (Gray-cheeks like forest floors); or by measurement (if you can catch one and measure the tail length and wing chord).

A couple days after Mt. Washington, we began a journey south to Cape Hatteras, North Carolina for a pelagic trip. On the way we had birds to find, of course.

One was a Gray-cheeked Thrush that had been reported at Mount Auburn Cemetery in Cambridge, Massachusetts. Gray-cheeked Thrushes nest in the Arctic regions and Alaska. Finding one that has paused its migration long enough to chase is a great opportunity.

When we arrived at the cemetery, it was raining pretty hard, but we hoped that the rain might keep our bird in place at its preferred location under a hedge of yews. We don't know this enormous cemetery well, and it took us quite a bit of time and a good deal of sleuthing to find the correct location.

Eventually the rain stopped, we found the yew and began to search. After 45 minutes, just when we were about to give up, the Gray-cheeked Thrush flew right between us and disappeared.

Fortunately, it began softly calling, and Ingrid found it foraging in leaves under an enormous bush. Ethan couldn't seem to get his binoculars on the bird, so we began our daily Big Year exercise of trying to describe where a moving bird is located.

Eventually, we were both able to find the Thrush, confirmed that it looked just like the Bicknell's Thrush from two days earlier, and got photos and diagnostic recordings. Back in the car we went and continued south toward North Carolina.

First, however, we made a two night stop in Virginia to bird at The Great Dismal Swamp National Wildlife Refuge. The Swamp is 750 square miles in size, of which the US Government manages 167.

People of a certain age may remember the jelly slogan, "With a name like Smuckers it has to be good." Well, any place named 'The Great Dismal Swamp' must be marvelous. And it is.

As we walked the trails through the swamp, we saw only one other person. However, there were so many birds singing, it was hard to keep track.

The foliage was very thick, and we almost never saw a bird for more than a few fleeting seconds. Still, we picked up three first of the year birds - Hooded Warbler, Swainson's Warbler and Acadian Flycatcher.

We left the Swamp impressed by the grandeur of the place and its historical significance. Washington camped there during the Revolution. The canals that criss-cross the swamp were dug by slaves under terrible conditions, and the Swamp was home to hundreds, perhaps thousands, of runaway slaves up through the end of the Civil War.

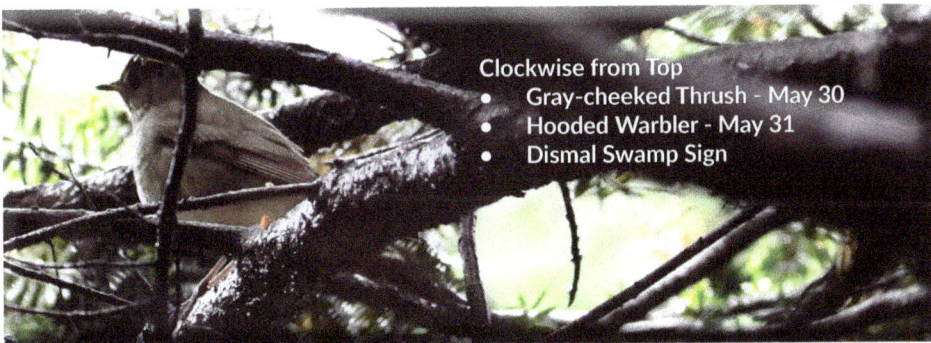

Clockwise from Top
- Gray-cheeked Thrush - May 30
- Hooded Warbler - May 31
- Dismal Swamp Sign

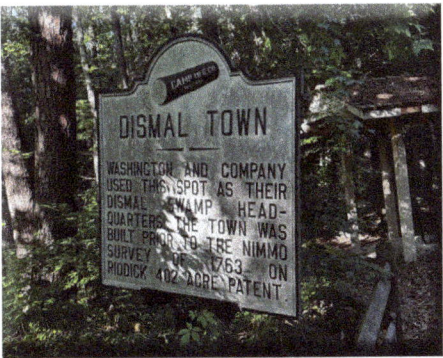
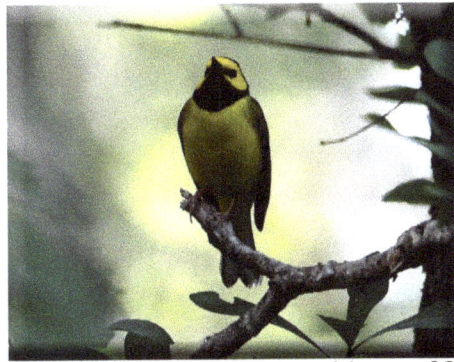

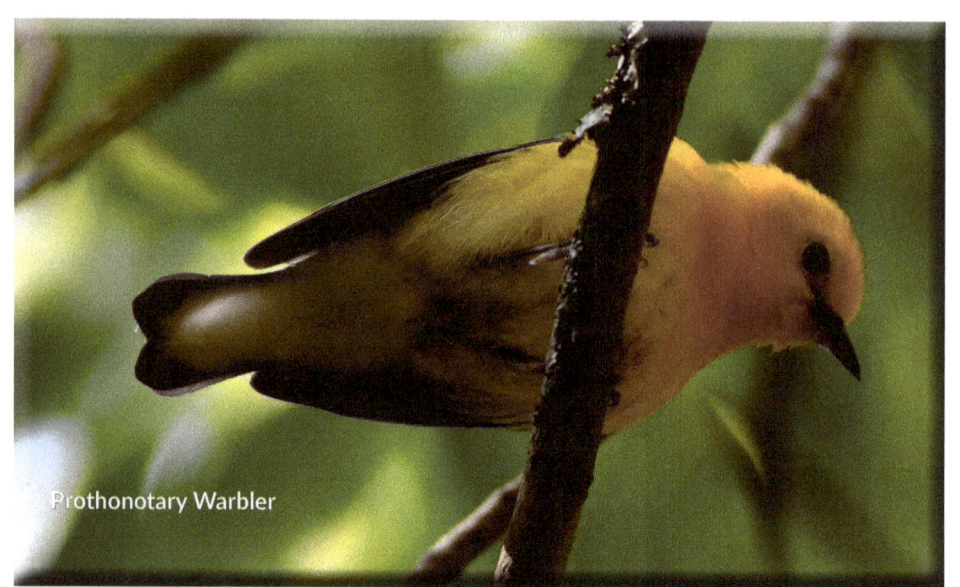

Prothonotary Warbler

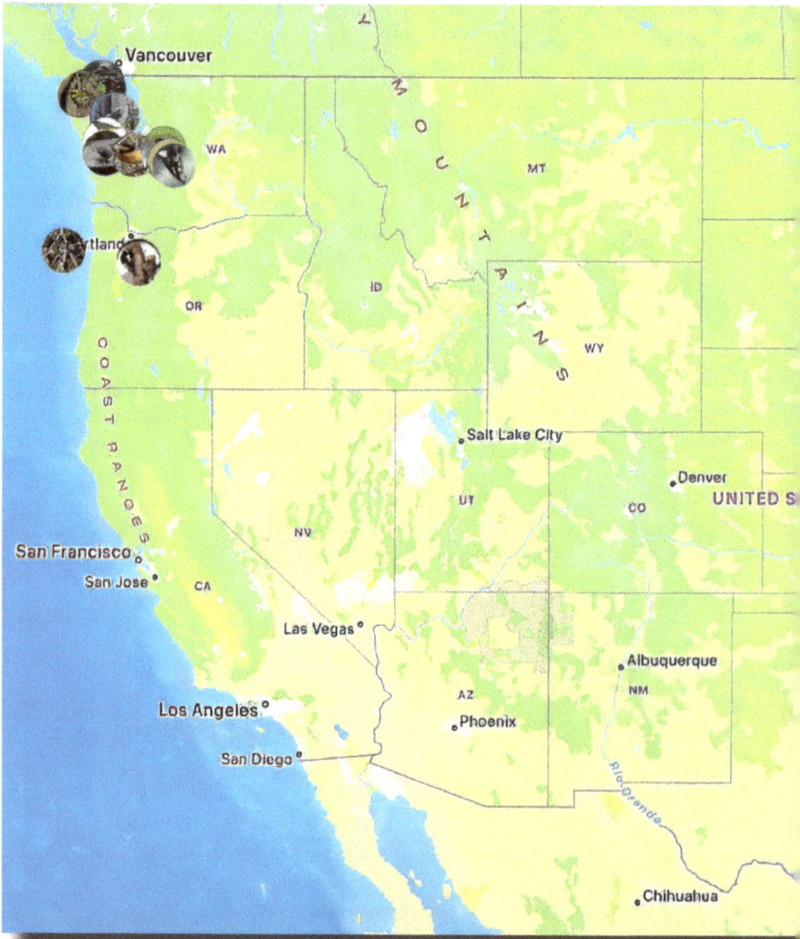

94 EVERY BIRD FROM SEA TO SHINING SEA

June

Travel	#
Plane Flights	4
Rental Cars	1
Nights Away	20
Boat Trips	3

State	Year Birds
Delaware	1
Maine	4
Michigan	3
North Carolina	10
Oregon	3
Virginia	2
Washington State	34
Total	57

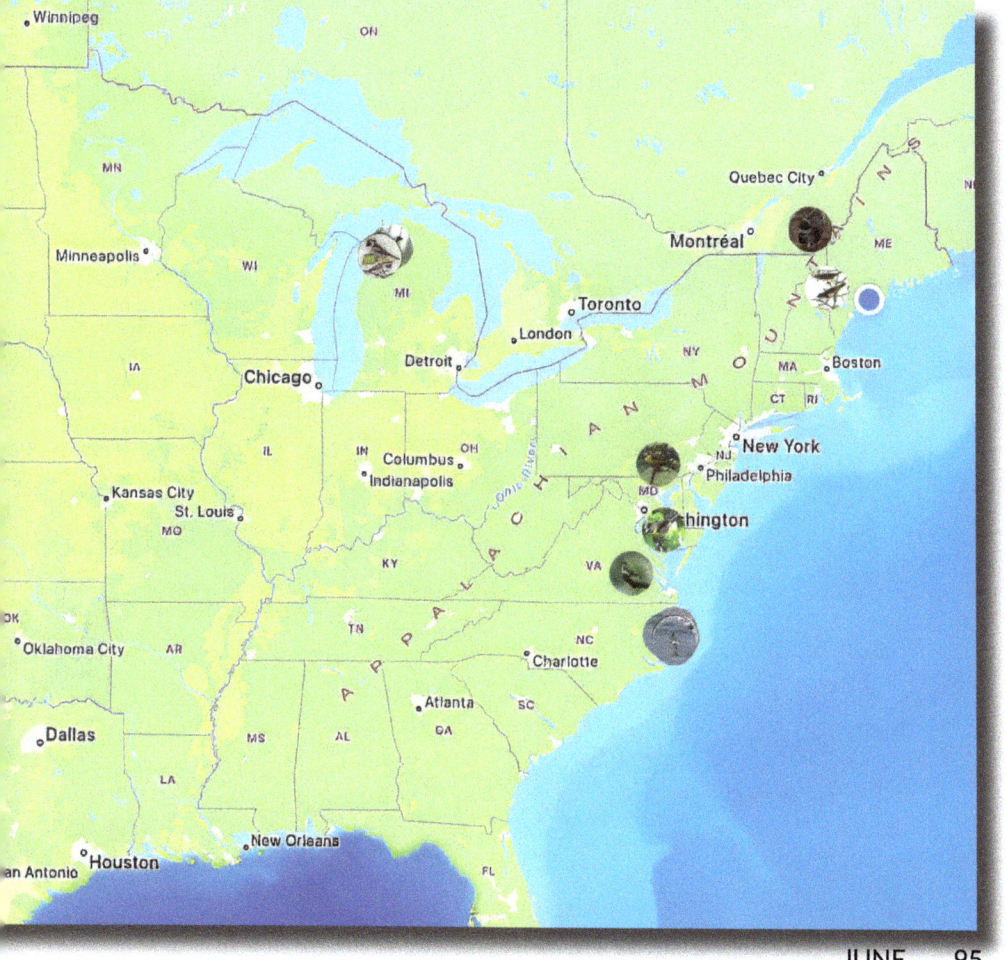

Hatteras Pelagic

"There is a life ring on the top deck. If someone falls overboard, tell me. Throw it, and we will go back and retrieve them." Was the captain joking about passengers falling overboard?!

These were the pre-trip instructions from Captain Brian Patterson as we stood on the deck of the Stormy Petrel II with 20 other birders in Hatteras, North Carolina. The sea was predicted to be choppy, and we were warned that we should expect to get wet on the ride out to the Gulf Stream.

Pelagic trips are key to a successful Big Year. There are dozens of seabird species that patrol the oceans of the world, only coming to land to nest and raise their young. The rest of the time they fly over or float upon the ocean.

As we began our eleven hour journey out into Pamlico Sound, the sunrise put on a stunning show. While we did not see many birds, nor did we expect to in our two hour motor out to the Gulf Stream, we didn't get bounced around too badly or get wet. That came later.

Shortly after reaching our target area, the crew, led by expert pelagic bird guide Kate Sutherland, began to chum the water. Chumming is the practice of luring seabirds with food that they love but that we would find revolting. A steady, slow drip

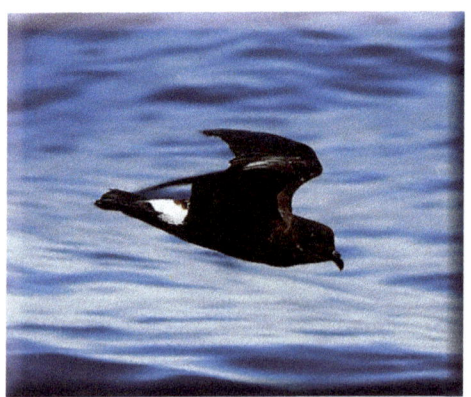
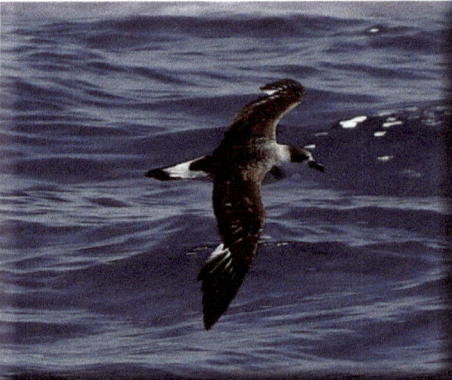
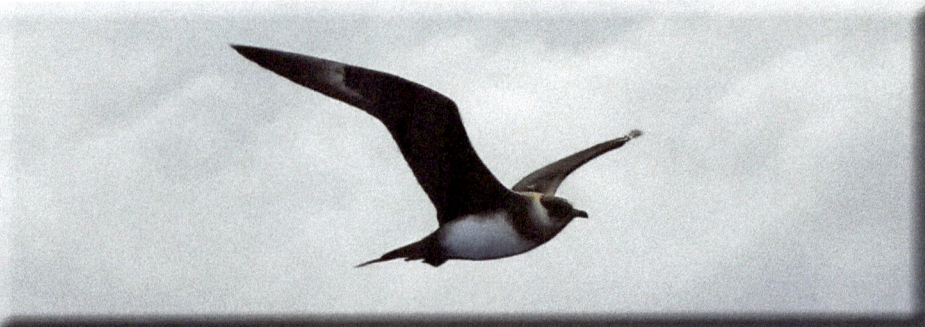

of menhaden oil and a block of frozen menhaden dragged behind the boat was the chum of choice. As it melts, the birds smell it and begin to circle the boat.

It wasn't long before we had our first sightings of Wilson's Storm-petrels and Audubon's Shearwaters. Gradually, interest built and more birds were coaxed - Band-rumped Storm-Petrels, Leach's Storm-Petrels and Black-capped Petrels among them. Over approximately 90 minutes we were treated to views of a wide variety of pelagic birds. Parasitic and Pomarine Jaegers stopped by. Cory's, Scapoli's and Great Shearwaters joined the mix. And then it stopped. As if the pause button was hit and never restarted.

Occasionally a bottle-nosed dolphin would swim close to the boat. Loads of flying fish were pretty entertaining, but the birds, other than the faithful Wilson's Storm-Petrels, disappeared. And, it was only 9:00 AM!

As we watched and waited, we enjoyed chatting with fellow birders, eating an early lunch and praying that the Bermuda Petrel that had made a brief appearance on yesterday's trip, would come flying by our boat. It did not.

Then came the return trip. During the three hour run in, we got more than a little bit wet. In fact, we were drenched! But we were determined to stay on deck in case any new birds should appear. We were rewarded with sightings of a Red-necked Phalarope and later a Sooty Shearwater sitting on the surf. In all, we got nine new birds for the year and one new lifer - the Band-rumped Storm-Petrel. Fortunately,

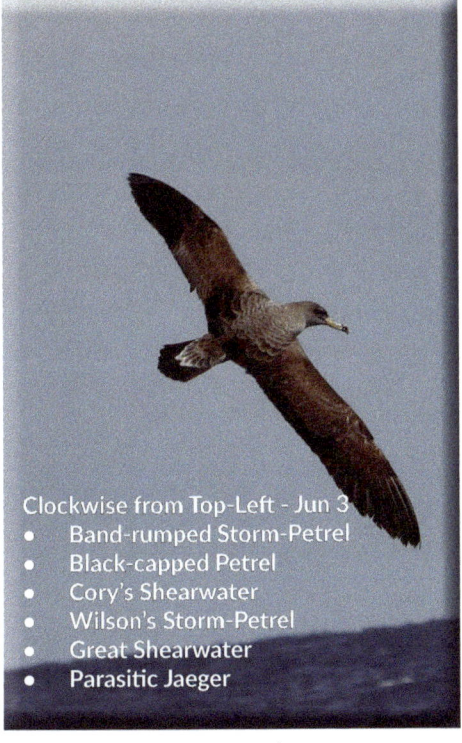
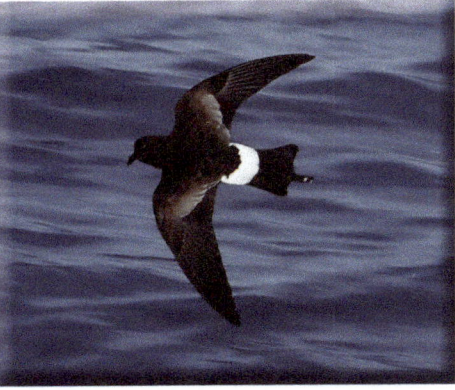
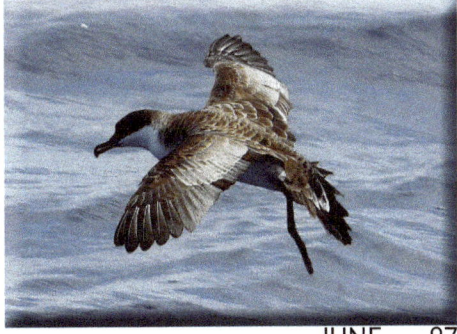

Clockwise from Top-Left - Jun 3
- Band-rumped Storm-Petrel
- Black-capped Petrel
- Cory's Shearwater
- Wilson's Storm-Petrel
- Great Shearwater
- Parasitic Jaeger

the life ring did not need to be deployed!

Over the next two days we made our way to Boston for a flight to Michigan. Along the way, we were happy to add two more birds to our year list - a Yellow-breasted Chat in Virginia and a Dickcissel in Delaware.

After arriving in Detroit early Thursday morning, we drove directly to a location where Golden-winged Warblers had been reported. This turned out to be a bit of a navigation nightmare as we searched for the "bushwhacked path leading to a boardwalk". After making a few wrong turns that led to soaking wet feet, we eventually found the boardwalk and a couple of singing males.

The next stop was the primary reason for this trip, the endangered Kirtland's Warbler. Nearly extinct 50 years ago, the Kirtland's Warbler has now recovered to about 2,000 breeding pairs. This habitat specialist only nests in northern Michigan and only in Jack Pine trees between 6 and 12 feet high, in a forest that has burned in the last 20 years. Fire is destructive for sure, but for some species of birds and mammals, it is life-sustaining. After a bit of hiking in light rain, we heard the song of a Kirtland's and found him moving among the Pines. We later found a second male. We enjoyed extensive views of this stunning life bird before the rain became heavy and chased us away.

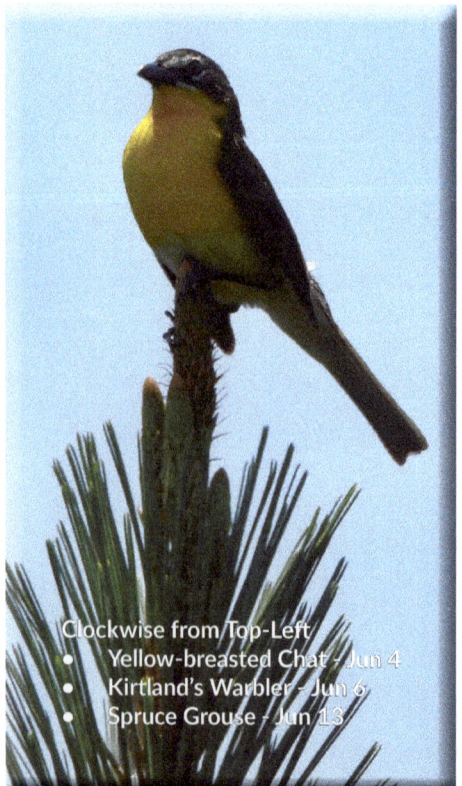

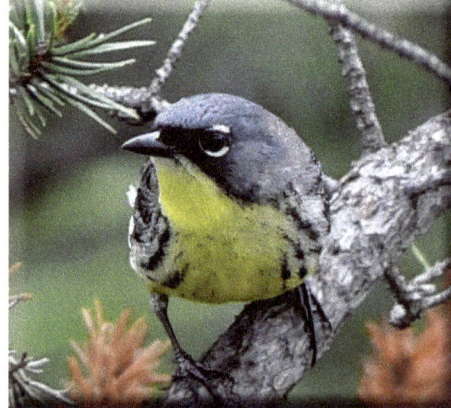

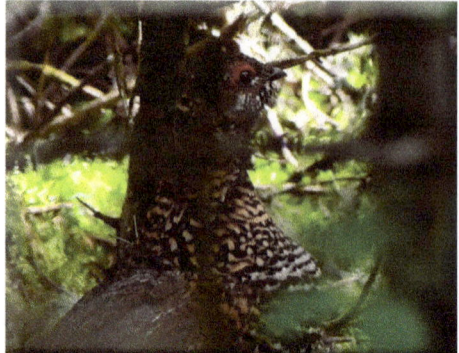

Clockwise from Top-Left
- Yellow-breasted Chat - Jun 4
- Kirtland's Warbler - Jun 6
- Spruce Grouse - Jun 13

Our next drive took us further north onto the Michigan Northern Peninsula to hunt for Spruce Grouse and Sharp-tailed Grouse. We failed miserably. But we did see Lake Huron, Lake Michigan and Lake Superior, and each of us was visited by at least 100 ticks climbing up our pant legs!

That evening we headed for Houghton Lake, about a half hour south of Grayling in hopes of finding a secretive bird that we had left off our Big Year plan when we drew it up last fall. The Yellow Rail is a tiny bird that rarely ever comes out in the daylight, instead hiding in thick, swampy, mosquito-infested reeds. Only after dusk will it sing sporadically, a faint song that sounds like two pebbles being tapped together. Unless you know what to listen for, you'd never notice the calling Yellow Rail, and they like it like that.

After dark, we were joined by a group of Mennonite birders from Indiana. Together we walked up and down the causeway hoping to hear the tapping song of the Yellow Rail and avoid getting hit by cars whizzing by a few feet away. Happily, our group all heard the Rails several times and got good recordings.

Spruce Grouse

Back home for a short stretch between birding in the Midwest and the Pacific Northwest we decided to chase a nemesis bird.

Every birder has a nemesis bird, a bird that eludes you regardless of how hard you try. For example, the bird that flew off just before you arrived or flew back in just after you got on the highway heading home.

Our nemesis bird was the Spruce Grouse, a relatively common bird in the enormous Boreal Forests of Canada and the northern edges of the continental USA. But it is a bird that seems to enjoy playing games with us. We had invested countless hours walking roads and trails in Northern Maine and Michigan looking for this annoying bird. All we ever got from our efforts is a few brief glimpses of the Grouse, and those were back in 2021.

Our friends in the Maine birding community are filled with advice:

"The Spruce Grouse is stupid and will walk right between your legs."

"Look at this photo of me posing with a Spruce Grouse."

"Oh, there's one hanging out by the parking lot. You can't miss it!"

On Thursday, we made another determined effort to conquer this nemesis, leaving the house at 4:00 AM headed for Boy Scout Road in Rangeley, Maine.

Rangeley is an ideal place to find Boreal birds because there the Canadian Spruce forest dips down into Maine and provides a southerly place to find Canada Jays,

Black-backed Woodpeckers, Olive-sided Flycatchers and Blackburnian Warblers.

At about 6:30 AM we turned our car onto rutted and muddy Boy Scout Road. After about a mile we saw two orange/brown blobs a couple hundred yards ahead in the road - a mother Spruce Grouse and a single chick. Our distant photos through the dirty windshield provided rather useless documentation for our Big Year, so we decided to get closer. After parking the car and approaching on foot, the birds scurried into the woods and disappeared. Curse you Spruce Grouse!!!

We spent the next hour exploring the Boy Scout Camp and identified forty-seven different species of birds, four white-tailed deer and a very confused turtle. As we walked down a quiet Spruce-lined trail with the forest floor covered with moss, Ingrid heard a cooing sound and then saw a handful of chicks running around a few feet away. The momma Spruce Grouse was calling to her young trying to get them away from the Big Year birders. Finally, after years of frustration we had good views of a Spruce Grouse, and Ethan got decent photos to boot. And we didn't see just one. We saw six!!

Pacific Northwest

Week 25 got off to a rather rocky start when the weather and travel gods conspired to thwart us once again. Little did we know when we arrived at Boston's Logan Airport on Thursday afternoon that we would be spending the night in nearby Medford and not Seattle. After three hours on the tarmac followed by another hour and a half back at the gate, that is exactly what happened. Our long night was followed by an earlier than usual return to the airport the next morning due to the crowds of celebrating fans descending upon the city for the Celtics' NBA championship Duck Boat parade.

Fast forward twelve hours and two more delayed flights, and we were finally in Seattle and on our way to Bainbridge Island. While most of our birding would need to wait until the next day, we did pick up a couple of first of the year birds from the ferry.

We reached Bainbridge as the sun was setting on our 10th anniversary. We had plans to celebrate in style, but our travel delays meant tacos at a pub just before closing. However, we remained cheerful - how many couples get to do a Big Year together? The next morning, we were happy to add a few more birds before leaving the island for Port Townsend in search of Puffins. Our finds included a life bird - the gorgeous Red-Breasted Sapsucker.

Upon arriving in Port Townsend, we found we had enough time for a little pre-Puffin birding - namely searching for West Coast Gulls. By the end of the day we had found and identified: Western Gull, Glaucous-winged Gull, California Gull, and a new life bird, the Heerman's Gull! We found dozens of Heermann's resting among hundreds of Glaucous-winged Gulls at the water's edge. The Heermann's Gull is one of the prettiest gulls with its soft gray and muted brown plumage set off by its white head and bright red bill.

While we love the adorable Atlantic Puffins we see in Maine, they aren't the only Puffins in the sea. A pelagic cruise to Puget Sound's Smith Island got us terrific views of their West Coast cousin, the Tufted Puffin - so named for the tufts on either side of its head. Other incredible birds feeding with the Puffins in the Kelp beds were Rhinoceros Auklets, who passed our high speed catamaran going 35 miles an hour on the way out, as well as Common Murres and Marbled Murrelets.

The next morning, in typical Pacific Northwest weather, we headed out to Olympic National Park and added a few more birds to our year list when the rain conveniently stopped upon our arrival: Sooty Grouse, Townsend's Warbler and Pacific Wren.

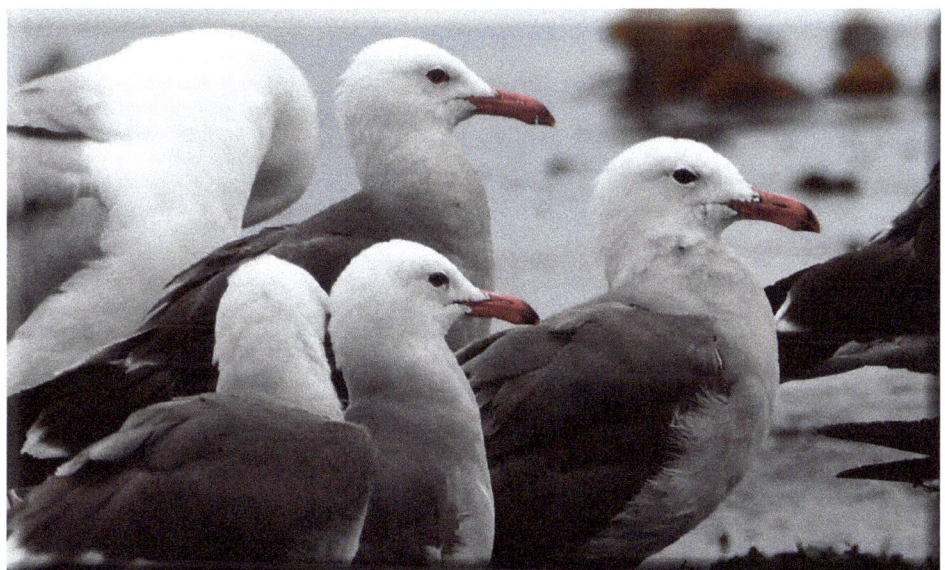

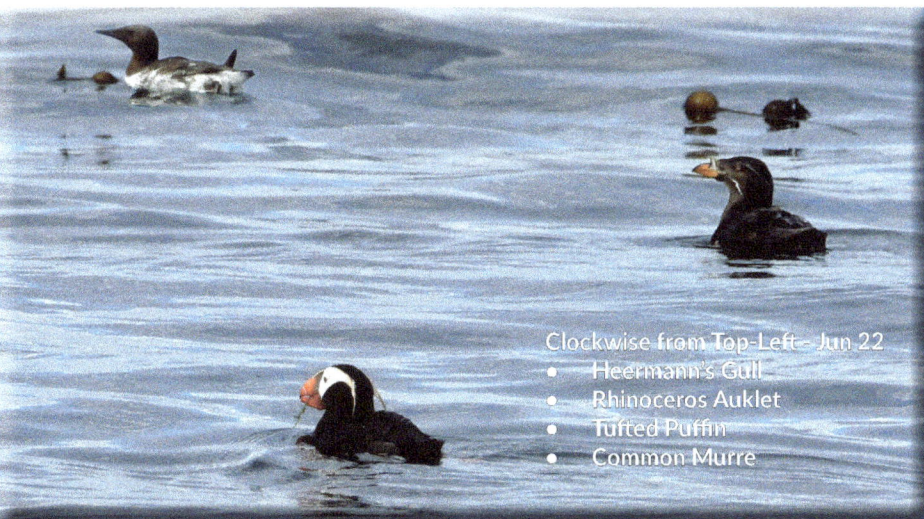

Clockwise from Top-Left - Jun 22
- Heermann's Gull
- Rhinoceros Auklet
- Tufted Puffin
- Common Murre

Dipper Day

It was another misty morning on the coast of Washington State when we pointed our car toward Olympia and began our quest to find an American Dipper. The American Dipper is unique among North American songbirds as it will dive underwater in search of its prey.

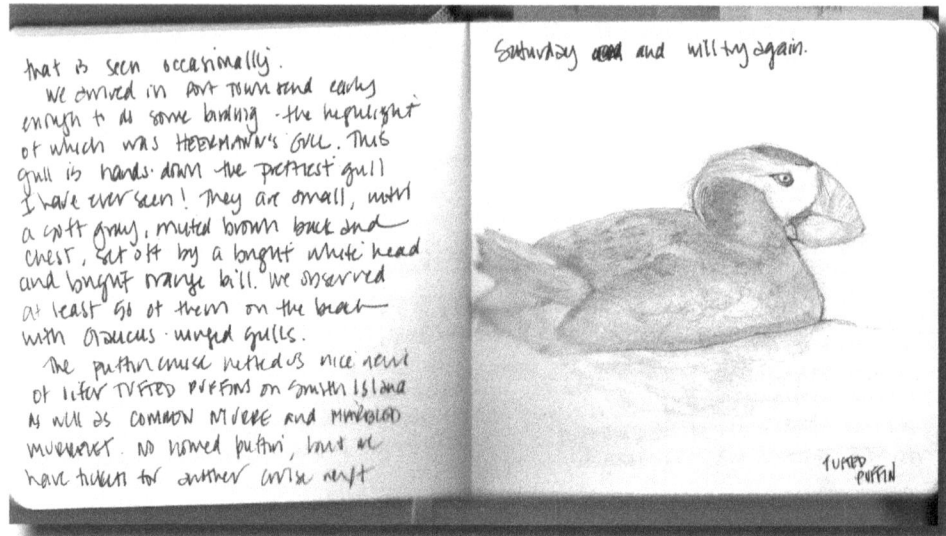

Not only would a Dipper give us another bird for the year, it would also be a life bird for us. We had searched for Dippers in Colorado in April to no avail and previously on a trip to the Northwest two years ago. Today would be Dipper Day!

We had learned of a nest at a fish hatchery and decided to start by checking the river across the road. While it looked to be a perfect habitat, with rapidly moving water, large rocks and ledges, we saw no sign of our bird.

Next, we tried the hatchery. The supervisor told us about a path to the river further along the road. Following his instructions, we made our way down to the river and did a thorough search of the cavities under the banks, waterfalls and downed trees hoping to find a nest. No luck. Our agreed upon deadline was fast approaching, and we feared that this was not going to be Dipper Day after all.

No sooner had this discouraging thought entered our minds when a gray bird zipped past Ingrid heading toward where Ethan was searching. "Dipper! There's a Dipper!" For the next several minutes, we watched this fascinating little bird wade, dive and feed on the river's edge.

After high-fives and hugs, we drove to a national wildlife refuge near Olympia, Washington where we added a MacGillivray's Warbler and a Cassin's Vireo to both our year and life lists.

On a trip to Seattle two years ago, we visited Mount Rainier National Park and came upon a flock of Varied Thrush in the Longmire area. Since the thrushes had been

600th Bird of the Year

American Dipper

June 24, 9:46 AM

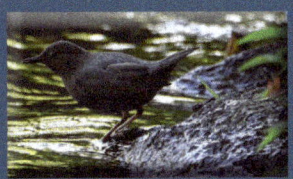

reported there recently, we decided this would be our next stop.

We were thrilled to return to this park. With its lush forest, beautiful trails, waterfalls, and well-managed facilities, it is chock full of stunning vistas, the highlight of which is majestic snow-covered Mount Rainier towering over it all.

As we reached the 5 mile mark outside of the national park, we noticed a sign stating that we needed to have a timed entry reservation to enter. Oh no, we were not aware of this! As you might imagine, a decent cell signal in this remote area was a hard thing to come by. Ethan frantically tried to make a reservation for our expected entry time, but the cell gods would not cooperate. What to do?

When we got to the gate, Ethan played a confused elderly gentleman baffled by the Internet and technology. The gate attendant took pity on him as he babbled about not understanding the website and how he didn't know how to use his phone, and let us pass.

About five miles later we arrived at Longmire and found zero Varied Thrushes in the parking area where we had found them before. We did spot a promising looking trail across the road, and lo and behold found exactly one Varied Thrush hopping along the moss-covered ground several feet off the trail.

After we left Mount Rainier and reached the eastern side of the Cascades, we were shocked at the change in landscape. Gone were the thick, lush green forests of Douglas Fir. Instead, we saw an arid, desert-like setting. We had no idea that there was such a stark contrast here!

As we reached Yakima, Washington, we stopped at a wildlife management area where Bullock's Oriole and Lewis' Woodpeckers had been reported, both in relatively high numbers. All we needed was one of each. Thanks to the generosity of the manager, who allowed us to walk into his yard to get a closer look, we found no fewer than four Bullock's Oriole and twelve Lewis's Woodpeckers, a bird Ethan notes looks dressed for Christmas. The Lewis's was a lifer for us!

The next morning, California Quail and California Scrub-Jay topped our list of most-wanted birds. After striking out at a local cemetery, we found a beautiful canyon trail where we heard the calls of three shy California Quail and saw one Califor-

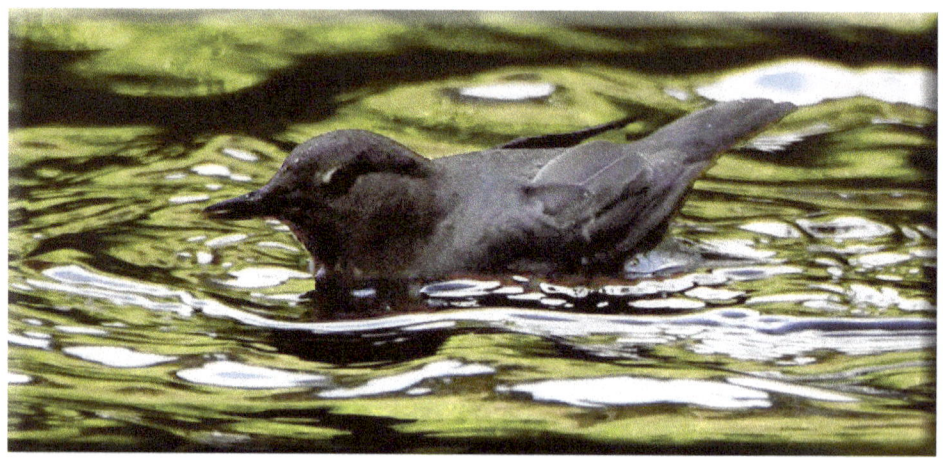

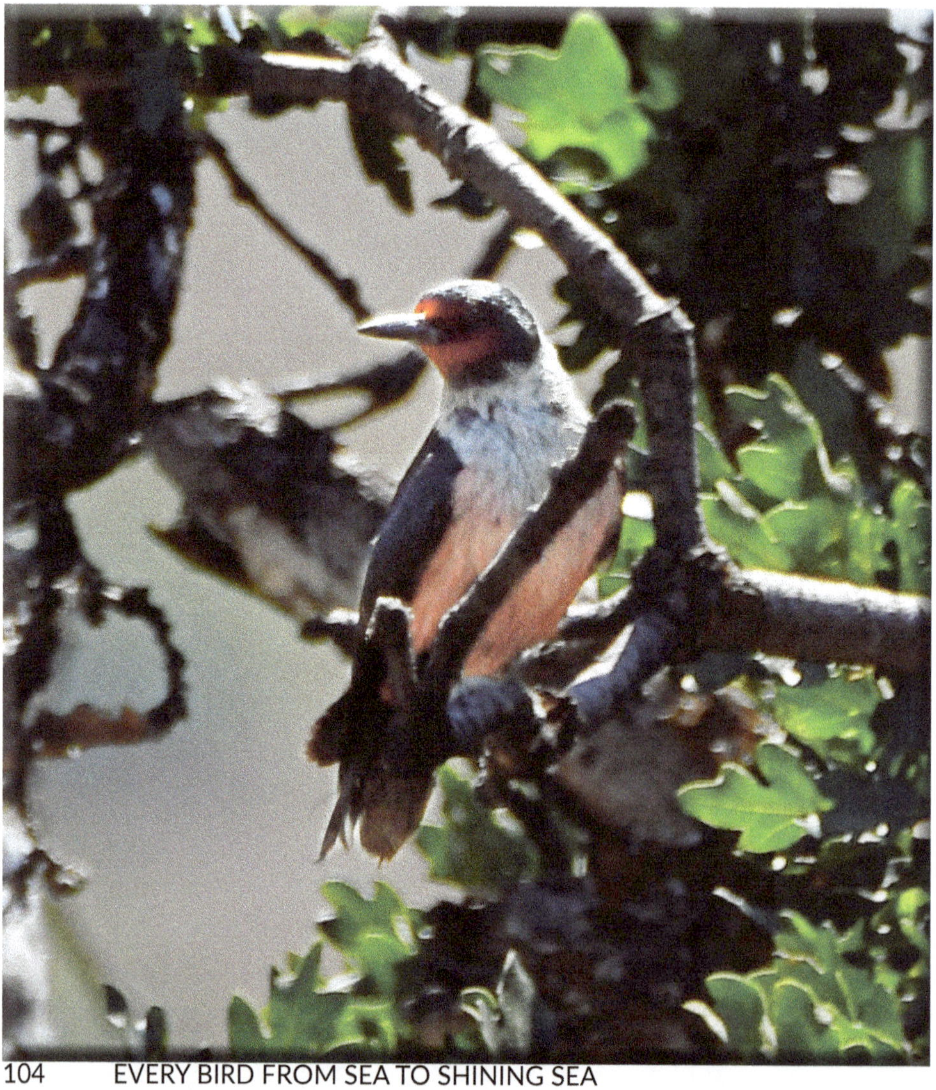

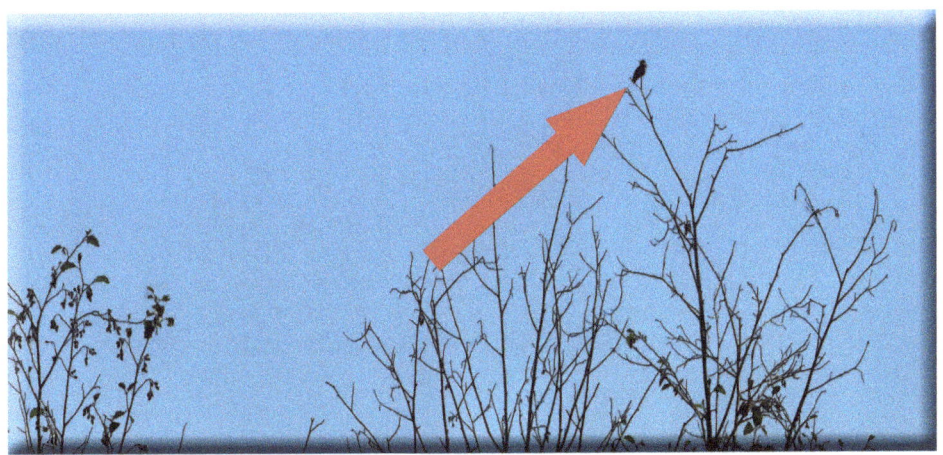

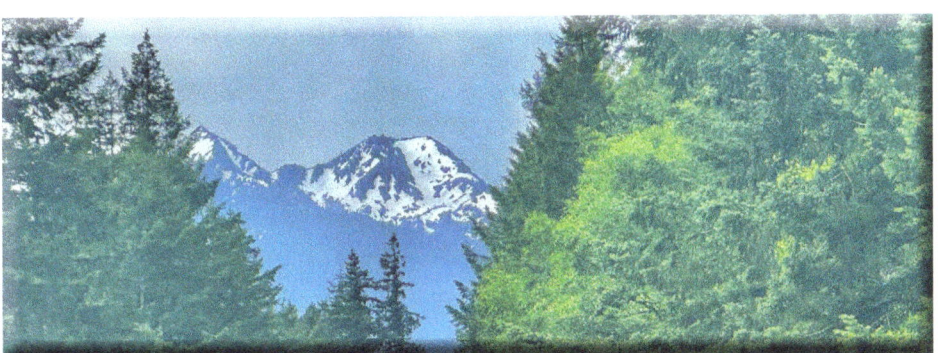

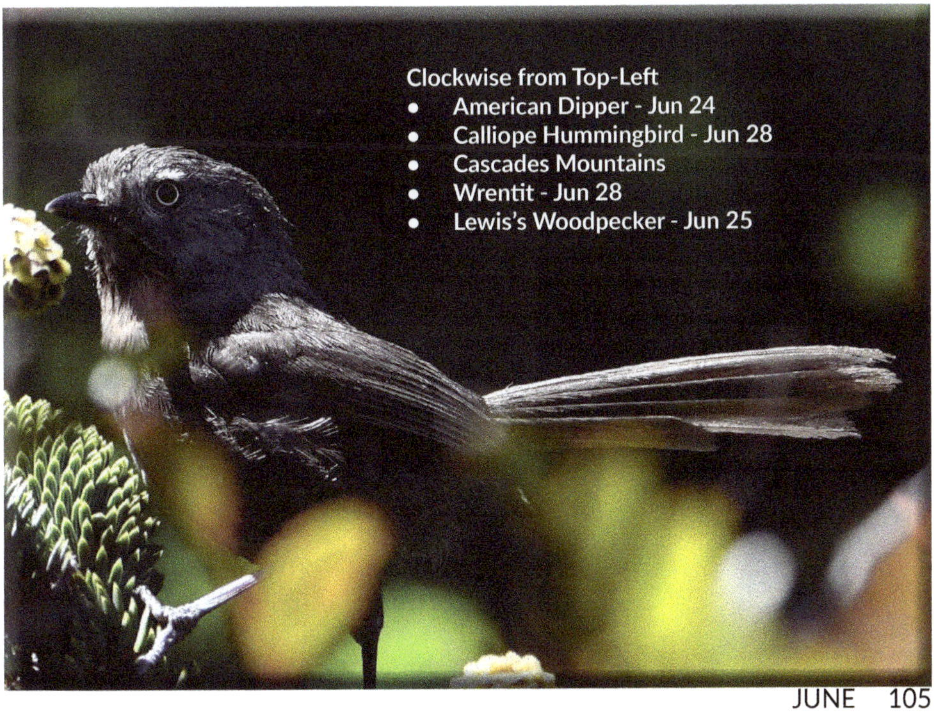

Clockwise from Top-Left
- American Dipper - Jun 24
- Calliope Hummingbird - Jun 28
- Cascades Mountains
- Wrentit - Jun 28
- Lewis's Woodpecker - Jun 25

nia Scrub-Jay. Our day was off to a great start!

After a further drive southeast, we reached a riparian area. A riparian area is a zone of land that occurs along the edges of rivers, streams, lakes or other bodies of water. Here we spent two hours walking a lovely gravel road with only each other, occasional cattle, and a diversity of birds to keep us company.

Through much of our time in Washington and Oregon we were the only birders, often the only people, on a trail. This is very different from what we experience at home. Over the course of our two hour hike, we added Red-naped Sapsucker, Dusky Flycatcher and, incredibly, a Flammulated Owl that called twice as we walked past. Thank you, owl, for sparing us a late night trip in search of you!

The next morning it was time to move on to Oregon, in search of a Wrentit. But that was not the only bird we hoped to see in the 34th state of our Big Year. On our route we stopped at the Deschutes National Forest Aspen Restoration Project in search of Williamson's Sapsucker and White-headed Woodpecker. This was the perfect place to find them among the Aspens and Ponderosa Pines they favor. And after a good bit of searching, find them we did! Not to mention the boisterous flock of Pinyon Jays that found us!

After a night in the charming western town of Prineville, where we really felt like we were on the Oregon Trail, we headed west through the Cascades once again. Our destination was the coastal city of Newport, Oregon. Before making that pass however, we decided to try once more for the Calliope Hummingbird we dipped on the previous day. Armed with better information about how to access Black Butte Swamp, we were determined to find this smallest of all North American birds before leaving one of its prime areas.

With the assistance of Google satellite maps and our knowledge of the bird's preferred habitat and its behavior, we eventually found a location that looked promising. Happening upon a bushwhacked trail, likely made by other Calliope seekers, we climbed over downed trees and through swamp grass to a place where we had a fairly open view.

Prepared to wait an hour or more for one to appear, we started scanning. Luckily our eyes quickly landed on a hummingbird perched at the top of a young Aspen tree. We were able to get our binoculars and cameras on it before it soon flew off. It was indeed a Calliope Hummingbird!

The small, noisy Wrentit lives only on the Pacific coast, where it can be found most often in chaparral - an area of shrubs and bushes. We had learned of a state park in Newport where they could be reliably found. But by the end of the trail they favored, we had not heard one. Maybe it was the time of day, or maybe not quite the right place.

As we turned around to retrace our steps, we noticed a sandy path leading into a very promising looking habitat. We had not gone far when one and then a second

A Bird By Any Other Name

The American Ornithological Society (AOS) is responsible for standardizing English bird names in North and South America. The AOS's North American Classification Committee (NACC) is responsible for:

- Arbitrating the official names of birds in North America
- Developing and maintaining English names for new or recently split species
- Considering proposals to change established names

As a result, each year bird names change for various reasons. Here are the changes that occurred during our Big Year:

Splits (A species was split into multiple species):
- Audubon's Shearwater changed to Sargasso Shearwater
- Barn Owl changed to American Barn Owl
- Brown Booby split adding Cocos Booby
- Cory's Shearwater split adding Scopoli's Shearwater
- Herring Gull changed to American Herring Gull
- House Wren changed to Northern House Wren

Hyphens removed or Added
- Black-crowned Night-Heron changed to Black-crowned Night Heron
- Blue-throated mountaingem changed to Blue-throated Mountain-gem
- Common Ground-Dove changed to Common Ground Dove
- Western Cattle Egret changed to Western Cattle-Egret
- Yellow-crowned Night-Heron changed to Yellow-crowned Night Heron

Parrots changed to Amazons
- Lilac-crowned Parrot changed to Lilac-crowned Amazon
- Orange-winged Parrot changed to Orange-winged Amazon
- Red-crowned Parrot changed to Red-crowned Amazon
- Red-lored Parrot changed to Red-lored Amazon
- White-fronted Parrot changed to White-fronted Amazon
- Yellow-headed Parrot changed to Yellow-headed Amazon

Lumps (Multiple Species merged into single species):
- Common Redpoll and Hoary Redpoll merged to Redpoll

popped up to the top of a bush, singing and calling loudly to match their reputation. We determined that we may have happened upon their nesting area, so we quickly took photos and said our goodbyes.

As the sun set on the second to last day of our trip and we enjoyed dinner at a local seafood restaurant in Newport, we celebrated the great success we had had on our Northwest journey. We had added no fewer than 37 birds to our year list and were thrilled. We looked forward to a meandering journey back to Seattle and our flight home. We would catch our breath and relax a bit on our last day. Not so fast!!

Back at our hotel room, we read an eBird report of sightings of a Horned Puffin at

Smith Island, where we had been searching for Puffins at the beginning of our trip. This bird had not been seen in days. We had tickets for a trip out the following evening, but had decided not to use them as the drive there and then back to the airport hotel we had booked for the night would be many hours long. But how could we leave without trying again?

To make the long journey north more palatable, we visited Columbia Ridge Winery in Vancouver, Washington for a rest and refreshment stop. We thoroughly enjoyed tasting this small vineyard's delicious wines while overlooking the vines on a rare dry, sunny day in the Columbia River Valley. Ethan made quick friends with the vineyard cat, aptly named Syrah!

We arrived in Port Townsend in a steady rain, not exactly the best weather for a boat trip. But the seas were calm, and pelagic birds do not pay rain much mind. At 7:30 PM, we set off in heavy drizzle toward Smith Island. Once near the island we began scouring the waters for our bird among flocks of Rhinoceros Auklets, Pigeon Guillemots, Common Murres and an assortment of gulls.

We spotted several Tufted Puffins, but no Horned Puffin. The time was getting late, the light quickly faded, and the drizzle morphed to a steady rain. And then a miracle happened!

As a large group of cormorants and gulls took flight from the tiny spit of land connecting Smith and Minor Islands, we kept our eyes on the water and saw a Puffin, with all of the markings of a Horned Puffin, dive under the water collecting fish in its bill! Ethan quickly captured photos that later confirmed what we saw, despite the low quality that could be achieved at dusk in the rain.

This very tired, but very happy birding couple returned to Seattle at midnight with bird 614 notched on their belts!!

The Patagonia Picnic Table Effect

In April, we stopped to visit the famous Patagonia Picnic Table on Route 82 in Arizona. The Patagonia Picnic Table Effect is a phenomenon associated with birding, when a rare bird is discovered at a particular location, soon other rare birds will be found nearby. The name is associated with this rest stop and picnic table where the phenomenon was first noted.

When we visited, there were no birds anywhere near this decrepit, broken down table ... such a disappointment.

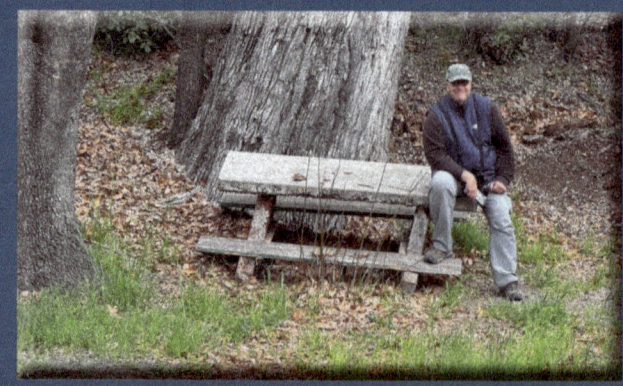

Weekly Recap

Our 2024 Big Year was a once in a lifetime adventure, so we decided to document it each week with a YouTube Video. Ranging from 2 minutes to 18 minutes each, the recaps required a lot of effort, particularly when produced in a hotel room after long days of birding.

But, we are very glad we made the effort as friends, family, armchair travelers and other birders all over the world got to travel along with us, at least vicariously.

On numerous occasions we had total strangers walk up to us and introduce themselves: "I've been watching your videos and …"

QR Code for our Recap YouTube Videos:

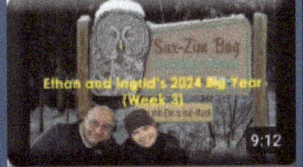
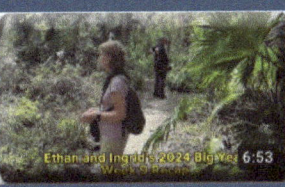
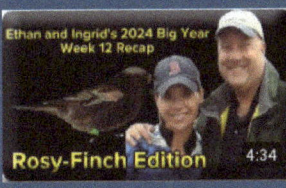

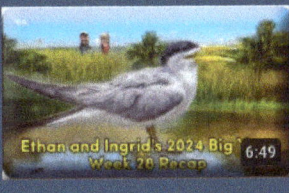
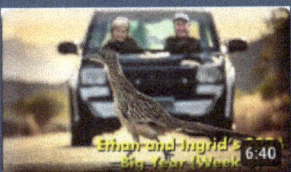
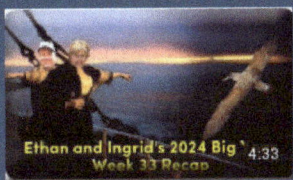
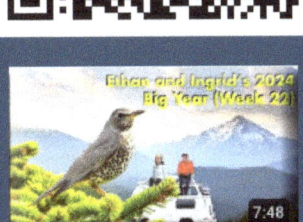

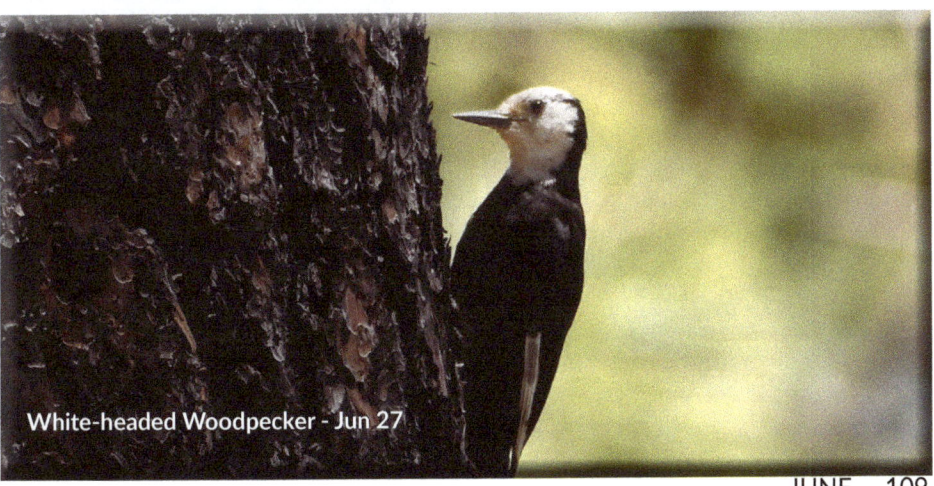
White-headed Woodpecker - Jun 27

JUNE 109

July

Travel	#
Plane Flights	4
Rental Cars	1
Nights Away	4
Boat Trips	2

State	Year Birds
Florida	4
Maine	4
Total	8

Florida Again

In the summer of 2023, a Large-billed Tern was seen in eastern Florida. A resident of inland freshwater ponds and lakes of South America, sightings of this bird in the United States are exceedingly rare (three times ever), making it a Code 5 Bird.

With our 2024 Big Year approaching, we resisted chasing the bird in 2023 and, naturally, the bird disappeared in December. Fortunately, the same bird rematerialized months later, around a group of freshwater ponds in Naples, Florida. It would appear and disappear for days at a time.

Also appearing in Florida were three other birds we did not have on our list. So, after a bit of consideration, we booked our flights and made a game plan for finding them.

As we stepped from the Fort Myers airport into a hot, humid mid-summer Florida, light rain was falling, and we feared our planned afternoon birding might be in jeopardy.

Fortunately, as we approached Naples to search for the tern, the rain stopped. And in a further "TERN" of good luck, the Large-Billed Tern was exactly where it was reported to hang out, and we saw it immediately upon pulling in the parking lot! This was our easiest Code 5 pick up ever, and one of those birds that makes up for the seemingly endless stakeouts for others!

The next bird up was the Rose-ringed Parakeet. The most widespread Parakeet in the world, the Rose-ringed is found across Africa, India, and Southern Asia. And, populations of escaped birds are established in California and Florida. A handful of these have found the Naples Zoo to be a favorable habitat.

The 'feels like' air temperature when we stepped out of our car at the zoo was a whopping 109 degrees, which may work for our friends in Florida or Texas but is simply inhumane for Mainers. We can handle snow, ice, cold and mosquitoes the size of Large-billed Terns, but this kind of weather is brutal. It was so hot, in fact, that a zoo visitor collapsed and had to be rushed away in an ambulance!

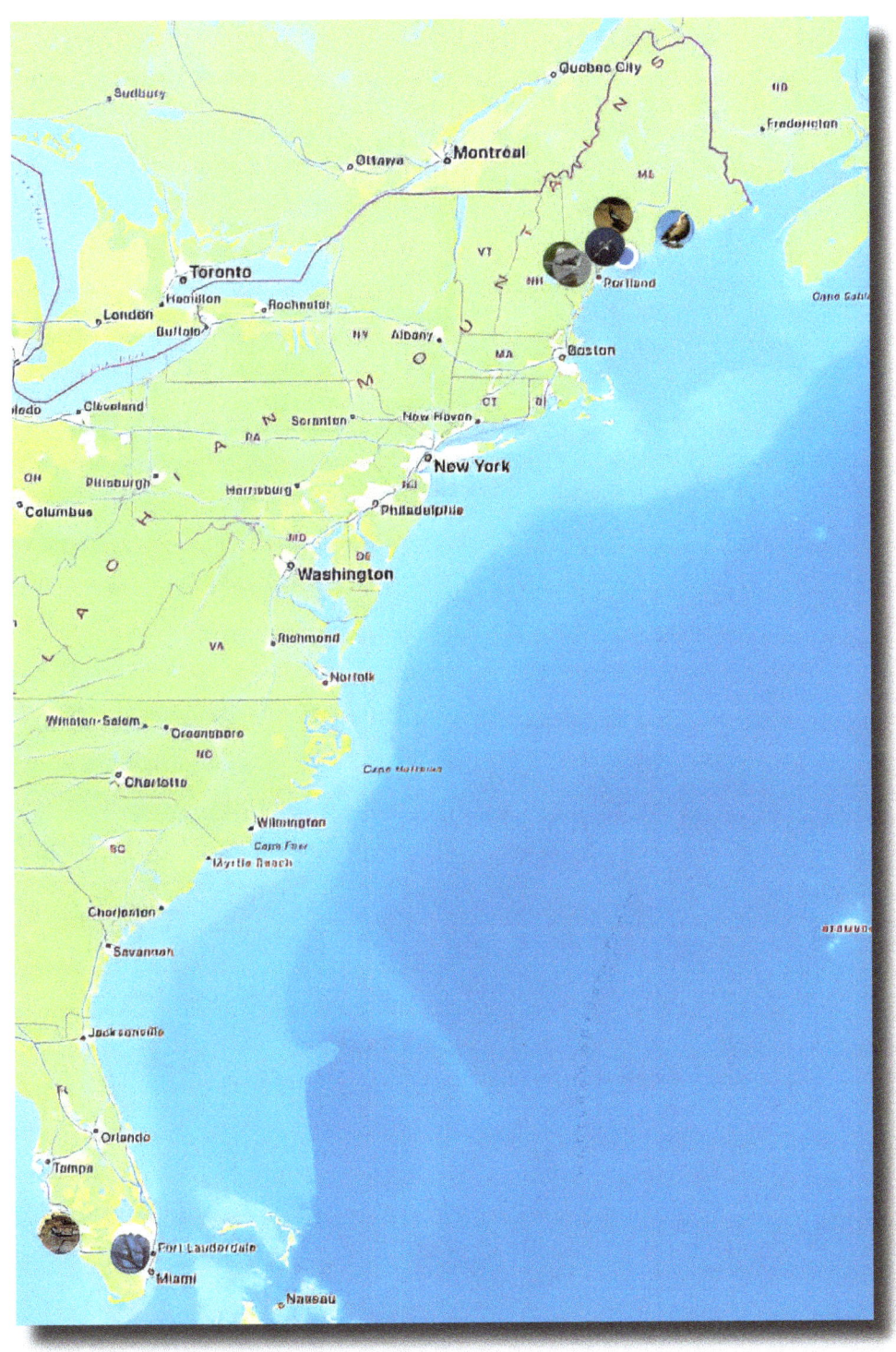

After about an hour of searching, we were wilting and with an afternoon thunderstorm rumbling in the distance we realized we only had a little time left to find the bird. Then, not far from the 'Honey-Badger Compound', we heard the characteristic high-pitched squeal of the Rose-ringed Parakeet as two flew from tree to tree in the dense canopy lining our path. We got quick views as they darted past us and then again a few minutes later. We ended the day with two new birds for the year and two ticks for our life lists!

Up and out early on Thursday morning, we made our way across the state to Miami on "Alligator Alley", the second coolest road name in America ... trailing "I Dream of Jeannie Way" in Cocoa Beach, Florida.

Our first stop was Bill Baggs Cape Florida State Park, where a Yellow-Green Vireo had been reported over the previous couple of weeks. Native to the Yucatan and Central America, this out of range bird had been frequenting a stand of dense foliage along a bike path in the park.

Armed with what we thought were excellent directions to the bird, we quickly learned what others before us had noted - the spot is not easy to locate. Eventually, we did find the bird. He was much easier to hear than see, as his yellow-green plumage camouflaged him well in the thick foliage.

Next we were off to Oleta River State Park where we dipped on the Yellow-headed Caracara in February. A Yellow-headed Caracara is an opportunistic scavenger who

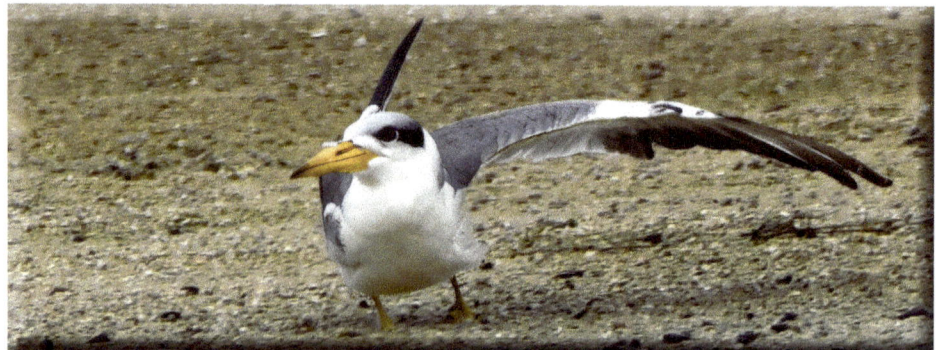

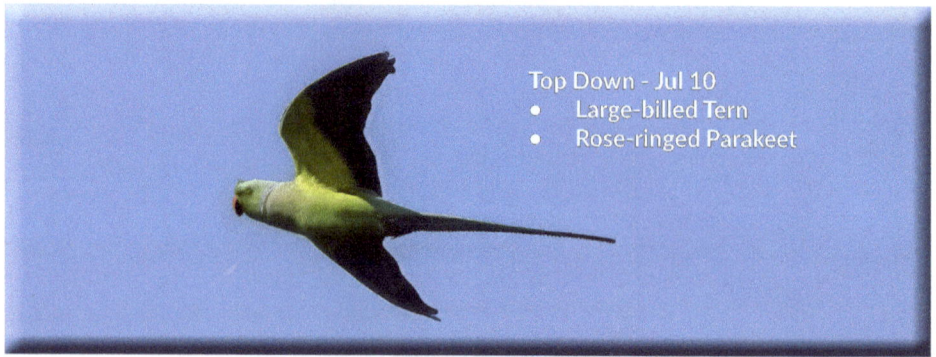

Top Down - Jul 10
- Large-billed Tern
- Rose-ringed Parakeet

will eat roadkill, human scraps, baby birds, seeds, fruit, and lizards. In other words, just about anything. A native of South America, sightings in the United States are extremely rare which make a single bird taking up residence in Miami quite exciting.

Since he had been seen more regularly of late, we arrived full of hope. But after more than two and half hours staking out his favorite location in the park, the dumpsters, heavy rain moved in and we moved out, dipping again.

The next morning we were up early to look for the Yellow-headed Caracara for the third time. We each took turns on dumpster-watch, while the other walked the pavilion circuit in this popular state park, making special effort to check every trash can and barbecue grill. We then crossed the sound and worked a marina and bait shack where the bird was seen last winter … still no Caracara.

We returned to the dumpsters only to find the local fire department doing ladder and hose tests in the same lot as the dumpsters, a distraction that would discourage any bird. So, we climbed into our rental car and reversed our journey on Alligator Alley.

Two and a half hours later, as we entered Naples, Ethan's phone buzzed - the Yellow-headed Caracara was at the dumpsters. Sigh…

Return to Dumpster Watch

After three visits and fifteen hours of fruitless searching for the Yellow-headed Caracara, we were frustrated, tired, stressed, hungry and had developed a real dislike for this bird! Despite our significant frustration, however, we weren't quite ready to be done with him yet.

On Saturday Morning, July 13, we were enjoying a leisurely breakfast. Our plan was to spend the day playing tourist - to visit Sanibel Island and other sights in the area, take a break from birding and decompress a bit. As we sipped our coffee and ate our pancakes, we both kept looking at our phones - the bloody Yellow-headed Caracara had been seen just a few hours after we left Oleta State Park the evening before. Were we really going to fly home to Maine without trying one more time?

The answer was of course no, so we packed up our bags and once again made the long drive across Alligator Alley, arriving at the park once again about noon.

Since it was a weekend, there were more beach-goers, kayakers and a few birders. We met Gordon Payne and Lisa Bonato, two experienced birders from Ontario, Canada, with whom we exchanged phone numbers and war stories.

Once again, the real-feel temperature exceeded 110 degrees, so we spent much of the next seven hours in the air conditioned car hoping our Yellow-headed nemesis would come into the dumpsters or one of the picnic pavilions around the park.

Finally at about 7:00 PM, sweaty, bored, frustrated once again and dreading the two hour drive back to our hotel, we said goodbye to Gordon and Lisa and headed out into Miami's Saturday night traffic. Twenty minutes later Ethan's phone jingled. It was Gordon. The bird was in the parking lot.

Should we go back? It was 7:20, the park would close at 8:00 and traffic was heavy. If we were going to go back, we had to turn around immediately if we had any chance of getting the bird. Let's go! Ethan did a U-turn that would have made Batman proud!

Driving as fast as possible, we wove through the traffic. Upon arriving at the park at 7:48 PM, the park ranger at the gate didn't want to let us in. But, we pleaded our case and, thankfully, she waved us through.

It took us about ten minutes of searching in the fading light until the Yellow-headed Caracara flew low over our heads near the dumpsters and disappeared into the woods. Not the most satisfying view but countable. After five months, four visits and over twenty hours of searching, we finally had our Yellow-headed Caracara tick!

After returning to Maine on Sunday, we were back out birding on Tuesday morning. This time, we were on a whale watch out of nearby Boothbay Harbor. Whale watches are an excellent way to find the incredible sea birds that patrol the world's oceans. Whales tend to find spots where plankton and krill are prevalent, the same places that the birds congregate.

Most of the folks on whale watches are tourists who are under dressed (it can be cold) and a little naive about whales (It can take several hours to find them). After a while these bored passengers start watching us call out and photograph various species, often asking us questions and helping point out birds. We'll let you in on a little secret - birders are actually hoping the boat crew does not find any whales. No whales means the boat will stay out at sea longer, and sometimes you'll get a free ticket for another whale watch.

By the end of the trip, we picked up two new birds for the year - a couple of Red Phalaropes moving south from their Arctic breeding area and two Northern Fulmars, bird #620 for the year.

Little Gull

Maine is a great state! We have the best lobster. We have great skiing, beautiful beaches in the south, a spectacular rocky coast in the north, and lakes in the middle. We have LL Bean and Stephen King.

Maine is also a great birding state with Spruce forest in the north, salt marshes along the coast, and it is located on one of the key migratory flyways. In the winters of 2022 and 2023, it was home to one of the more remarkable birds ever seen in the United States ... the Steller's Sea Eagle. Maine is also our home and the place where we did lots of birding.

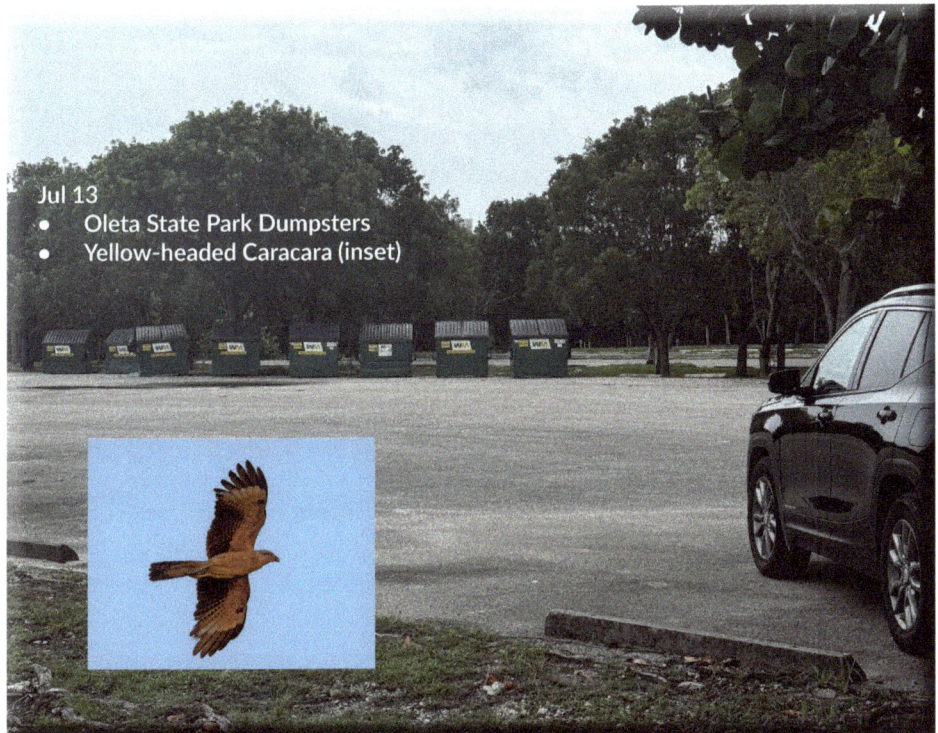

Jul 13
- Oleta State Park Dumpsters
- Yellow-headed Caracara (inset)

One of the challenges of doing a Big Year is balancing birding with other things in life. Various appointments for eye glasses, checkups, dental visits and car maintenance all need to happen as they normally do. So does family time and important events in the lives of those close to us. Such was the case with our little grandson's first birthday. We were not going to miss this, even when tested by the fact that a hard-to-find Little Gull had showed up on a beach forty-five minutes south of our birthday party beach. Naturally.

Little Gulls breed in Central and Eastern Europe and winter in small numbers in eastern North America. Since these gulls are not easy to get, we hoped this one would decide to stick around and enjoy the nice Maine weather and the ample beach snacks until we could get there. So after pizza, cupcakes, presents and games, we said goodbye to our little birthday boy and headed for the Little Gull.

When we arrived and made our way to the beach, the tide was low but rising. While there were decent numbers of shorebirds scattered about, many were far out of viewing range. Moving about the beach with our spotting scope in tow, we scoured the groups of gulls hoping to turn up the Little Gull amongst flocks of Terns and Bonaparte's Gulls, many of them juveniles appearing all too similar to a Little Gull.

Over time, we were joined by other birders looking for the same celebrity bird, but none of us was having any luck. As we had visiting family awaiting dinner, we abandoned our search and headed home. And then, as so many times before, twenty-five minutes later, a Little Gull was reported, followed, incredibly, by another.

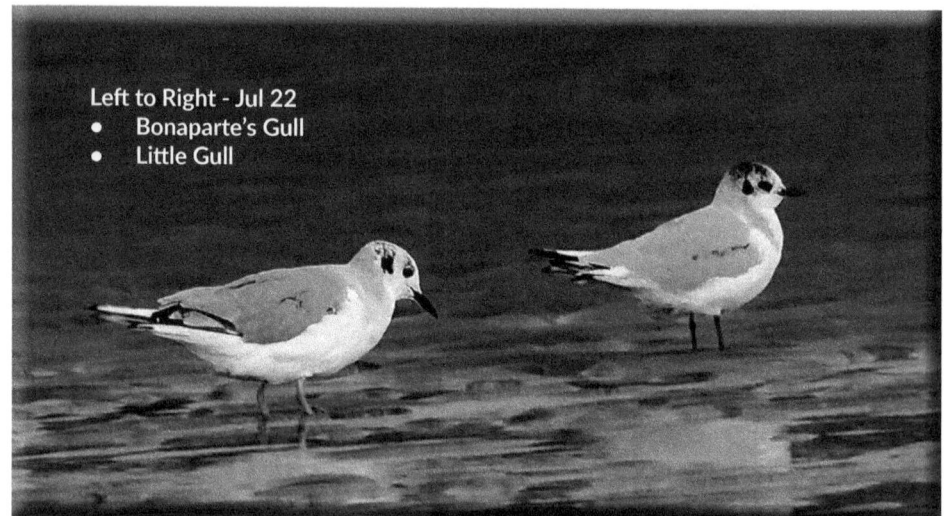

Left to Right - Jul 22
- Bonaparte's Gull
- Little Gull

Once again, the sun was setting and there was no choice but to continue our journey. No Batman heroics this time. No way we could make the drive and the one mile walk back in time.

After dropping our daughter off at the airport the next afternoon, we headed directly to Hills Beach, determined to remain there until we found a Little Gull. A few of our birding friends were already on watch and more joined us as time passed. Although no Little Gull was present yet, we were hopeful that with this many trained eyes on the lookout, if one came in, it would not go unnoticed.

And that is exactly what happened when our friend Tova Mellen was scanning with her scope. Ingrid's phone rang. "Definitive Little Gull in between us!" she exclaimed and described where it was. She quickly made her way over and got us on this adorable little bird. Birding friends really are the best! Bird number 621 for our Big Year!!

Saturday we boarded a Whale Watch out of Bar Harbor with one target bird in mind ... the South Polar Skua. A Skua is a large, barrel-chested seabird that makes its living chasing Gulls and Shearwaters until they regurgitate their food, thus providing the Skua with a nice meal. Yuck! The South Polar Skua breeds during our winter near Antarctica and roams over the world's oceans the rest of the year, showing up in the Gulf of Maine each summer and fall.

After a couple of hours out on the ocean picking out the Shearwaters and Phalaropes, we saw two birds in the distance that looked to be good candidates for Skuas. As we raised our binoculars to get a better look, the boat abruptly turned to the left toward a Humpback Whale, blocking our view of the birds.

Ethan raced to the back of the boat, through the inner seating cabins, no doubt knocking over several small children! When he reached the stern he was able to reacquire one of the birds and get a lousy but diagnostic photo - definitely a South Polar Skua and bird #622 for the year. We spent the night in Bangor to shorten the distance to the Maine North woods and Sunday's target bird, the American Three-toed Woodpecker.

An inconspicuous woodpecker of Spruce forests or bogs with many dead trees, the American Three-toed Woodpecker is a very challenging bird as it prefers remote locations, often at altitude in the mountains. We had hoped to see one in our earlier travels through the Rockies and the mountains of New Mexico and Washington State, but no luck. So on Sunday we went to the place where we had found our one and only Three-toed, back in 2021, on the Umbazookus Road in the Maine North Woods.

To get to Umbazookus Road, one first has an hour of pleasant highway driving north to Millinocket. From there you head west for thirty miles on the Golden Road, a dusty combination of washboard gravel, incidental pavement filled with potholes and ruts, not to mention huge lumber trucks hauling tons of harvested trees out of the woods. The lumber trucks have absolute right of way and reportedly will not stop for anything. Great Northern Paper, owner of the road, allows private drivers access. It is a major thoroughfare into the North Woods for sportsmen, paddlers and people looking for the American Three-toed Woodpecker.

After an hour of teeth-rattling driving on the Golden Road, we turned north onto the Telos Road for another twenty miles. The Telos Road is notorious for shredding one's tires, and a friend who drives it regularly carries a full spare, a can of 'fix a flat', a portable air compressor and a breaker bar. We survived the Telos Road unscathed, thanks to driving at twenty-five miles per hour.

Finally, we reached Umbazookus Road, Maine's only somewhat reliable place to find the American Three-toed Woodpecker. We had detailed intelligence from friends who had gotten the bird earlier in the summer, and after surviving Golden Road and Telos, we were confident of victory. Unfortunately, all we got was the agony of defeat. We searched for five hours and never found the bird, and we came pretty darn close to hitting a moose when we turned a bend on a very narrow road.

The Birds We Skipped

The Colima Warbler and the Himalayan Snowcock are celebrity Big Year birds found on remote mountains in Texas and Nevada, respectively. It seems that every birder that has chased these species has a story to tell about the arduous hike required by the chase. We made a strategic decision to skip the Colima and Snowcock as each represented a significant detour away from dozens of other birds ... a strategic but difficult decision.

Sapsuckers

Sapsuckers are a unique group of woodpeckers that get their name from their specialized feeding behavior: they drill shallow rows of holes, or "sap wells," into trees to drink the sap that flows out. This behavior distinguishes them from other woodpeckers that mainly forage on insects hidden within tree bark. Sapsuckers also feed on insects attracted to the sap, as well as on fruits and tree cambium.

There are four species of sapsuckers found in the United States. Each has its own unique range, appearance, and behaviors. Yet, all share a dependence on tree sap as a primary food source.

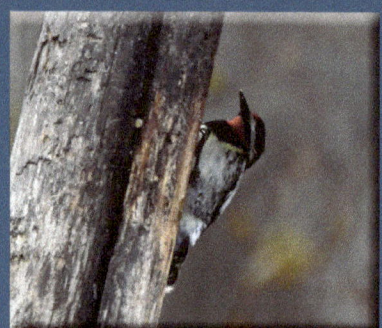

The Yellow-bellied Sapsucker is the most widespread of the group, breeding across much of Canada and the northeastern United States and wintering in the southeastern U.S., Mexico, and Central America. True to its name, it has a faint yellowish tint on its belly, along with a striking red cap and, in males, a red throat. Yellow-bellied Sapsuckers create rows of sap wells on a variety of deciduous trees, especially birch and maple, which helps sustain them throughout the year. They are known for their migratory behavior, making this sapsucker the only one regularly found east of the Rockies.

The Red-naped Sapsucker primarily inhabits the interior western United States, from the Rocky Mountains through parts of the Great Basin, as well as southern Canada. It closely resembles the Yellow-bellied Sapsucker but has a red patch on the nape of its neck, distinguishing it from its eastern counterpart. Red-naped Sapsuckers are commonly found in mixed conifer and Aspen forests, where they drill sap wells in trees like Aspen, Pine, and Willow. Unlike some other woodpeckers, they are somewhat quieter, relying less on drumming and more on subtle vocalizations, a trait that adds to their unique charm.

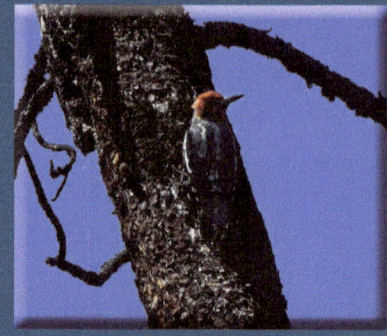

The Red-breasted Sapsucker is found along the Pacific Coast, from Alaska to central California. It is easily identified by its completely red head and breast, which give it a more vibrant appearance compared to the other species. Red-breasted Sapsuckers prefer coniferous and mixed forests, often choosing to drill sap

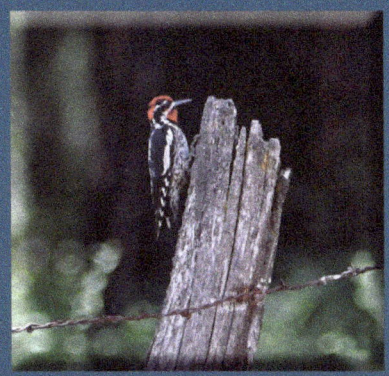

wells in trees like Hemlock, Pine, and Cedar. An interesting behavior of this species is that it maintains its sap wells meticulously, ensuring that sap continues to flow and provide a reliable food source. These wells attract various insects and even hummingbirds, which benefit from the sapsucker's work, creating a mini-ecosystem around the sap wells.

The Williamson's Sapsucker is a striking and somewhat mysterious species that lives in mountainous areas of the western United States, particularly in high-elevation forests of pine and fir from the Rocky Mountains to the Sierra Nevada. Unlike the other sapsuckers, Williamson's Sapsuckers exhibit pronounced sexual dimorphism: males are primarily black with a bright yellow belly, while females are brown with a barred back, making them look almost like separate species. Williamson's Sapsuckers drill sap wells in conifers, especially Douglas Fir, and are known to nest at higher elevations than other sapsuckers, preferring cooler mountain habitats.

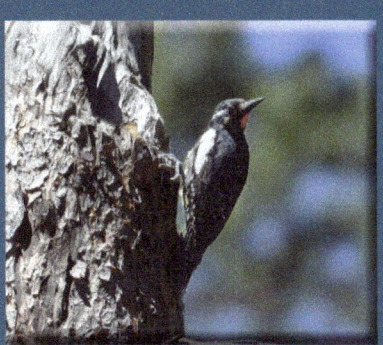

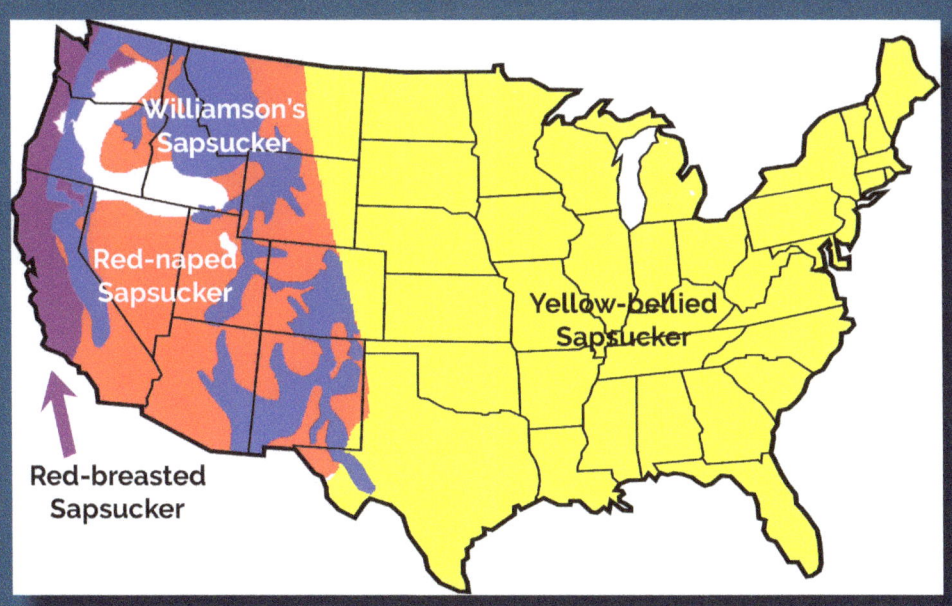

August

Travel	#
Plane Flights	2
Rental Cars	1
Nights Away	9
Boat Trips	0

State	Year Birds
Arizona	18
Maine	1
Massachusetts	1
New Mexico	1
Total	21

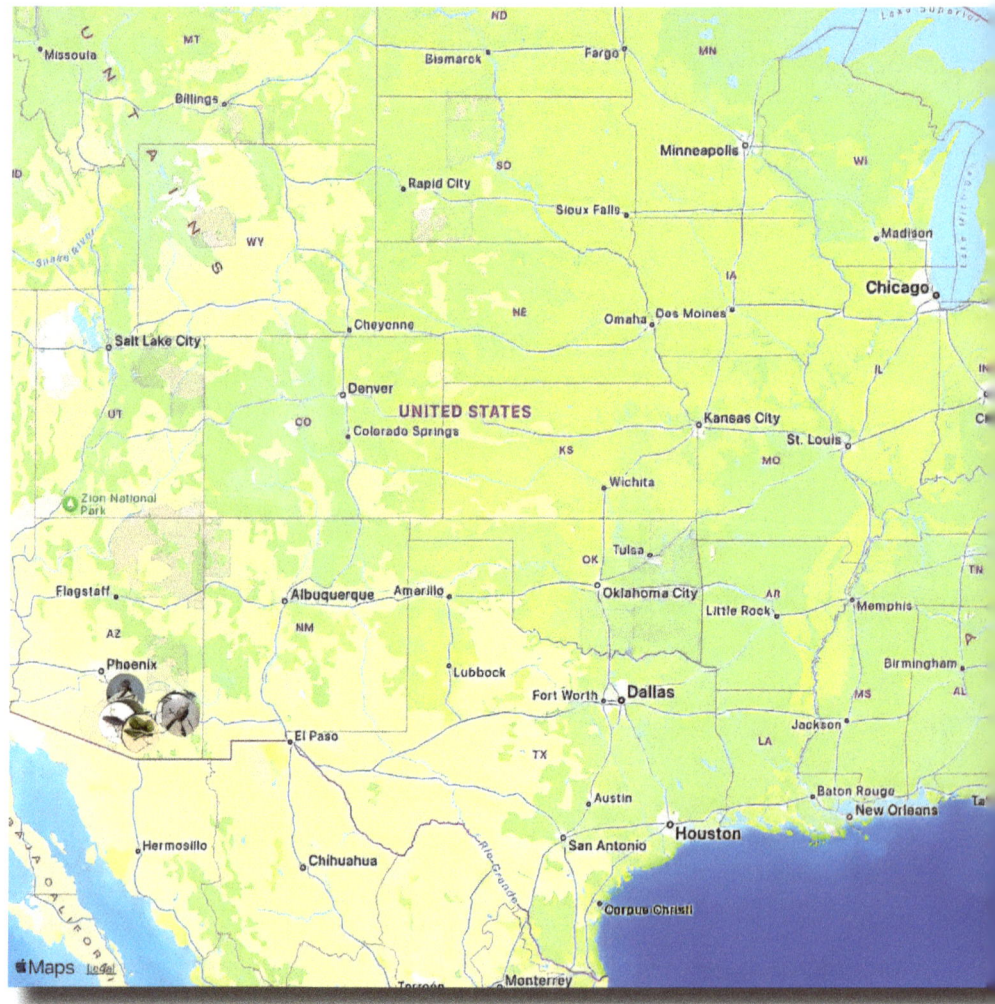

Arizona in August???

Each year, Arizona goes through a rainy or monsoon season in late July and early August. This causes things to green up, flowers to bloom and insects to hatch, drawing birds from Mexico and the Great Plains into Arizona for the feast.

As part of Arizona's second spring, Tucson Audubon puts on a birding festival where guides drive vans of birders into remote canyons to find these late summer birds. Having had our fill of navigating rocky washboard roads, violent switchbacks, with steep drop-offs we decided to take advantage of the transportation at the festival.

Flying out four days early, we did a little birding on our own. We spent the first few nights at an inn in Madera Canyon, a well known birding spot near the top of the canyon at 5,000 feet. A Rivoli's Hummingbird, North America's largest and most aggressive hummer patrolled the trees around the patio driving off all other hummingbirds from the inn's feeders. And an Acorn Woodpecker spent much of the day stashing acorns in the holes he drilled in the siding of the inn.

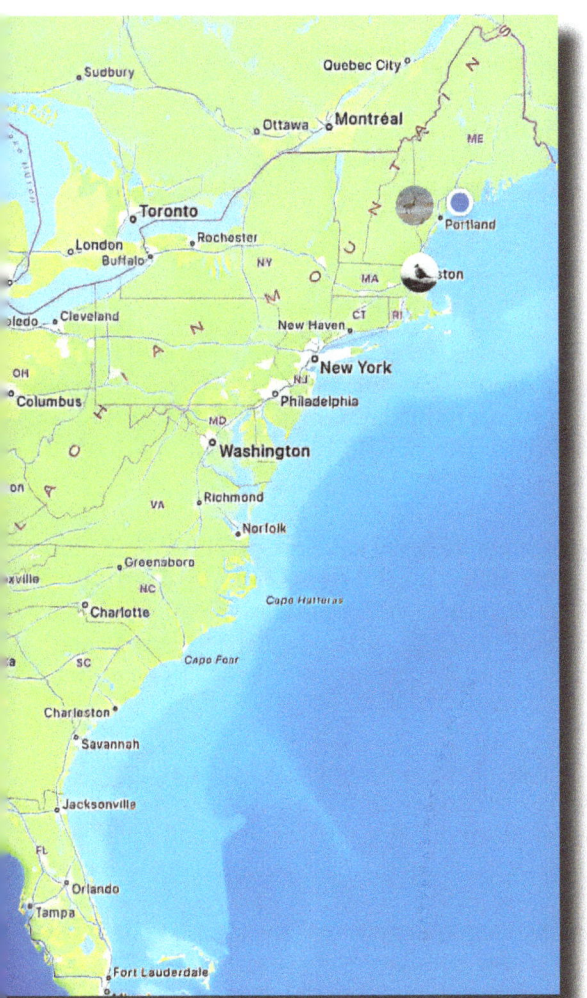

The first evening we sat out on the patio well after dark waiting for the song of the Mexican Whip-poor-will, bird #623 for the year and a life bird for us both.

August birding is pretty much over in Arizona each day by noon as the temperatures and afternoon rains drive birds and birders to shelter. Thus, we were up at 3:00 AM the next morning, as we had a two hour drive to Miller Canyon and wanted to be there near sunrise. Our early start was rewarded with a Flame-colored Tanager, Buff-breasted Flycatcher and Sulphur-bellied Flycatcher, all life birds for the Whitakers.

Ash-Canyon Bird Sanctuary was our next visit. Once a bed and breakfast with lots of bird feeders, the owner eventu-

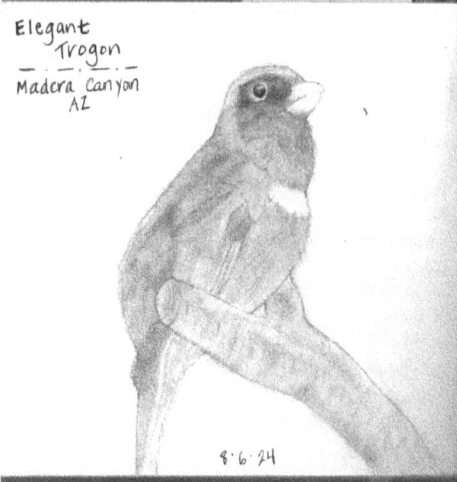

ally gave up renting rooms to concentrate on renting chairs to birders. When owner Mary Jo Ballator passed away in 2019, the Southeastern Arizona Bird Observatory purchased the property and built additional blinds and observation platforms. While 223 species of birds have been documented at Ash Canyon, we were hoping to see a single bird, the Lucifer Hummingbird, a Mexican bird that occasionally crosses the Rio Grande during the summer.

We explained to the Ash Canyon volunteers that we were doing a Big Year, and needed a Lucifer. They enthusiastically told us exactly which feeder it liked to visit and exactly where to sit. After ninety minutes of watching other species of hummers visit the feeders, a volunteer alerted us to the Lucifer chowing down near the center of the facility. Ethan took a few quick photos before it flew away ... Bird #628 for the year.

On Tuesday morning we decided to do something we hadn't done much during the Big Year - sleep in and have a leisurely coffee on the patio. The morning before, when we were visiting Miller and Ash Canyons, a good sized Black Bear had visited the patio and were hoping for an encore. Instead, we had something equally cool happen (at least for birders) when an Elegant Trogon began calling in the distance, lower in the canyon.

While not particularly rare, the Trogon is generally silent except during the spring, and we were well past spring. Trogons also tend to sit quietly in the cover of trees making them extra difficult to find. We heard our Elegant Trogon calling again, this time closer. Then again, even closer.

Finally, after ten minutes of waiting, the Trogon appeared at the top of a dead tree on the outskirts of the property. Not a new bird for us this year, but it is always a thrill to see this stunning creature. We then packed up and headed to Tucson.

Before the festival began, we had a day to chase the White-eared Hummingbird in

Paradise, in the southeastern corner of the state. Another rarity from Mexico, this bird had been coming to feeders at the George Walker House.

The proprietors of the George Walker House were amazing hosts, showing us the ideal spot to see the White-eared Hummingbird, describing its habits, where to get the best photos, and even offered us bug spray.

Unfortunately, no one told the Hummingbird about us, and it never showed up. We spent three and a quarter hours waiting, hoping and enjoying the other avian visitors, but our target never arrived.

On the three hour ride back to Tucson, we picked up two more first of the year birds - a Bendire's Thrasher and a Brown-crested Flycatcher - bringing our total up to 630.

At dinner we learned that the White-eared Hummingbird had returned to the George Walker House around 5:15 in the evening.

Southeast Arizona Birding Festival

When we made our Big Year plan and tried to balance the goal of seeing as many birds as possible with grand-parenting, professional responsibilities and simple sanity, we hoped that the Southeast Arizona Birding Festival would be an efficient way to tick off the rainy season birds that hide in remote locations throughout southern

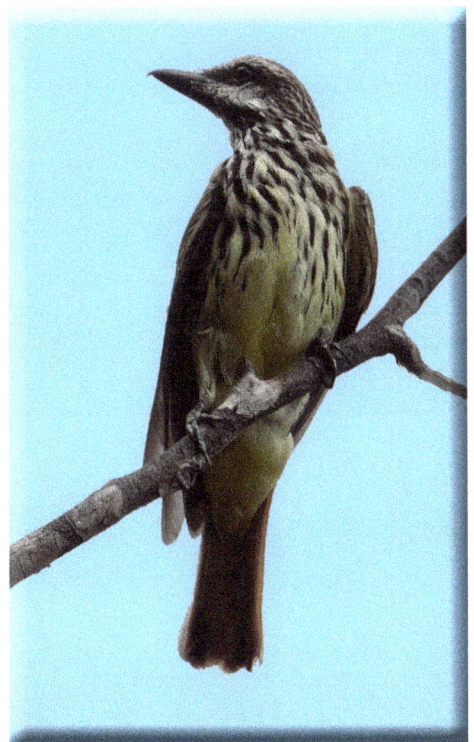

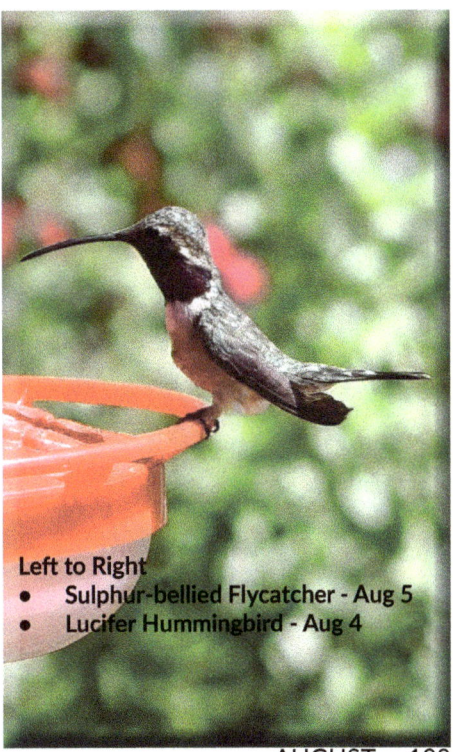

Left to Right
- Sulphur-bellied Flycatcher - Aug 5
- Lucifer Hummingbird - Aug 4

Arizona. Thanks to volunteer guides who are familiar with the birds and the challenging terrain, we had one of the more successful weeks of our Big Year.

On our first trip of the festival, we traveled south of Tucson to Montosa Canyon guided by Sharon Goldwasser. As the sun rose and we approached the canyon, we had our fingers crossed that we would find our two target birds - the Five-striped Sparrow and Varied Bunting. No sooner did we step out of the van when we heard the call of the Sparrow, and almost as quickly, the Bunting. Soon after, we were treated to extended views of both! Birds 631 and 632 for our Big Year.

Fellow Mainer and expert birder Alex Lamoreaux was our guide for Friday's trip to Las Cienegas Grasslands southeast of Tucson. Las Cienegas encompasses 45,000 acres of grasslands, woodlands, riparian zones and a wide variety of species. Our target for the day was the Botteri's Sparrow. And once again, we heard and then saw it within minutes of arriving. Big Year Bird #633.

The base of Mt. Lemmon is located about forty minutes northwest of Tucson, our destination for an all day birding trip on Saturday. Reaching 9,000 feet, Mt. Lemmon offers habitats spanning from Saguaro cactus forest at its base to alpine krummholz at the top.

Jake Molhmann, our guide for the day, began by asking for everyone's target birds, and after hearing the extensive list, devised a plan. Since most of the birds would be found near the top, we started the trip up the mountain. At 7,000 feet, amidst a diverse habitat of both coniferous and deciduous trees, we experienced a 'warbler

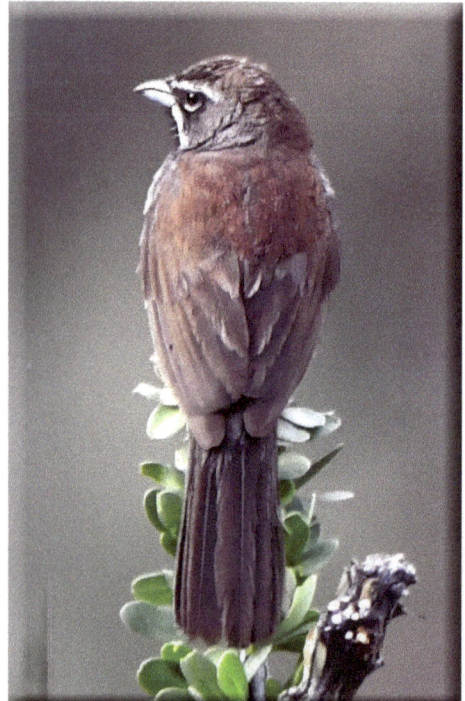
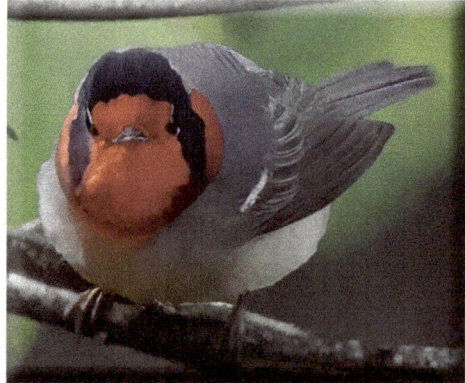
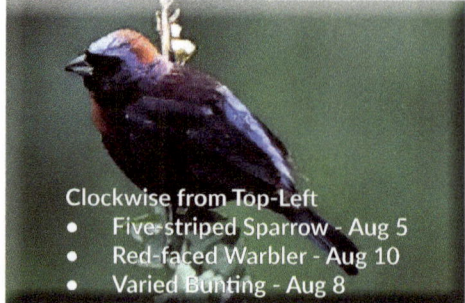

Clockwise from Top-Left
- Five-striped Sparrow - Aug 5
- Red-faced Warbler - Aug 10
- Varied Bunting - Aug 8

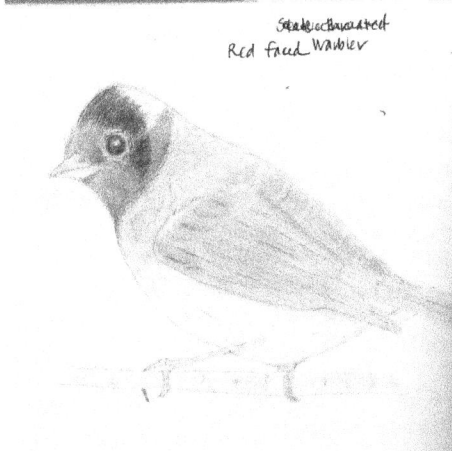

explosion'!

Along with numerous Hermit Warblers were a plethora of others, including a Grace's Warbler, Black-throated Gray Warblers, Painted Redstarts, and a bird we were both most excited to see - the Red-faced Warbler, a stunning bird that isn't particularly shy. Missing from the party was an Olive Warbler, which we found at the top of a Pine tree at a lower elevation. Another lifer, thank you very much!

Next was an attempt to get a bird that eluded us when we were in Arizona in April, the Black-chinned Sparrow. At Geology Vista, we were able to find two after a bit of searching. Unfortunately, our last target of the day, a Gray Vireo, was nowhere to be found. Mid-afternoon heat and tourist traffic didn't make things any easier, but who can complain after getting four lifers in one day?

Our Big Year total increased to 637.

Sunday morning found us on our way to Box Canyon southeast of Tucson in the Santa Rita Mountains close to Madera Canyon. Here grasslands are nestled in expansive basins between steep canyon walls. We had visited Box when we came to Arizona in April. This time we were here with guide John Yerger. Today's target birds were Thick-billed Kingbird and Montezuma Quail.

Shortly after stepping from the van, we were greeted by a singing Varied Bunting, followed quickly by a Five-Striped Sparrow who refused to be upstaged! While we had multiple views of the species when we were in Montosa Canyon, this outgoing sparrow treated us to close, extended views. While attempts to coax a Monetzuma Quail were unsuccessful, we did locate two Thick-billed Kingbirds. Big Year Bird #638. With the festival over, we bid our new friends goodbye and began to plan our final full day in Arizona.

Out the door before dawn once again, we were determined to find the three birds that had eluded us so far - the Gray Vireo, Montezuma Quail and White-eared

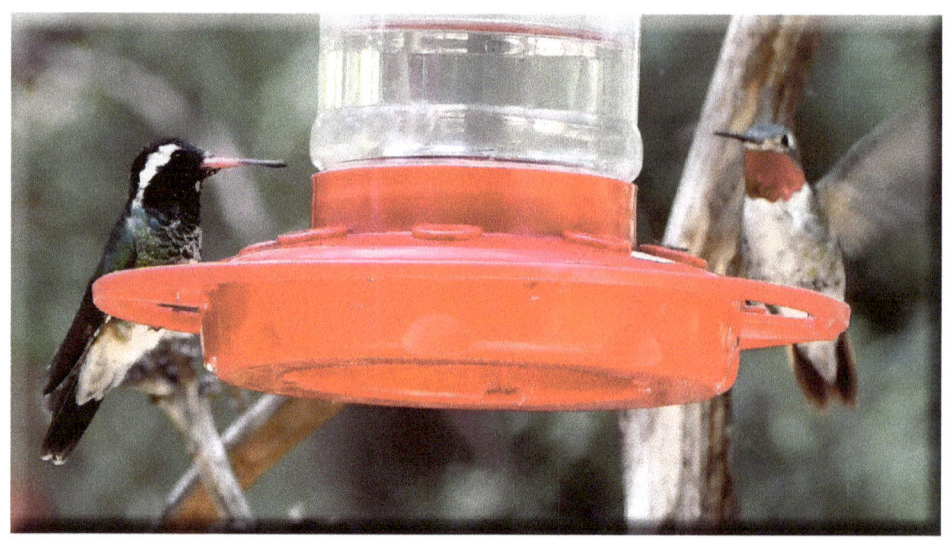

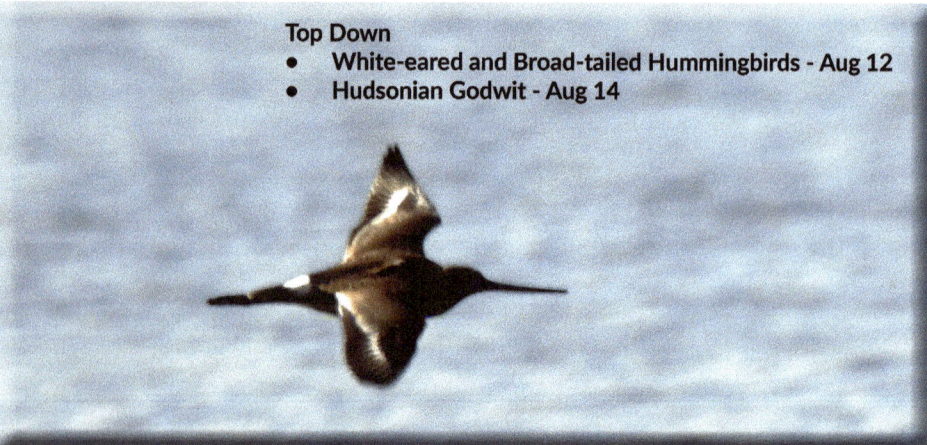

Top Down
- White-eared and Broad-tailed Hummingbirds - Aug 12
- Hudsonian Godwit - Aug 14

Hummingbird. Forty minutes later we were back in Molino Basin at Mt. Lemmon, where we dipped on the Gray Vireo two days before. We hoped that arriving first thing in the morning when it's cooler, the birds are more active and the road noise substantially quieter would give us a better shot at finding this bird. Our plan paid off when we located one singing thirty minutes after we arrived. Back in our rental car, we trekked three hours east to the George Walker House in Paradise, AZ and our second chance to see the rare White-eyed Hummingbird.

As we arrived and walked up to the porch overlooking the feeders, two birders passed us with smiles on their faces. This had to be a good sign! Sure enough, they reported they had seen the White-eared just ten minutes before. We anxiously took our seats with homeowners Jackie and Winston. The hummingbird feeders were more active than the previous week and with a greater diversity of hummers. Black-chinned Hummingbirds, Broad-tailed Hummingbirds, Broad-billed Hummingbirds, Rivioli's Hummingbirds and Rufous Hummingbirds zipped in and out.

Then it happened, Ingrid got a quick glimpse of the White-eared Hummingbird as he entered the yard only to be chased off by another hummer. We moved to the edge of our seats and waited. Two long minutes later, a black-headed bird with a white ear stripe flew in for a quick snack before disappearing into a nearby tree to rest. A few minutes later, he emerged and stayed long enough for us to get more photos and a video. A rare White-eared Hummingbird, a real thrill!!! We got our final bird of the trip a couple hours later - a Montezuma Quail, at the Southwestern Research Center thirty minutes away in Portal.

When we arrived back at our Tucson hotel that evening, we had spent seven hours in the car, a significant portion on unpaved, narrow and challenging mountain roads. We were exhausted but had nailed our three target birds, all of them lifers.

On our summer Arizona adventure, we added 19 new birds to our Big Year tally, bringing our total to 641 birds.

Hudsonian Godwit

The Mayo Clinic defines jet lag as: "A temporary sleep disorder. It occurs when the body's internal clock is out of sync with cues from a new time zone. Fatigue and difficulty concentrating are symptoms."

On our trip to Arizona we were up and out the door before 6:00 AM for nine straight days, and when we landed in Portland, Maine at 11:00 PM, our internal clocks were all screwed up. So naturally, a Hudsonian Godwit, a bird that had eluded us for eight months, showed up the next day just ninety minutes away. Neither of us felt like chasing it, but we knew this might be our only opportunity.

Arriving in Biddeford Pool, we realized we had miscalculated the tides for the 400th time this year and were trying to find a fifteen inch tall shorebird hiding in the grass while it waited for the water to recede and the mudflat to reappear. We set up our scopes and scanned the high tide line, back and forth, while the no-see-ums, a particularly voracious insect of the Maine summer, ate us alive. Finally, we found the Hudsonian Godwit, with its upturned pink bill, snapped a few distant photos and headed home.

Cape Cod

Cape Cod is a hook-shaped peninsula extending from the easternmost point of southern Massachusetts into the Atlantic Ocean. Race Point lies at the very tip of the peninsula, where the water is deep and teeming with fish, drawing pelagic birds close to shore.

We ventured out on a number of pelagic offshore birding trips over the course of our Big Year and were very successful with them. However, one bird that had escaped us was the Long-tailed Jaeger. That changed when we saw reports of two juveniles regularly observed at Race Point Beach, four and a half hours from our home in Maine.

A Jaeger is a gull-like bird with a ravenous appetite. Aggressive and agile, Jaegers will harass the dickens out of terns and gulls in an effort to steal their food. There are three species of jaegers seen in the Lower 48 - the larger Pomarine and Parasitic Jaegers, which we saw off of the coasts of Maine and North Carolina earlier in the summer, and the smaller and less common Long-tailed Jaeger.

By the time we arrived at Race Point Beach, we had done our homework - carefully reading sighting descriptions in eBird for specific location clues and consulting maps of the beach. Thus, we began our search of this very expansive beach, which wraps itself around the tip of the Cape, at Herring Cove.

Fortunately, it did not take very long before we spotted a pair of Jaegers harassing a Common Tern. Unfortunately, with the sun setting over the ocean, the lighting was not in our favor. Even with two powerful spotting scopes on them, we struggled to identify which species of Jaeger we were looking at. Then, technology stepped in to help.

After having had multiple failures with his camera due to high heat and humidity in Florida and Arizona, Ethan tried out and bought a new one at the Southeast Arizona Birding Festival. Olympus's OM 1- Mark II is a mirrorless digital camera. Coupled with target-finder technology, it can locate the bird and focus on the eye. It cut through the setting sun, focused on the bird, and once back at our hotel room, we were able to confirm we had seen Long-tailed Jaegers. Bird #643 for the year.

Mammals

While birding we occasionally ran into some interesting mammals.

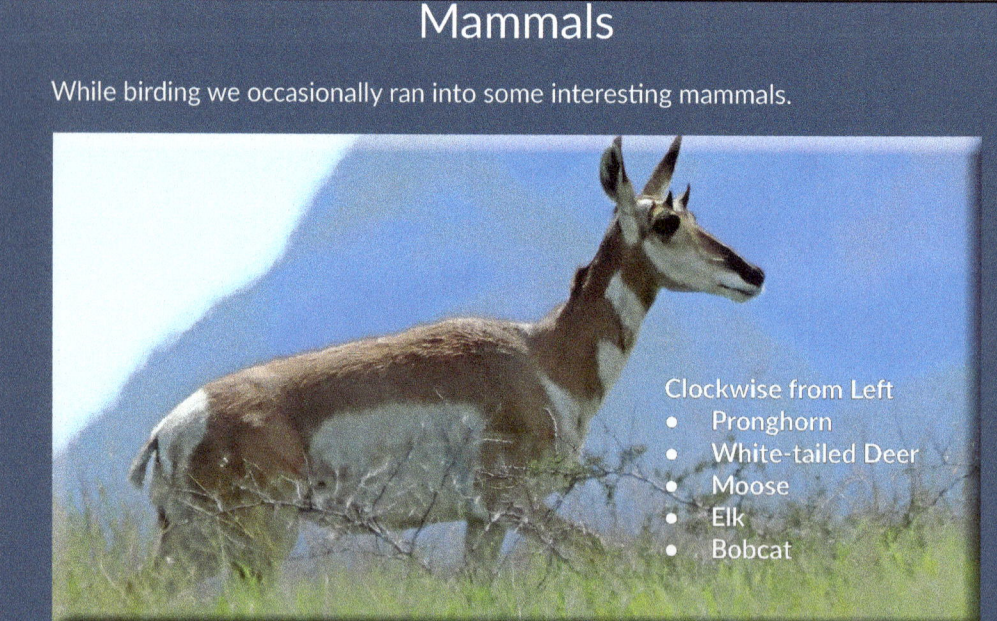

Clockwise from Left
- Pronghorn
- White-tailed Deer
- Moose
- Elk
- Bobcat

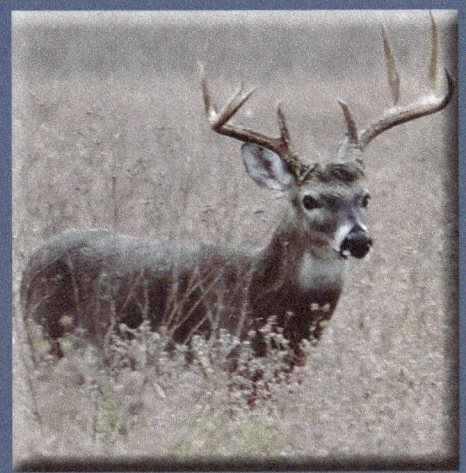
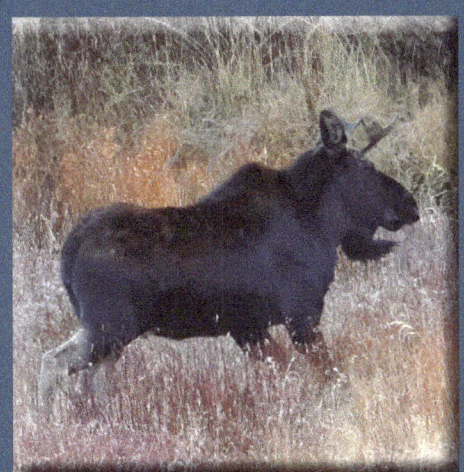
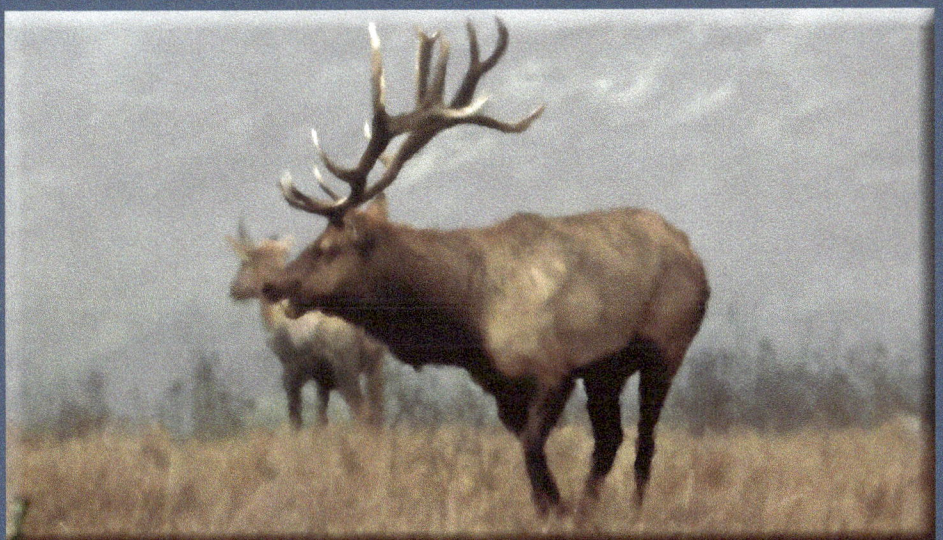
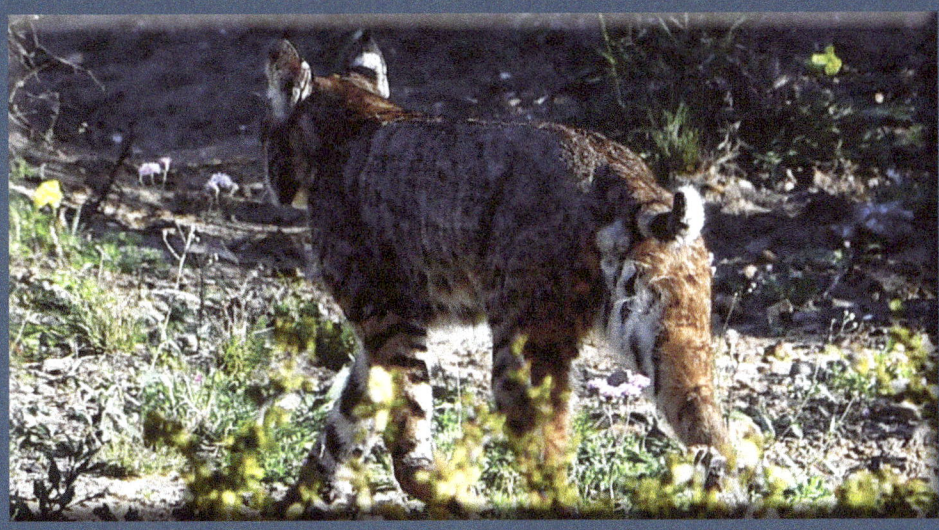

Clockwise from Top Right
- Gray Squirrel
- Red Squirrel
- Ground Squirrel
- Antelope Squirrel
- Fox Squirrel
- California Ground Squirrel
- Black Squirrel

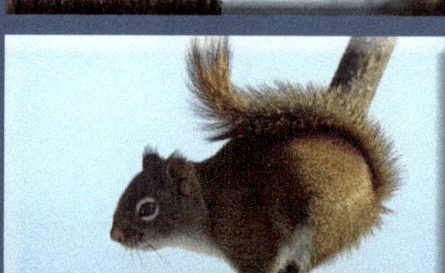
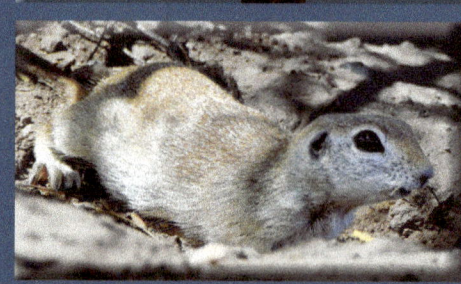
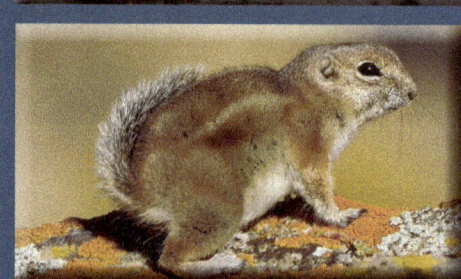
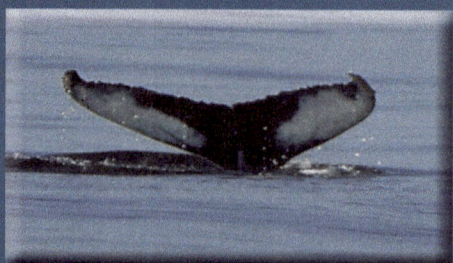
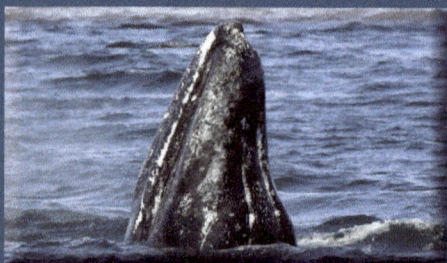
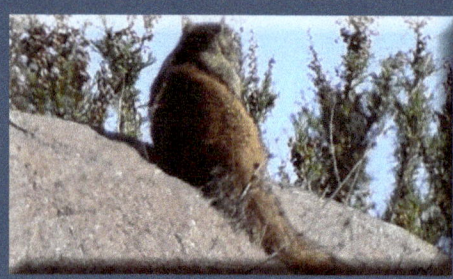
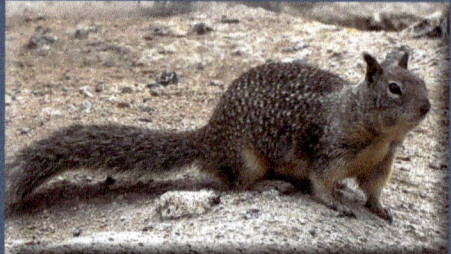
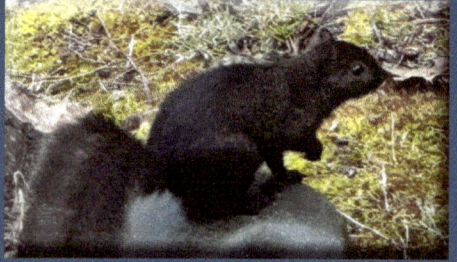

From Left
- Gray Whale
- Humpback Whale

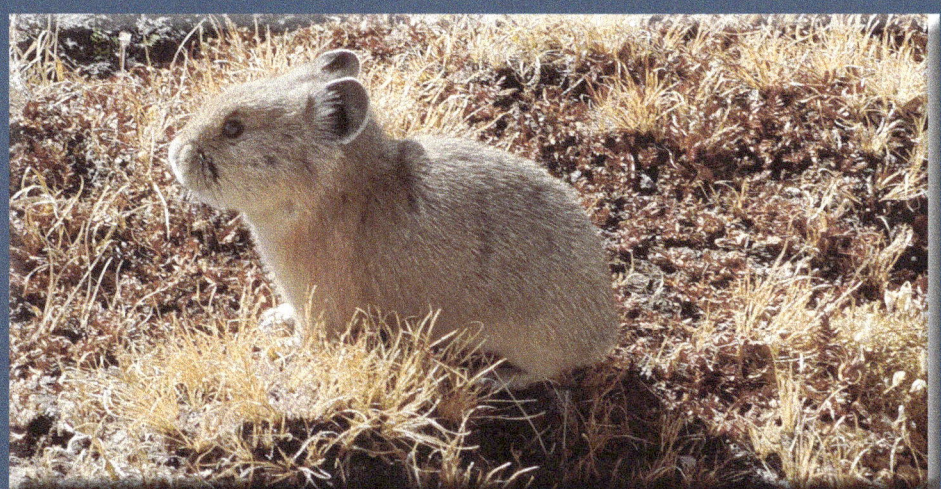

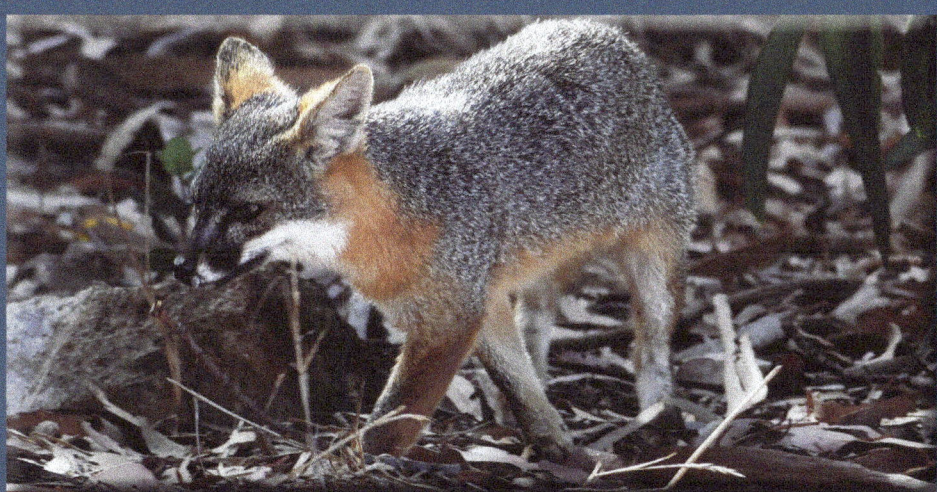

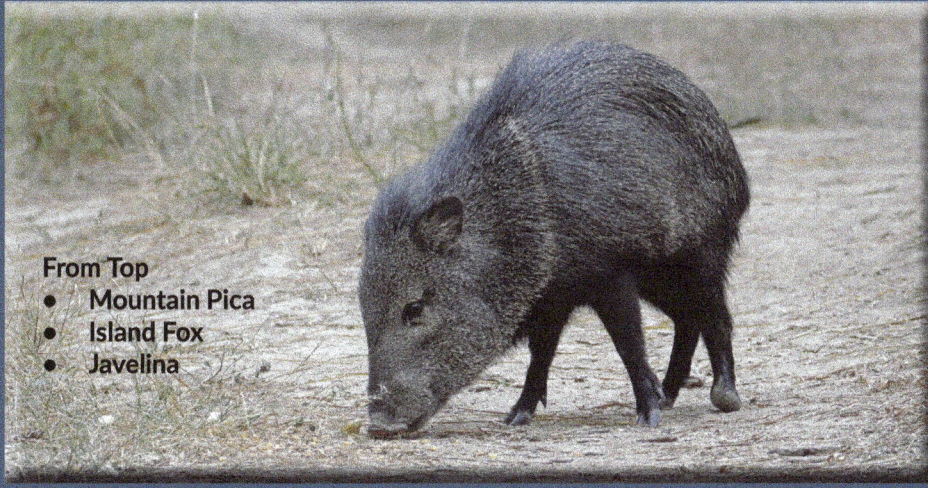

From Top
- Mountain Pica
- Island Fox
- Javelina

September

Travel	#
Plane Flights	2
Rental Cars	1
Nights Away	14
Boat Trips	3

State	First of Year Birds
California	44
Massachusetts	2
New Hampshire	1
Total	47

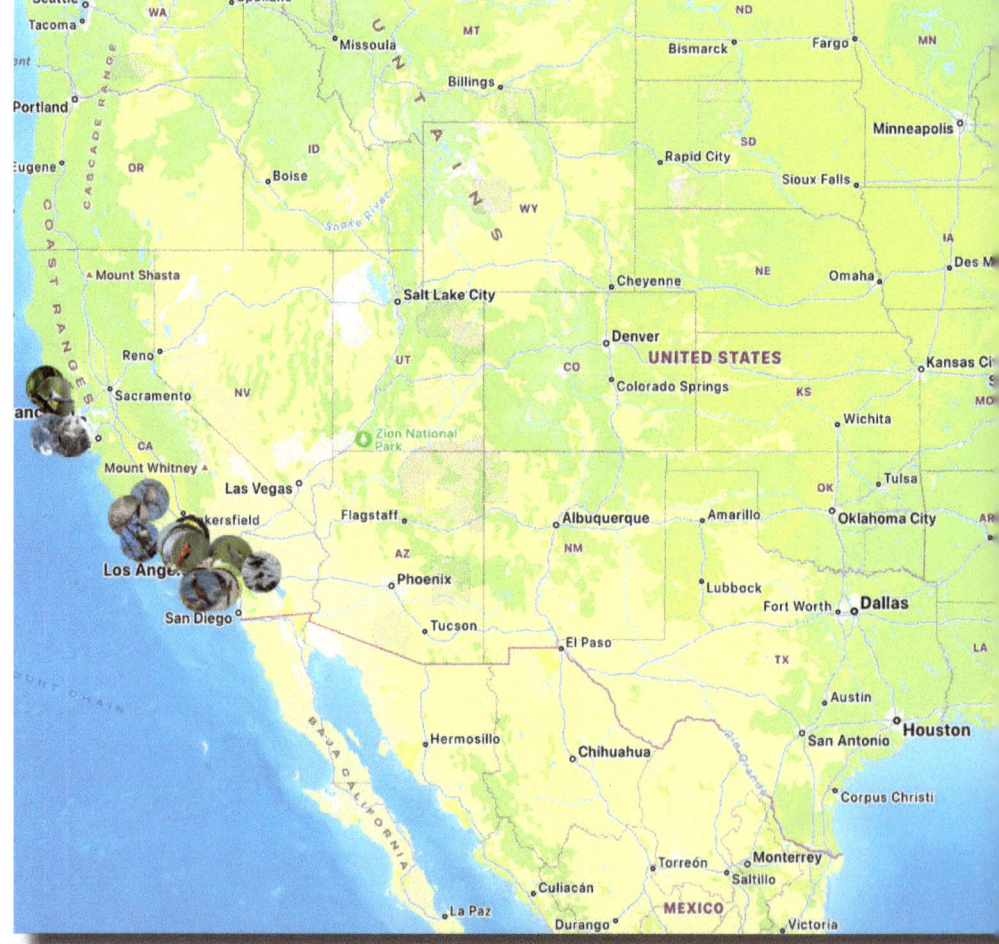

California

We left our home in Maine on the morning of Wednesday, September 4 headed for Boston's Logan Airport, after making a brief stop at Pease Airport in New Hampshire to look for a Buff-breasted Sandpiper that had been foraging between the runways for the previous few days. We set up our spotting scopes and cameras on a bluff looking out at the runways and scanned until we found the tiny 8-inch bird wandering around the freshly cut grass a quarter mile away. A nice start for a long day and bird #642 for the year.

Ten hours and 3,046 miles later we identified bird #643 of the year, an Elegant Tern, not far from the Queen Mary in Long Beach, California. The next morning we went to the San Pedro Fishing Pier and ticked off another seven birds, highlighted by a Wandering Tattler. We had almost given up on a key bird reported there, a Scripp's Murrelet. It is an adorable black and white alcid. As we headed to our car, we decided we couldn't leave without one more look further down the beach.

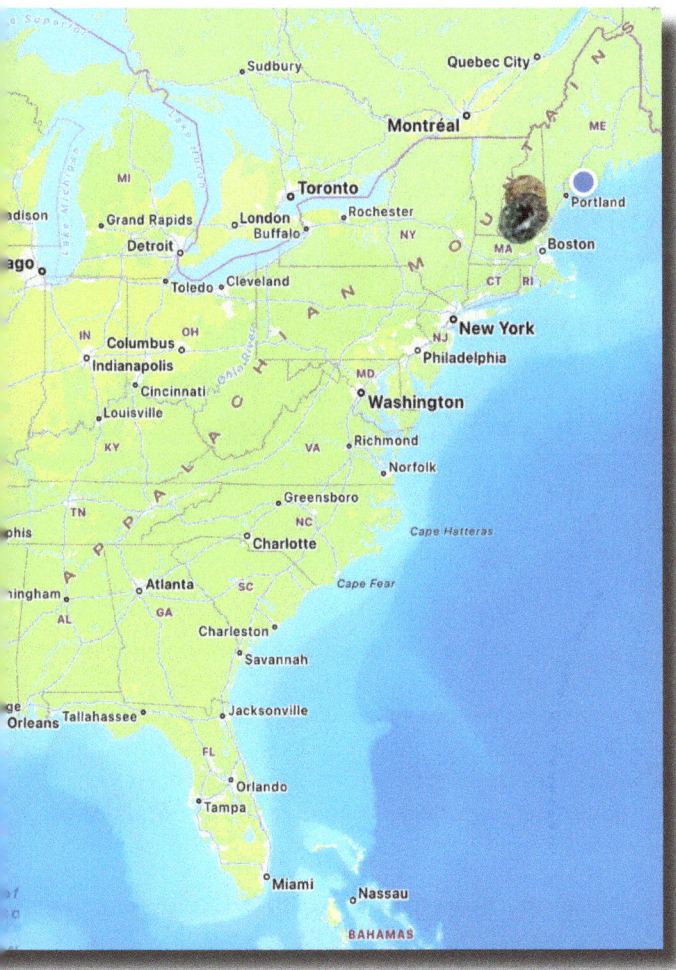

Just then, Ingrid caught sight of a small, dark bird not far from shore. Oddly enough, we initially thought it was a Dovekie, a bird we see off the Maine Coast. But of course, we were off the Pacific, and it wasn't a Dovekie. It was our hoped-for Scripp's Murrelet, not 20 feet from us! One second he was there and then was almost as quickly gone, after a Cormorant harassed him. This was a lucky moment, and we were thrilled to have been in the right place at exactly the right time to see this lifer.

At another stop at a nearby park we picked up a California Towhee and a Pin-tailed Whydah. And it was only 10:00 AM. But, California was getting hammered by a crunching heat wave at the time. This was the first day that the temperature had cracked 100 degrees in the last two years, great timing!

Our next stop was at the Los Angeles River, the 51 mile route that drains water out of the city. Here we hoped to find the White Wagtail that had been seen occasionally near Rosencrantz Avenue. The White Wagtail gets its name from its habit of constantly bobbing its tail. A common resident of Europe and Asia, it occasionally shows up in Alaska and sometimes on the West Coast. Getting one during our California visit would be a real coup.

650th Bird of the Year

On the San Pedro Fishing Pier in Los Angeles, CA we picked out a Surfbird life bird foraging and dodging waves.

September 5, 10:30 AM.

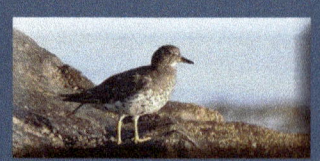

We walked up and down the cement paths overlooking the river for an hour while our skin baked (actually seared, sizzled and even charred) as the sun pounded down on the sidewalk. Like a thirsty man lost in the desert, we saw numerous mirages - a Wagtail feeding in the river two hundred yards away, but over and over it ended up being an extremely common Killdeer.

San Diego Pelagic

On September 6, we checked out of our Long Beach Hotel and headed south toward San Diego. After ticking off the Northern Red Bishop along the Santa Ana River Trail in Orange County, we visited a local park where we were happy to locate a flock of California Gnatcatchers and a California Thrasher before photographing Burrowing Parakeets in National City. Lots of driving and lots of year birds had us exhausted when checking into our San Diego Hotel. We needed to rest and prepare for the next day's pelagic trip offshore.

Legacy Whale Watch runs several pelagic trips every year. These trips are very popular with birders, offering the opportunity to see annual Southern California pelagic birds as well as the chance for a rarity or two. Over eleven hours at sea, covering miles of the Eastern Pacific, chances are pretty good. San Diego was draped in a thick blanket of fog when we arrived at the Legacy's dock before dawn. As we listened to pre-trip instructions from the head guide, we all hoped the fog would soon burn off.

Not far off shore we found our first new birds for the year, all lifers - Cassin's Auklet, Black-vented Shearwater (surprisingly small compared to East Coast Shearwaters)

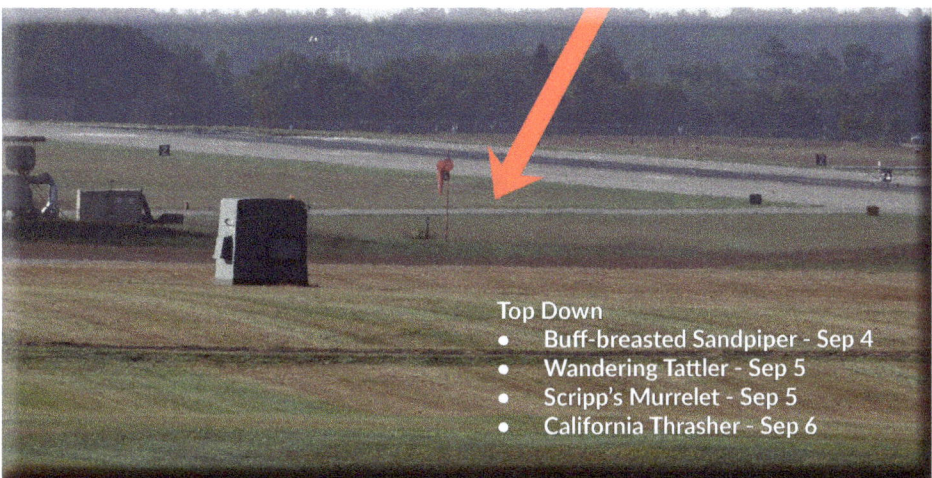

Top Down
- Buff-breasted Sandpiper - Sep 4
- Wandering Tattler - Sep 5
- Scripp's Murrelet - Sep 5
- California Thrasher - Sep 6

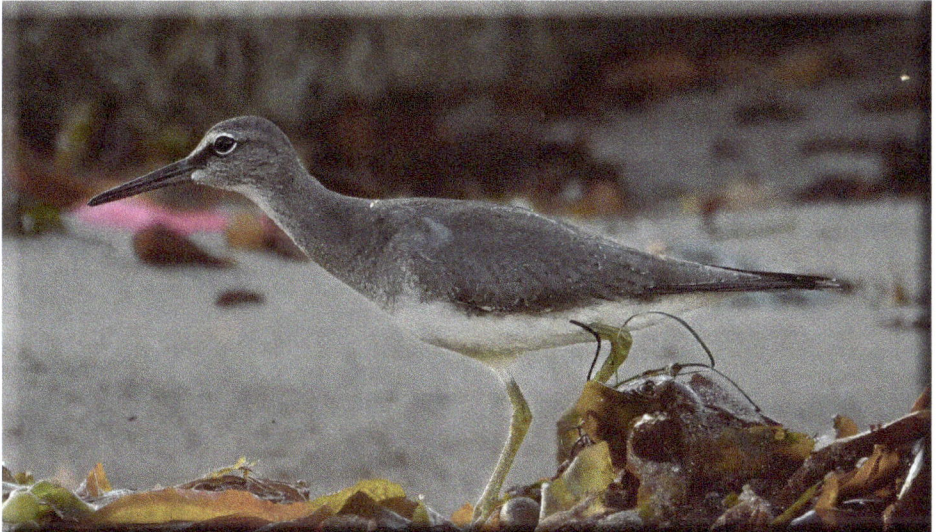

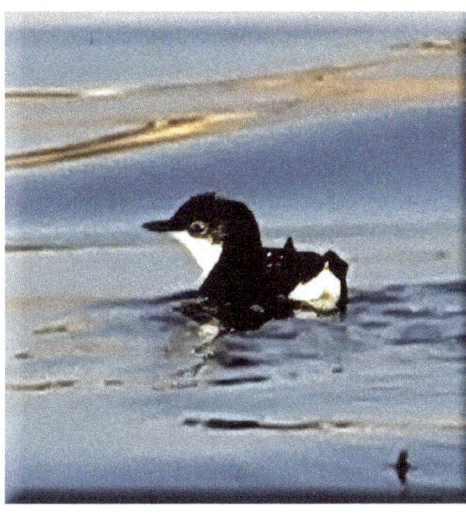

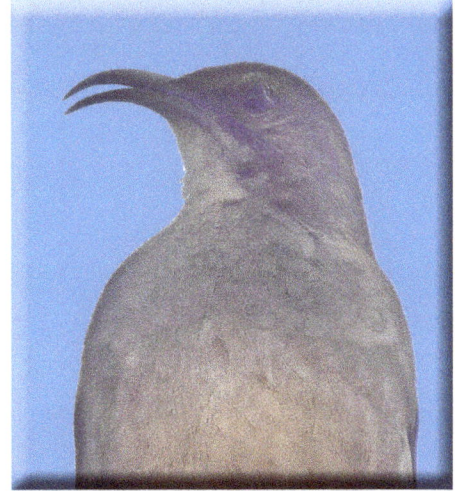

and Black Storm-Petrel. This was a great start to a day that was about to get even better.

As we reached deeper waters, Pink-footed Shearwaters, Townsend's Storm-Petrels and a Least Storm-Petrel all appeared. Three more year birds and three more lifers!

On every pelagic trip one can expect hours of staring out to sea with few, if any, bird sightings. We chat and scan, chat and scan, chat and scan some more, have a snack, maybe even nod off to sleep, grow quiet and yes, even bored. But then, suddenly, on a very lucky day, someone spots something that brings the entire boat into a frenzy!!!!

"Tropicbird!" shouted a passenger. "Tropicbird!" He had spotted a Red-Billed Tropicbird sitting on the water in the distance. Although found periodically off of Southern California during migration, Red-billed Tropicbirds are infrequent visitors, and this was the first report of one in the Lower 48 in the past month.

The boat went crazy, and so did we. When things finally calmed down, a birder from Arizona asked if this was a life bird for us. When we told him that we had had one in Maine a few years ago, his mind was truly blown. Yes, a Red-billed Tropicbird returned every summer to an island off of Maine for 17 years. He was last seen in 2021.

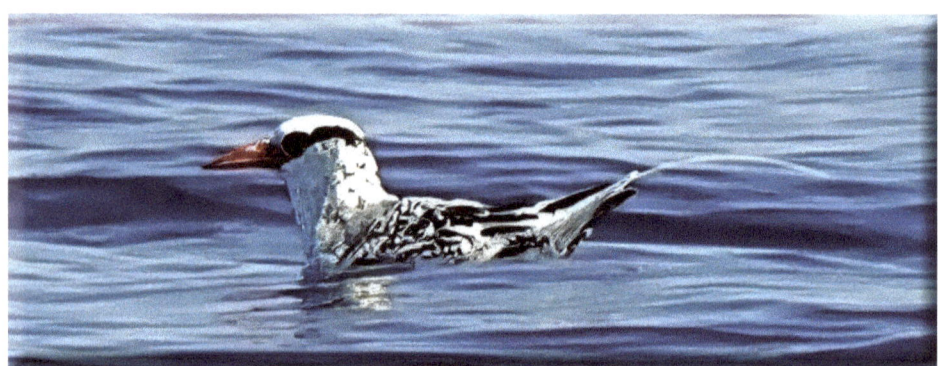

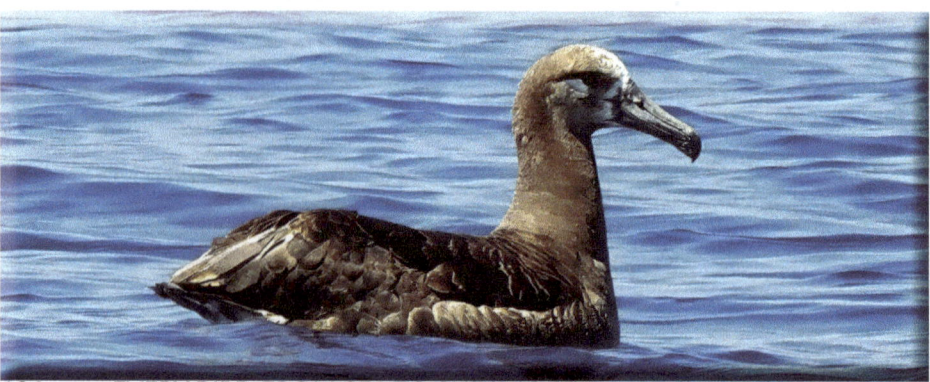

Our incredibly successful day was topped off with several sightings of Black-footed Albatross (the very size of this bird is remarkable), a Cocos Booby, several pods of delightful Short-beaked Dolphin and a couple of impressive Elephant Seals. We ended the trip having gained ten new birds for the year and nine lifers.

Sunday dawned extremely hot in Southern California, so hot that by the time we reached Lindo Lake at 11:00 AM, the temperature was already 105 degrees. Fortunately, there was a little bit of shade, and it did not take us too long to find our target Tricolored Blackbird. This Blackbird looks just like the ubiquitous Red-winged Blackbird, except it doesn't have a yellow stripe on its wing. Onto our next stop - the even hotter Salton Sea.

The Salton Sea is a shallow, landlocked and highly salty lake in southeast California. It was accidentally created in 1905 when an irrigation canal broke during spring floods. For two years water flowed into an ancient dry lake bed, creating the Salton Sea.

In the 1950s and 1960s, the Salton Sea became a tourist attraction with hotels and vacation homes. Its location on the Pacific Flyway attracts migrating birds and the crazy people that follow them. It is also located on the San Andreas Fault, yikes!

Slowly, the lake began to dry up and become increasingly toxic due to agricultural runoff. It is currently about 15 miles long and 35 miles wide. However, its boat

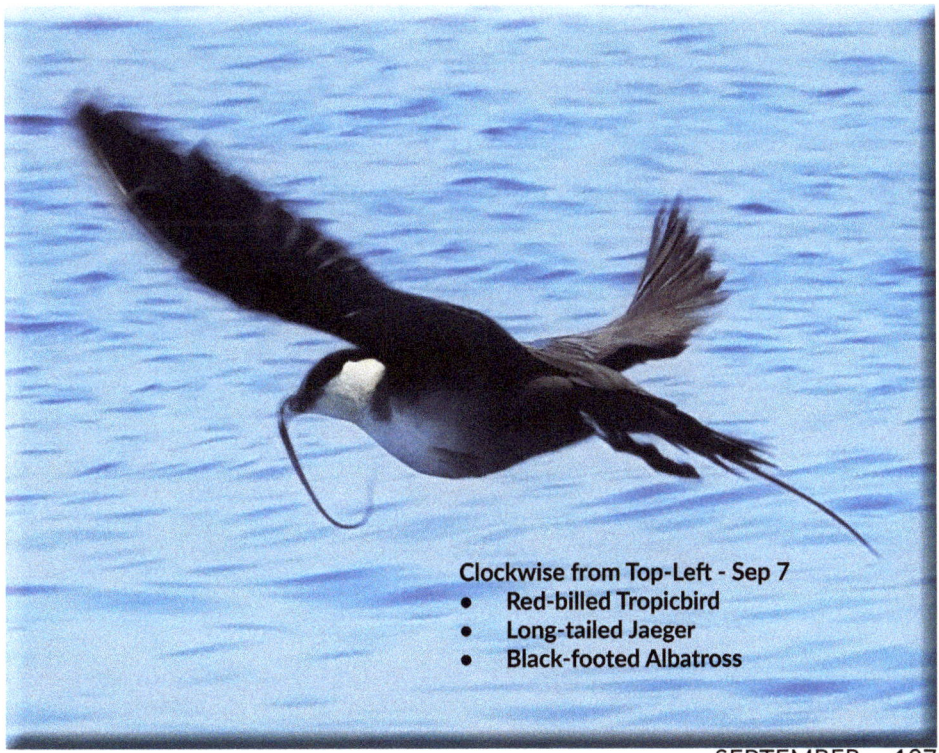

Clockwise from Top-Left - Sep 7
- **Red-billed Tropicbird**
- **Long-tailed Jaeger**
- **Black-footed Albatross**

launches sit miles from the current shore and massive die-offs of fish and birds happen on occasion.

We made the two and a half hour trek from San Diego to the Salton Sea and stood on a clay bluff in 113 degree heat looking for one particular bird, the Yellow-footed Gull. The Salton Sea is the only place in the United States where they are found. When we arrived, the lake was shimmering in the heat, and it was filled with other Gulls, Stilts and shorebirds. Our spotting scopes quickly became hot to the touch.

Finally, we spotted one gull bigger than the rest, with a bright white chest, dark black wings and yellow legs. We took a few photographs and got back in our air conditioned Renta-Jeep. We had our Yellow-footed Gull.

The heat continued on Monday, reaching 111 by the time we arrived in Pasadena. We made a birding stop in the mountains where it was only 90 degrees, positively refreshing!

As dusk arrived Monday night, we raced through residential Arcadia and Pasadena chasing a flock of Amazons (Parrots). The birds would land in a tree or on a power line, and we'd jump out and take photos. After a few minutes, the squawking birds would take off in unison and fly a few blocks over. And, we'd track them down while traversing a tangle of one way streets and cul-de-sacs and get a few more photos in the dark. Rinse and repeat. Rinse and repeat.

Why all the photographs? The flock was primarily Red-crowned Amazons (Parrots), a species we'd seen in Texas in February, but we hoped that there might be a few Yellow-headed Amazons buried in there someplace. After reviewing our photos, we had, in fact, seen three Yellow-headed Amazons.

Another life bird on Tuesday morning, the Pacific-Golden Plover, brought our year total up to 675.

Suddenly 700 birds for the Big Year began to look possible.

Finishing Up in California

Planning our Big Year was quite a challenge for us both. First we needed to decide what type of Big Year we were doing. Initially, we were planning to do a full ABA, which encompasses all of the United States and Canada - including Hawaii and Alaska. Another option was the ABA Continental which leaves Hawaii out of the mix. After lots of discussion, we decided to do a Lower 48 State Big Year which would cut back on the expensive and time-consuming plane flights. But, there is still a lot of ground and a lot of birds to cover. We read a bunch of books on Big Years, talked to birding friends and Googled "How to Do a Big Year" several hundred times.

The birdiest state in the country is California, where 711 species have been identified over the years. Did we begin our Big Year there or in the very birdy states of

Florida, Texas or Arizona? No, we ignored everything we had learned and spent most of January birding at home in Maine. When we finally hit the road on January 28, we were in about 2,000th place in the country. We did not panic, however. We had a strategy, one that we felt confident would work, and California waited until September.

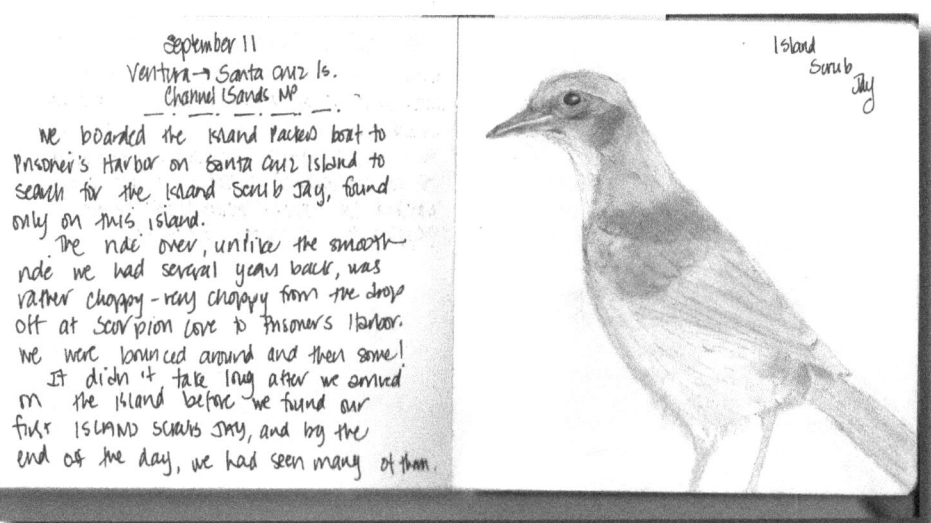

By the 8th day of our California adventure, we had found many of our target birds. Some, however, required a special effort. On Wednesday, the 11th, we took a ferry out of Ventura to Santa Cruz Island, one of the Channel Islands and the only place in the world to find the Island Scrub-Jay. A close relative of the California Scrub-Jay, the Woodhouse's Scrub-Jay and the Florida Scrub-Jay, the Island Scrub-Jay is a little larger than its mainland cousins.

It's also really easy to find, and we saw our first one sitting in a tree over the island's outhouses, only about 5 minutes after we were dropped off at Prisoners Harbor. Unfortunately, the return ferry didn't leave for 6 hours. A fellow birder quipped, "They must call it Prisoners Harbor because you are basically an all day prisoner on the island!" But we had planned for this and had brought a picnic. We ate it while staring at the mainland coast twenty miles away - where a dozen rare birds were out of our reach. To ease our suffering, we were kept entertained by the adorable and endemic Island Fox which wanders about with no fear of human visitors.

The next day brought us to San Francisco to look for a rare Warbler that had been hanging out at Pine Lake Park for over a month. On our way we swung through an agricultural area in search of the beautiful Yellow-billed Magpie. We are not sure how popular these birds are with the vineyard owners, but Magpies were on fences, trees and power lines.

After working our way through Bay Area traffic, we arrived at Pine Lake Park and made the short walk to the end of the pond where the Slate-throated Redstart had

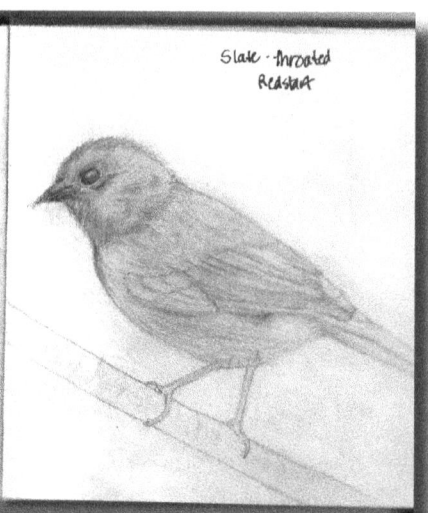

been seen. A resident of Mexico and South America, this very lost bird was first reported on July 29 to great excitement in the birding community. The fact that it was still being seen in the same general area a month and a half later was very fortuitous for us. A small army of birders helped us find the Redstart, and we stuck around for quite a while to get better looks and photos.

On Friday, we drove north of the city to a legendary birding hotspot, Point Reyes, targeting an early Golden-crowned Sparrow. A summer resident of Alaska, mid-September is still a bit early to find one in California where they winter. Port Reyes was fogged in during our visit, making it difficult to see anything. During one brief break in the weather, we came upon a magnificent Elk and his harem.

We eventually found a couple of Golden-crowned Sparrows traveling with a mixed flock of Western Bluebirds, Song Sparrows and Pine Siskins. The pea soup fog continued to thicken, and we decided to drive south to Muir Woods and its famous Redwood trees. This was Ethan's first visit to the Redwoods.

On Monday, we climbed on yet another birding boat, a pelagic out of Monterey Bay. We hoped this trip would be half as good as the San Diego Pelagic eight days earlier, and it almost was. We picked up four new birds, highlighted by Buller's Shearwater and Flesh-Footed Shearwaters. While not a new bird, the Sooty Shearwaters, a bird we see only sporadically on the East Coast, were migrating. The counters on board our boat reported 9,950 of them! We also saw 28 Black-footed Albatrosses, an incredible day on the water.

Our final bird in California was the White Wagtail that had eluded us earlier in the trip. We found it cavorting in the Los Angeles River an hour before catching our flight back to Boston. Just in the nick of time!

After our red-eye to Boston, we stopped on a beach in Massachusetts to tick off a juvenile Common Ringed Plover. Unfortunately, it looked almost identical to the more than four hundred Semipalmated Plovers that were all over the beach. It took us three hours and five miles of walking on sand to find it!

Exhausted and finally home in Maine, our belated California trip added forty-six new birds to our year list. Maybe we should have gone earlier in the year, but we were pretty happy with our progress thus far. 687 birds, within striking distance of 700.... if we got very lucky.

Connecticut Warbler

Warblers are small, colorful bug-eating birds that typically fly and hop rapidly from branch to branch. In most of the United States they are observed during spring and fall migration as they move from their wintering grounds to breeding grounds and back. Birders cherish the warbler season as, under the right conditions, a dozen different species of these colorful gems can be seen in a single morning.

There is one particular warbler that is set apart from the rest, the evasive and somewhat mysterious Connecticut Warbler. It prefers to walk around in heavy, often impenetrable thickets. It sings only for a few weeks in late May and early June on its nesting sites in upstate Minnesota. That particular area is boggy and is legendary for mosquitoes that can chase even the toughest adventurer out of the woods.

The bird was named 'Connecticut Warbler' because the first specimen of the spe-

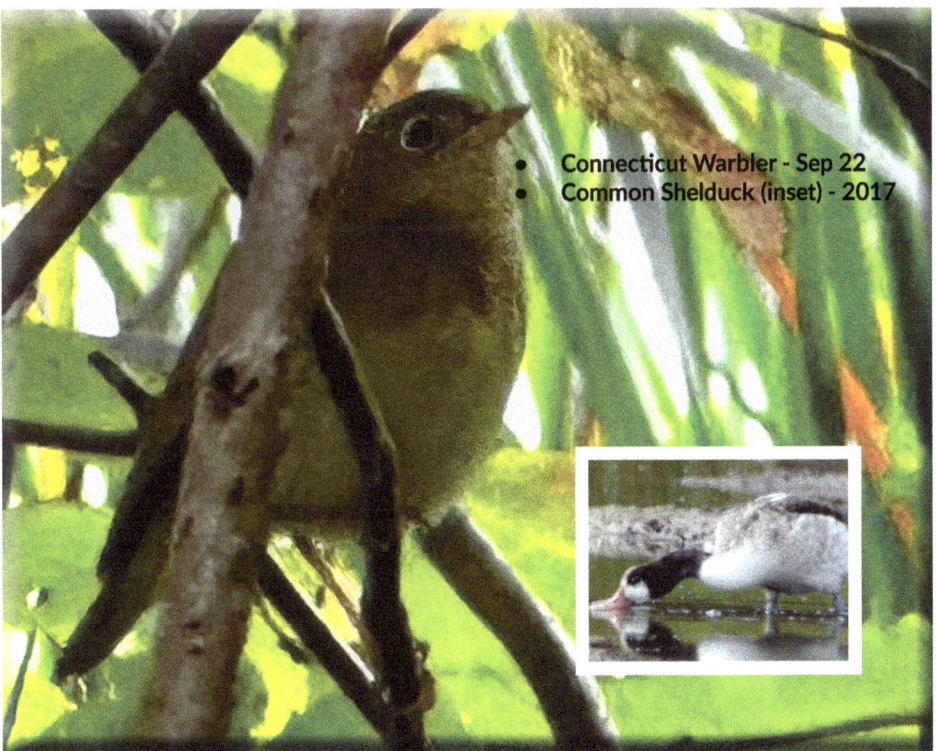

- Connecticut Warbler - Sep 22
- Common Shelduck (inset) - 2017

cies was collected in Connecticut. Despite the name, the bird is rarely seen in Connecticut or any other New England state. Ethan saw one briefly in September 2020. It popped up onto a bush before dropping back into a thicket never to be seen again.

Since then, we have spent many, many fall hours searching bushes for a Connecticut Warbler. We've read that they like pumpkin patches, and Ethan asked a number of farmers for permission to peruse their fields. He found exactly the same number of Connecticut Warblers as Linus's Great Pumpkins!

And it's not just us. There are a lot of very good birders that have never seen a Connecticut Warbler. It's not really chaseable. When one hears about a Connecticut Warbler sighting, you'd better be nearby and ready to go because it will disappear into the brush in minutes.

On Sunday morning, we heard about this nemesis bird being seen in Melrose, Massachusetts, just outside of Boston. The same bird had been reported twice the day before. A Connecticut Warbler that was staying in place? This might be our chance! We jumped in our car and made the two and a half hour trip at somewhat faster than legal speed limits allowed.

Ell Pond sits in a lovely suburban park. Along the edges of the pond, large sections are roped off to allow trees and bushes to grow naturally.

As we jumped out of our car in the parking lot, we ran into a gentleman who we had met when chasing the Common Ringed Plover. He smiled at us and said, "A bunch of birders are watching the Connecticut Warbler down that path." He was pointing at a trail not 50 yards away. Was it really going to be that easy?

It was! We watched this hyperactive little bird walk in and around the shoreline scrub. He would appear for ten seconds and disappear for thirty. Then, he'd materialize ten feet away before dematerializing just as quickly. Ethan's expensive new camera was useless. The bird was so close but so hidden behind grass and sticks, he couldn't get it to focus. Incredibly though, his iPhone was able to focus on the whirling dervish bird.

Finally, after 45 minutes, we high-fived our fellow birders and headed home. Bird #688 of the Big Year. One step closer to 700.

This Connecticut Warbler sighting reduced the gap

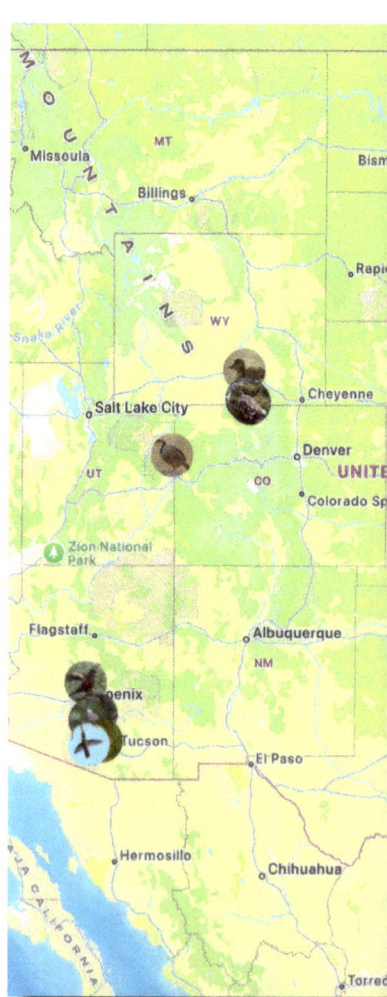

October

Travel	#
Plane Flights	4
Rental Cars	2
Nights Away	9
Boat Trips	0

State	Year Birds
Arizona	6
Colorado	3
New York	1
Wyoming	1
Total	11

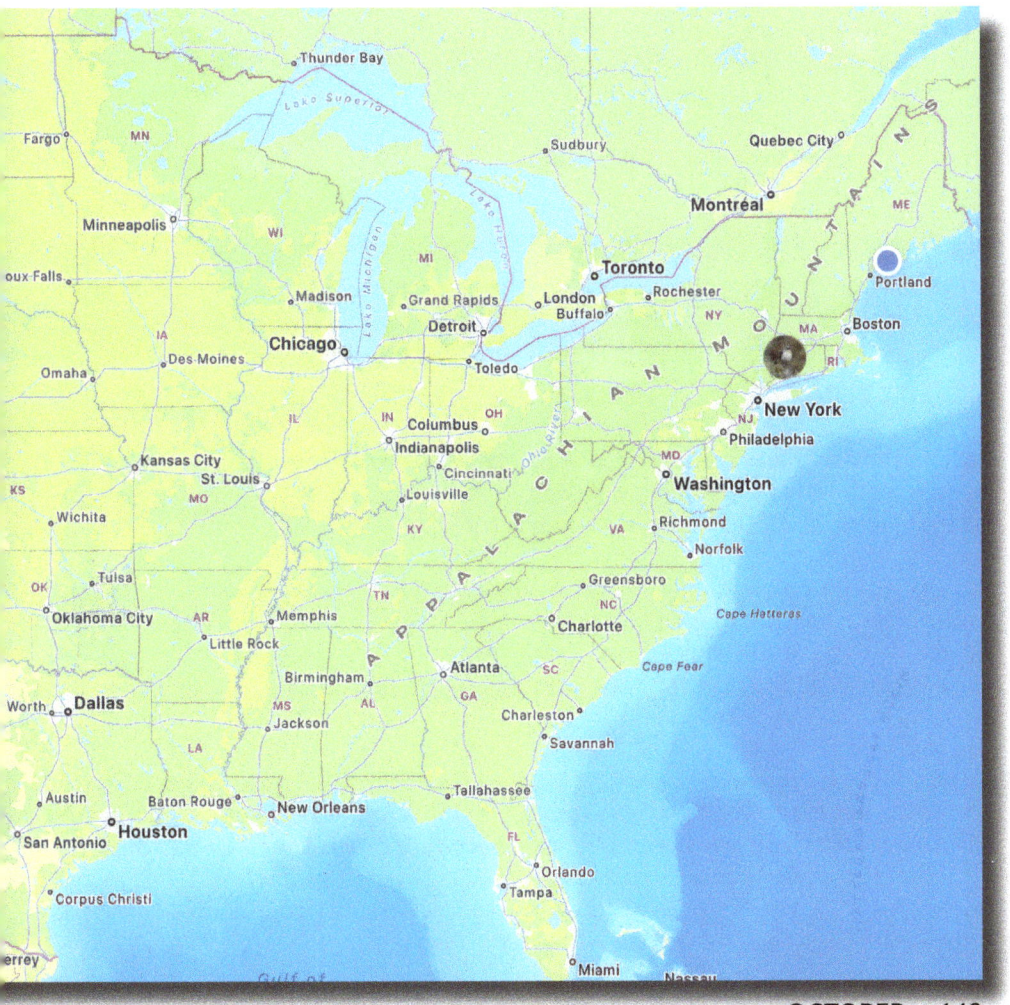

between us on US life birds to one. The only bird Ethan has that Ingrid doesn't is a Common Shelduck, a bird he saw in New Hampshire in August 2017. Ingrid was working that day, and apparently Ethan called in sick.

Waiting for Vagrants

With our Lower 48 State Big Year over three-fourths complete, we spent the week at our home in Maine planning our final push to get to 700 birds before the year ends. With ZERO new birds for the week, we remained twelve birds short of 700. We did do a bit of local birding, but that was more to enjoy the beautiful fall foliage and the suddenly cooler temperatures.

We kept overnight bags packed and sitting by the door all set to chase anything that showed up in New England, New York or New Jersey as winter approached. Top of that list was a Snowy Owl, a winter bird that in some years is remarkably easy to find, but neither of us had seen one since 2022.

Snowy Owl irruptions are influenced by their primary nesting area food source, the Arctic Lemming. Lemming populations contract and expand cyclically from year to year. During a boom year for the little critters, Snowy Owl parents may successfully raise multiple young. During a bust year, they may not nest at all. The winter following a boom year, the adult Owls will chase the young south, and that is when we see lots of Snowy Owls.

Other vagrants that we hoped would appear were Northern Lapwing and Northern Wheatear, both species that we'd seen in recent years and hoped we would again before January 1st.

Long Island Ferry

Late in the afternoon on Sunday, October 6, as we were recovering from another embarrassing defeat by our beloved New England Patriots, we heard about a Northern Wheatear being seen on the eastern tip of Long Island, New York!

A Northern Wheatear is an American Robin-like thrush that summers from Greenland across Eurasia to Alaska. In the fall, Wheatears migrate to Sub-Saharan Africa, where they spend the winter. Each year a few will turn the wrong way and be observed along the East Coast of the United States for a few days. A couple of years ago, one appeared on a beach in southern Maine for about a week, the only time we had seen this species.

Was this Long Island Wheatear chaseable, we wondered? It was already getting late in the day, and the more than eight hour drive to the bird from Maine would get us there after dark. Further complicating matters, we had appointments scheduled for Monday. So, after some discussion, we decided to wait and see if the Northern Wheatear would hang around until Tuesday.

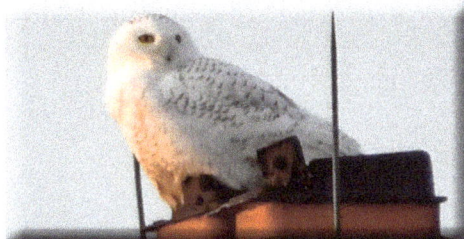
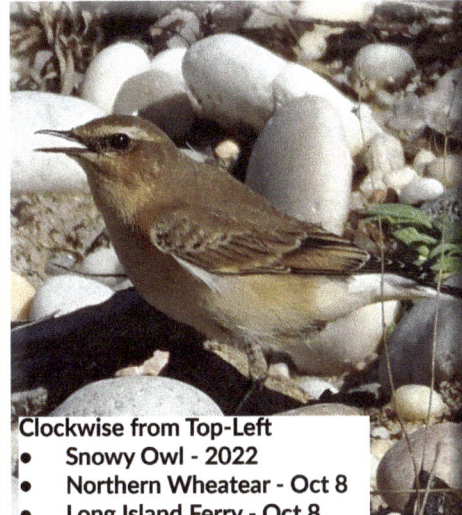
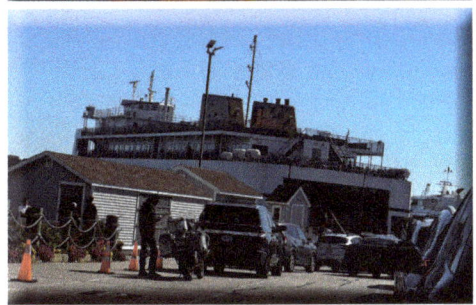

Clockwise from Top-Left
- Snowy Owl - 2022
- Northern Wheatear - Oct 8
- Long Island Ferry - Oct 8

Up early Tuesday morning, we packed the car for an overnight trip and waited. At 8:41 AM, a report came through on eBird; the bird was still there. Ten minutes later, we were driving south.

On our drive we began to text with Ezekiel Dobson. Ezekiel is a 19 year old birder who was also doing a Lower 48 State Big Year. While we were currently tied for second place in the 2024 competition, we were an incredible forty birds behind Ezekiel. He needed another twenty birds to break the Lower 48 State record. Ezekiel had flown in from Los Angeles to see the Northern Wheatear, and we were exchanging notes on our respective progress.

Fortunately, traffic was extremely light, and we made the 1:00 PM ferry from New London, Connecticut to Long Island in time for the 80 minute crossing. Fittingly, Ezekiel beat us to the Wheatear but was kind enough to hang around for a half hour for us to arrive so he could point out the bird.

This was the first time we had actually met Ezekiel, even though we had been in the same towns chasing the same birds throughout the year and had texted many times. While Big Years are a competition, it's all done in a friendly manner and most folks are happy to help others get on a bird or give advice about logistics. Birding superstars David McQuade and Tammy McQuade, a married couple from Florida, have seen 700 birds in a year, six consecutive years. We have never met in person, but they were a great help to us all year long.

When our ferry arrived at Long Island, it was only a 5 minute drive to the Northern Wheatear beach, where the bird was happily chowing down on crickets. We got great photos and videos and enjoyed visiting with Ezekiel, Hanyang Ye, who was also doing a 50 State Big Year, and local New York birders.

We then turned around, caught the ferry back across Long Island Sound and drove back to Maine. We enjoyed learning that the ferry we were on, the Cape Henlopen, was built as a landing craft for the D-Day Invasion.

Colorado

There are two strategies for doing a Big Year:

Option 1: Watch for rare bird reports and then rush by plane, train or automobile to find the rare bird. The more common birds will take care of themselves.

Option 2: Schedule trips around the country to see all of the common birds and hope you are lucky enough to find a few rarities along the way. Ethan refers to Option 2 as the "win the lottery" method. When we had completed our eight day trip to Colorado, Wyoming and Arizona, this approach was paying off.

On Sunday October 13th, we left home before 3:00 AM, as we had an early flight from Boston to Denver. Upon landing in Colorado, we made a diversion to Laramie, Wyoming and the shallow lake where a Yellow-Billed Loon had been reported. Wyoming was the 37th state we visited during our Big Year, and we enjoyed seeing the many ranches with cattle, horses and pronghorn on our race to the loon.

Normally found nesting in the high Arctic and wintering in southern Alaska, this was a bird we never expected to get on a lower 48 Big Year. Luck is a great strategy!

When we arrived, the Yellow-billed Loon was on the distant corner of the lake but visible in our spotting scope. We took a few documentary photos and headed back to Denver. The next morning, Ryan Dibala, an experienced birding guide, picked us up in his Jeep to help us find the handful of Colorado birds we missed when we were there in April.

Our first stop was at Loveland Pass on the Continental Divide and a search for the White-tailed Ptarmigan. This Ptarmigan lives its entire life above the tree line, turning all white in the winter and partly brown during the summer, needed camouflage from predators on this barren landscape.

We live literally at sea level along the Maine coast. When we suddenly thrust ourselves onto a mountain at 12,000 feet, our breathing became difficult and walking up a simple incline made our hearts beat out of our chests. Ryan led us for several miles across the boulder-strewn 'moonscape', looking for the little critters, but we had no luck. We did enjoy the comical Mountain Picas, a rabbit-like rodent that can be seen scurrying about the rocks all while emitting a panicky squeak.

We were also amazed by Ryan's billy-goat-like stamina. As we stood panting in a gully, he would race up and over a nearby peak looking for the Ptarmigans. Finally though, we called it quits and headed west toward Grand Junction, a town we had stayed in last spring. The following morning we were chasing Chukars.

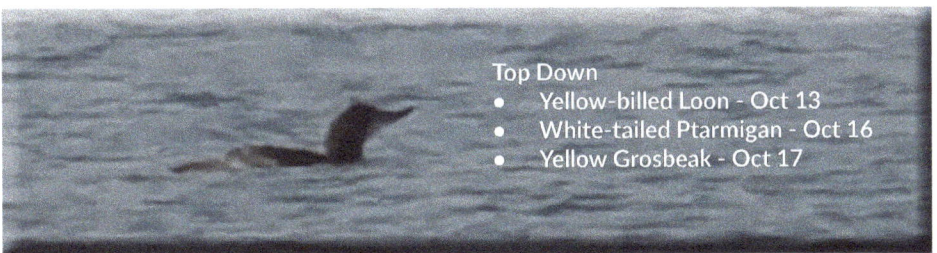

Top Down
- Yellow-billed Loon - Oct 13
- White-tailed Ptarmigan - Oct 16
- Yellow Grosbeak - Oct 17

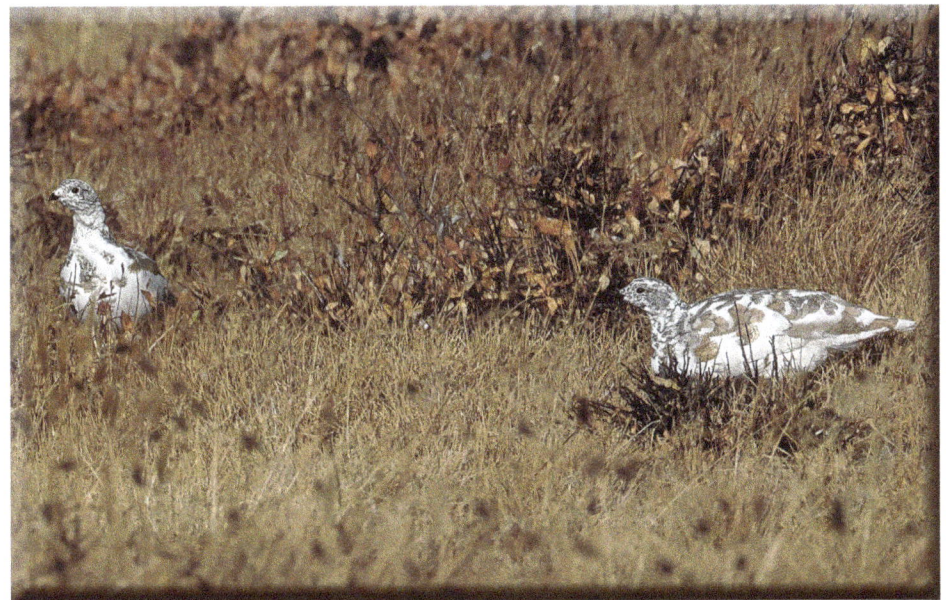

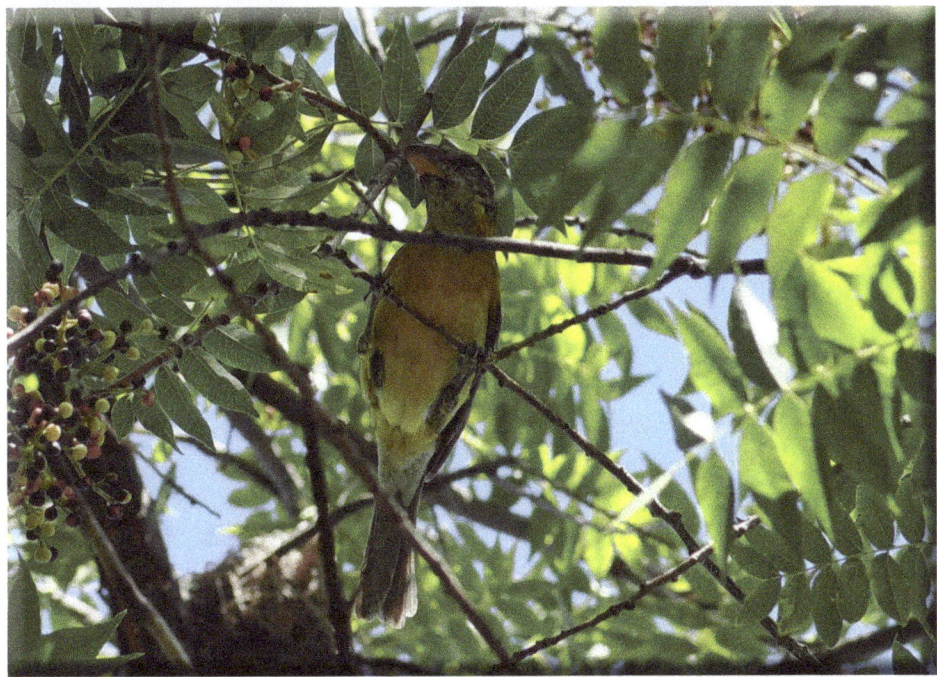

The Chukar is not native to the United States. It is a Eurasian game bird introduced to North America by sportsmen who use them to train hunting dogs. Some of these imported Chukars escaped, established breeding populations in parts of the US and are now countable during a Big Year. But not everywhere.

We often see Chukars near our home, but the population in Maine is virtually all escaped birds. So, the Chukar walking down the road in front of our house isn't countable. But, the one we heard singing in Coal Canyon was.

That evening, Ryan took us owling. When our trip began, we had seen ten of the fourteen species of Owls regularly observed in the Continental US. The tiny and elusive Boreal Owl was tonight's target. On our fourth stop, we heard one and then a second.

The following morning we were in Rocky Mountain National Park at Medicine Bow Curve, on a mountain that normally would have been covered with snow by now and inaccessible. Luck smiled on us once again and allowed us a second shot at the elusive White-tailed Ptarmigan.

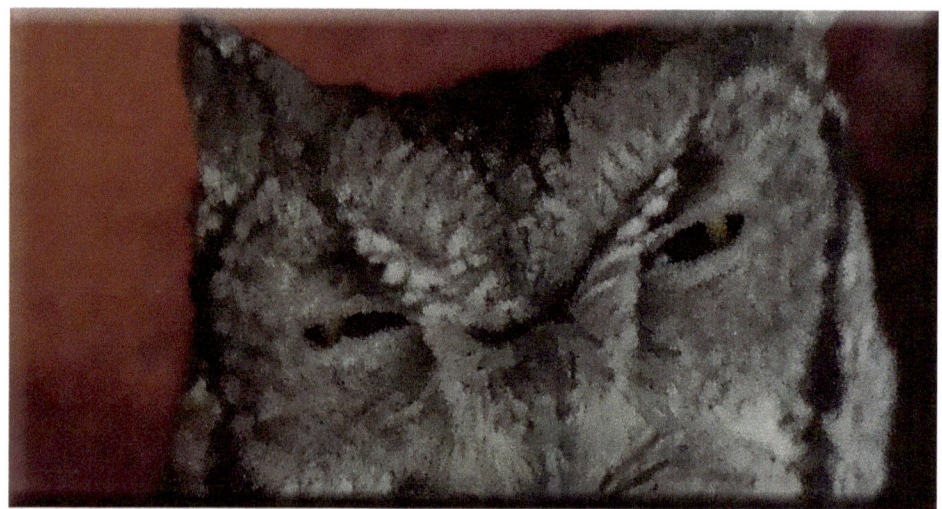

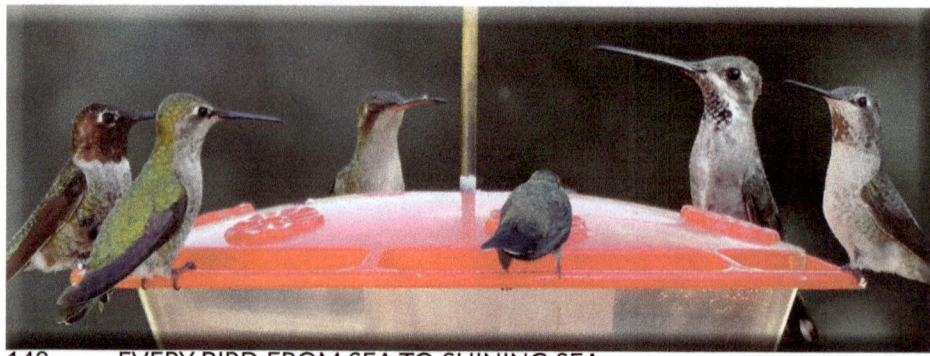

Well above the treeline, the views were spectacular as the three of us split up to search. After ninety minutes, we were exhausted (the altitude was brutal), and we waved Ryan over. We were ready to give up. While waiting for Ryan, we both suddenly heard a Ptarmigan call. A few minutes later, Ethan, out of the corner of his eye, saw a bird fly behind a distant boulder. By now Ryan had arrived, and he pointed about fifty yards down the mountain. Eight beautiful White-tailed Ptarmigans were walking toward a recently melted stream.

High-five and hugs all around ... a beautiful, unique bird, and we had really worked for it.

Arizona

Twenty-four hours later, we arrived in Phoenix, jumped in our rental car at the airport and raced east toward the Boyce Thompson Arboretum, an hour away.

Why the hurry? A Yellow Grosbeak had journeyed up from Mexico and was feeding in a Pistache tree. How lucky was that? Upon arriving, a birder was pointing up into the tree and there was the Grosbeak ... Yellow with a huge beak. Our twelfth Code Four bird of the year.

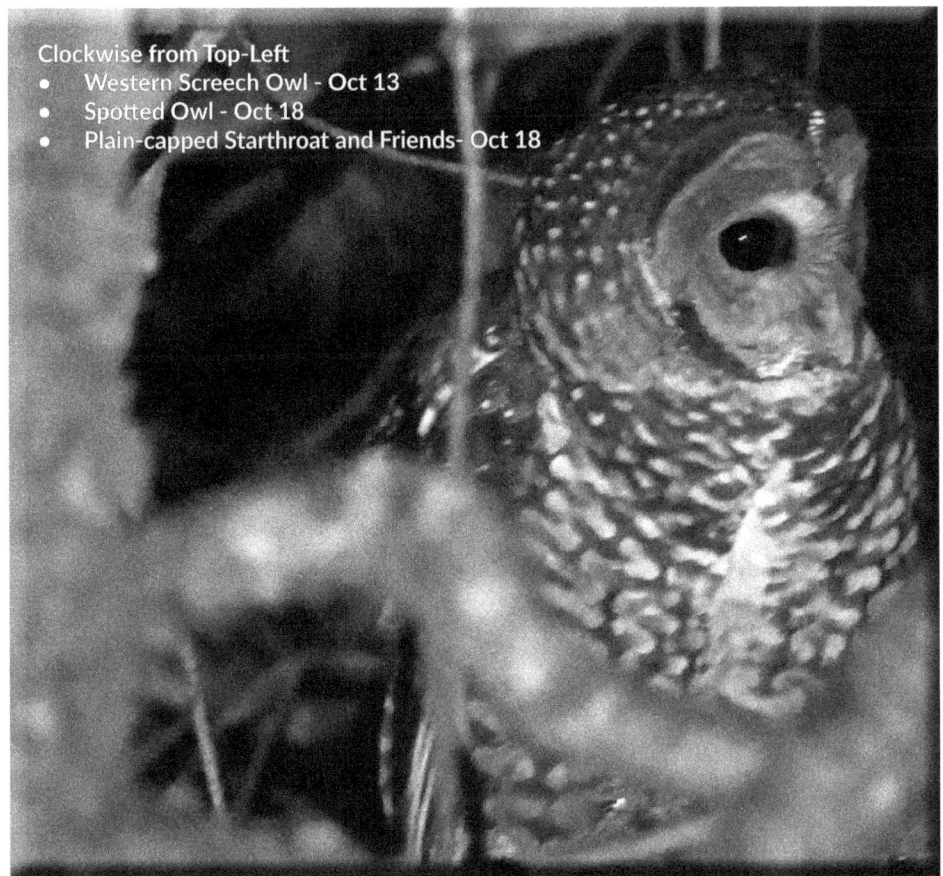

Clockwise from Top-Left
- Western Screech Owl - Oct 13
- Spotted Owl - Oct 18
- Plain-capped Starthroat and Friends- Oct 18

About fifteen minutes later a Code Three Rufous-backed Robin flew in to join the Yellow Grosbeak. A Code Three AND a Code Four in the same tree?! When we planned this trip the month before, we never predicted that. And then, that night Arizona was hit by heavy winds, and the Yellow Grosbeak moved on.

After staying in four different hotels over four nights in Colorado, we checked into a lovely Tucson ranch house for three nights, a nice change from packing and unpacking. We were charmed by the Western Screech-Owl that slept above the front door. At night he would sing from the backyard.

While on the subject of Owls, we had been looking for a Spotted Owl all year, striking out on earlier trips to Arizona, California and Washington State. Friends had raved about birding guide Kadynn Hatfield's ability to find these secretive birds, and we contracted with him to take us up nearby Mt. Lemmon on the night of October 18.

But before our Spotted Owl excursion, we had a rare Hummingbird to chase.

About an hour south of Tucson, there is a small residential community called Tubac. A significant portion of the town is made up of folks of retirement age. The homes are lovely, well maintained, and a significant number of them have hummingbird feeders. A friend who had been helping us with our Big Year learned that a Plain-capped Starthroat was coming to a feeder at a private home in Tubac. He did some public relations work for us, and the homeowners extended an invitation to come see the bird.

The Plain-capped is a large Hummingbird, perhaps 50% bigger than the Anna's, Ruby-throated and Rufous Hummers seen throughout the country. It ranges from Northwest Mexico south to Panama. We'd seen reports of Starthroat sightings in Arizona in the fall, but most seemed to be one day wonders.

We arrived at Tubac in the early afternoon, rang the doorbell of the homeowners and were invited through their house and out on their expansive patio. These folks were remarkably welcoming and generous.

They had arranged four deck chairs to give us optimal views of their three Hummingbird feeders and water fountain. And boy, did they have hummers - Black-chinned Hummingbirds, Anna's Hummingbirds, Costa's Hummingbirds, Rufous Hummingbirds, and Broad-billed Hummingbirds flew in and out, fought with and chased each other, and fed and fed and fed.

The homeowners told us that the Plain-capped Starthroat had been coming to their feeder for eighteen days in a row, but they were keeping it secret, as they had had a bad experience with over zealous bird chasers in the past.

They pointed out what tree he liked to sit in; that he favored the left-most feeder; and that he was so big he had to bend his body backwards to reach the nectar holes designed for much smaller birds.

We were warned that while this particular Starthroat was quite reliable, returning every hour to feed, he sometimes went to other feeders in the neighborhood...so no guarantees.

We only had to wait about fifteen minutes when one of the homeowners pointed, and declared, "There he is!" And no joke, this was a large Hummingbird, dwarfing the smaller Hummingbirds around it. This giant among Hummingbirds came in three times over the next 15 minutes giving us wonderful views. He then took off on his hourly respite, and we promised the homeowners that we would keep the sighting embargoed from eBird for a week.

We were back in Tucson long enough to have a quick dinner before meeting Kadynn in a shopping center parking lot north of the city.

After a twenty-mile drive up Mt. Lemmon's twisting cut-back roads, we reached a small turnoff. Together we stood on a cold, windy, remote, and dark point on the mountain and began to wait and listen. After about five minutes Ethan heard the first hoot. Then we all heard it. Ten minutes later the bird was sitting in front of us, hooting away, posing for photos, simply incredible!

On the drive down the mountain, Kadynn told us how to find a Baird's Sparrow. It was an adventuresome hike across the grassland the next day, but his directions were spot on, and we got the bird. The Baird's Sparrow was our sixth life bird in Arizona as we also picked up a Ruddy Ground Dove.

The Spotted Owl and the other birds we picked up in Arizona brought us to 700 birds for the year. Seven-hundred has long been considered a Big Year milestone. In recent years, due to eBird and social media, getting to 700 has become somewhat easier and fifteen people have cracked 700 in the Continental US/Lower 48 States. There are also quite a few more birds to chase as a number of species have been 'split' when DNA evidence showed that regionally separated sub-species were actually different species altogether.

For example, in July 2004 the American Ornithologists Union split the Canada Goose into two species: the smaller Cackling Goose and the larger Canada Goose. They also occasionally 'lump' species together ... combining multiple species into one, but there are generally more splits than lumps. On Monday, eBird rolled out

700th Bird of the Year

Spotted Owl

October 18, 7:22 PM

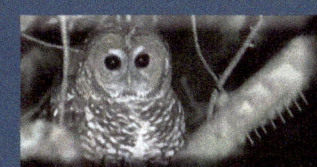

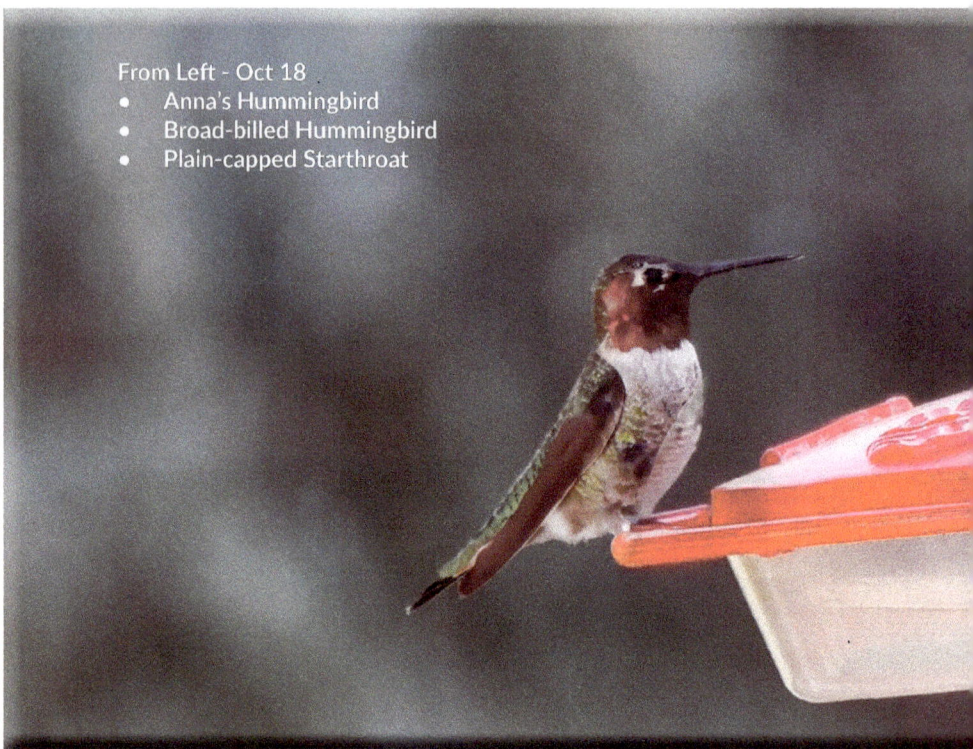

From Left - Oct 18
- Anna's Hummingbird
- Broad-billed Hummingbird
- Plain-capped Starthroat

their 2024 'splits' and our year count anticlimactically jumped to from 698 to 700.

We knew the splits were coming and hugged when we saw the new Scopoli's Shearwater in June and Cocos Booby in September, but it would have been nice to have the Spotted Owl put us over the top instead of an accounting method. But hey, we never thought we'd get anywhere close to this many birds, and we did it!

The Birds That Got Away

While we had a very successful Big Year, we still dipped on (or missed) a number of birds:

We searched for the American Three-toed Woodpecker in Northern Maine, Washington State, Oregon and Colorado but only saw signs where this bird had flaked bark off trees.

On one ridiculous effort, we heard a Woodpecker tapping deep in the woods off a Colorado trail. After bushwhacking for 20 minutes, we found that the tapping was the wind blowing a branch against a tree.

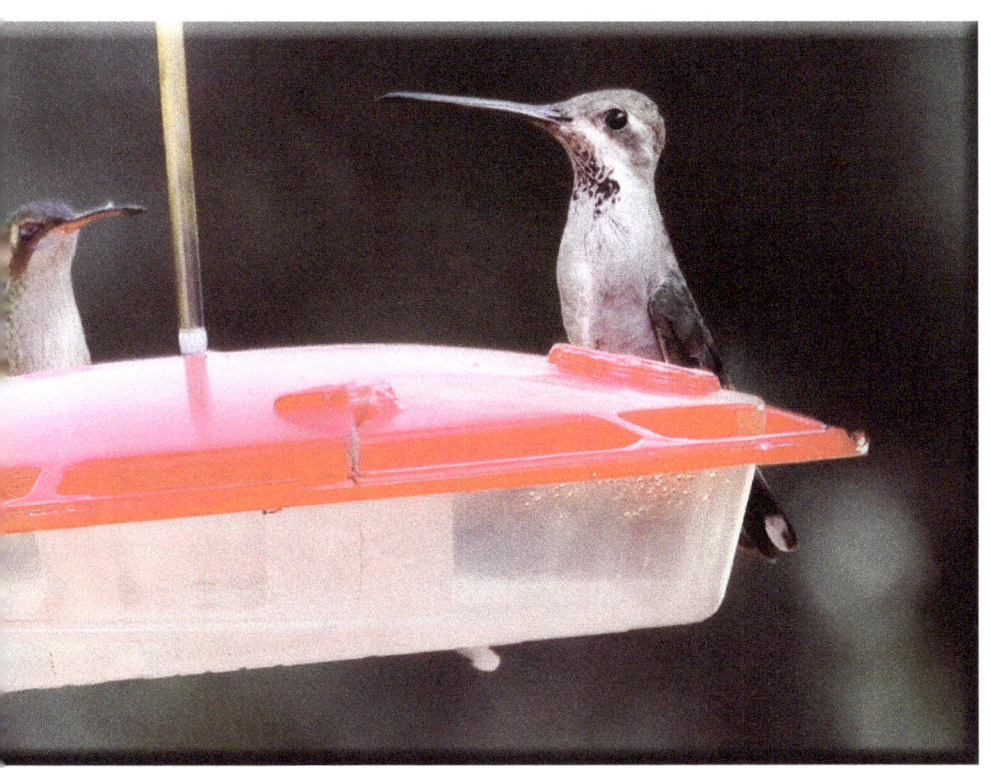

The Mountain Quail is a relatively common bird that we had seen in previous trips to the west coast, but it eluded us this year ... despite many hours searching in the mountains.

One morning we were driving up a steep road in ideal Mountain Quail habitat when Ingrid remarked, "Wouldn't it be great if a Mountain Quail ran across the road in front of us?" As if on cue a minute later, Ethan slammed on the brakes to avoid the Quail that had suddenly darted into the road. Much laughter and hugs followed; we had our Mountain Quail! Then the car got very quiet, as we both without conferring opened up our field guides to Mountain Quail ... and then California Quail. Sadly, the bird had been a California Quail.

Other problematic birds: Sharp-tailed Grouse, Dusky Grouse and Gray Partridge.

Orioles

Orioles are colorful songbirds whose regional distributions in the Lower 48 United States reflect their preferences for habitat and climate.

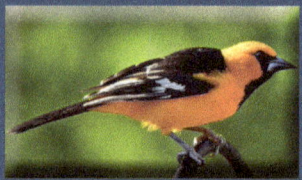

The Altamira Oriole is largely confined to southern Texas, particularly in the Rio Grande Valley, where subtropical woodlands and scrub provide a their preferred habitat.

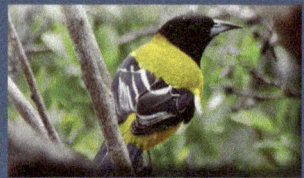

The Audubon's Oriole, similarly limited to the southernmost regions of Texas, is found in dense thickets and woodlands, often in areas with mesquite and live oak. Both species reach the northernmost part of their range in the U.S. and are common targets for birders visiting southern Texas.

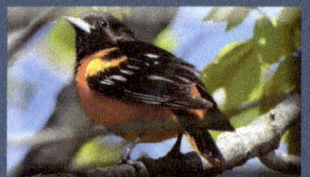

The Baltimore Oriole is widespread across the eastern and central United States during the breeding season. Its range extends from the Great Plains eastward, and the bird is often seen in parks, backyards, and woodlands with deciduous trees.

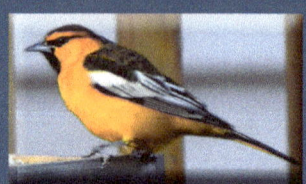

In contrast, the Bullock's Oriole occupies the western half of the United States, favoring riparian areas, open woodlands, and urban spaces.

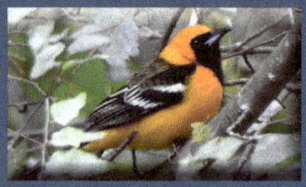

The Hooded Oriole is predominantly a southwestern species, with a range that includes parts of Arizona, New Mexico, California, and Texas. These birds favor desert regions, gardens, and areas with palm trees, often nesting in urban areas.

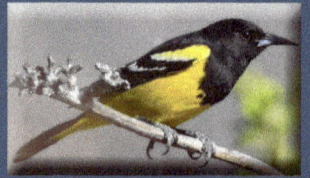

Similarly, the Scott's Oriole is a bird of the arid Southwest, commonly found in scrub lands, yucca-dotted deserts, and grassy areas from southern California through Texas. Both species' affinity for dry environments sets them apart from other orioles.

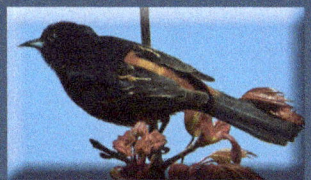

The Orchard Oriole, the smallest of the group, breeds across much of the eastern and central U.S., occupying open woodlands, orchards, and riverbanks.

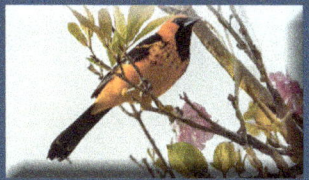

The Spot-breasted Oriole, on the other hand, is restricted to southeastern Florida, where it was introduced and has since become established in suburban areas and parks.

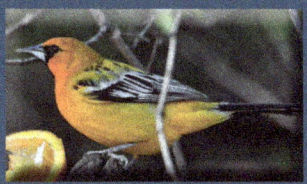

Finally, the Steak-backed Oriole, is a Mexican species, rarely seen in the Continental USA.   We were lucky enough to see a pair in April, just east of Phoenix.

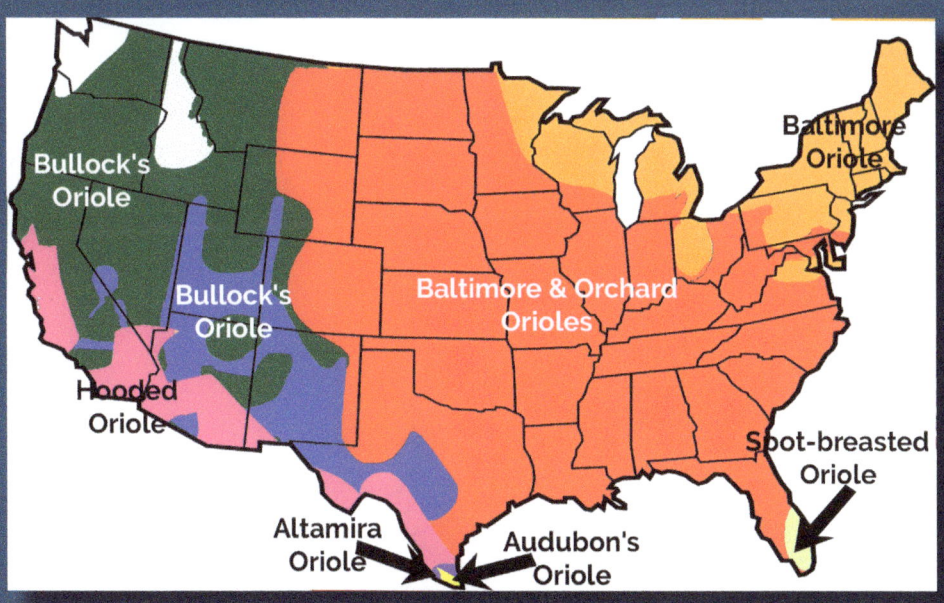

November

Travel	#
Plane Flights	2
Rental Cars	1
Nights Away	8
Boat Trips	0

State	Year Birds
Massachusetts	1
Texas	4
Total	5

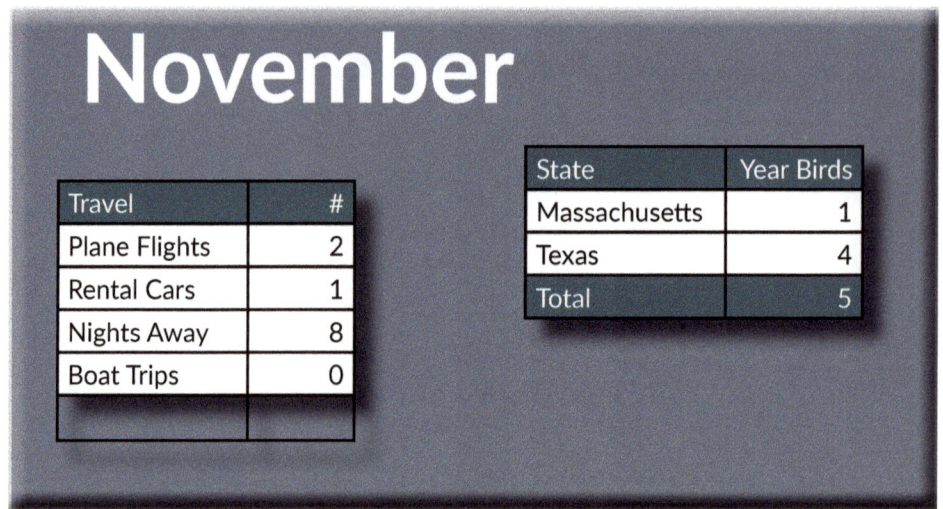

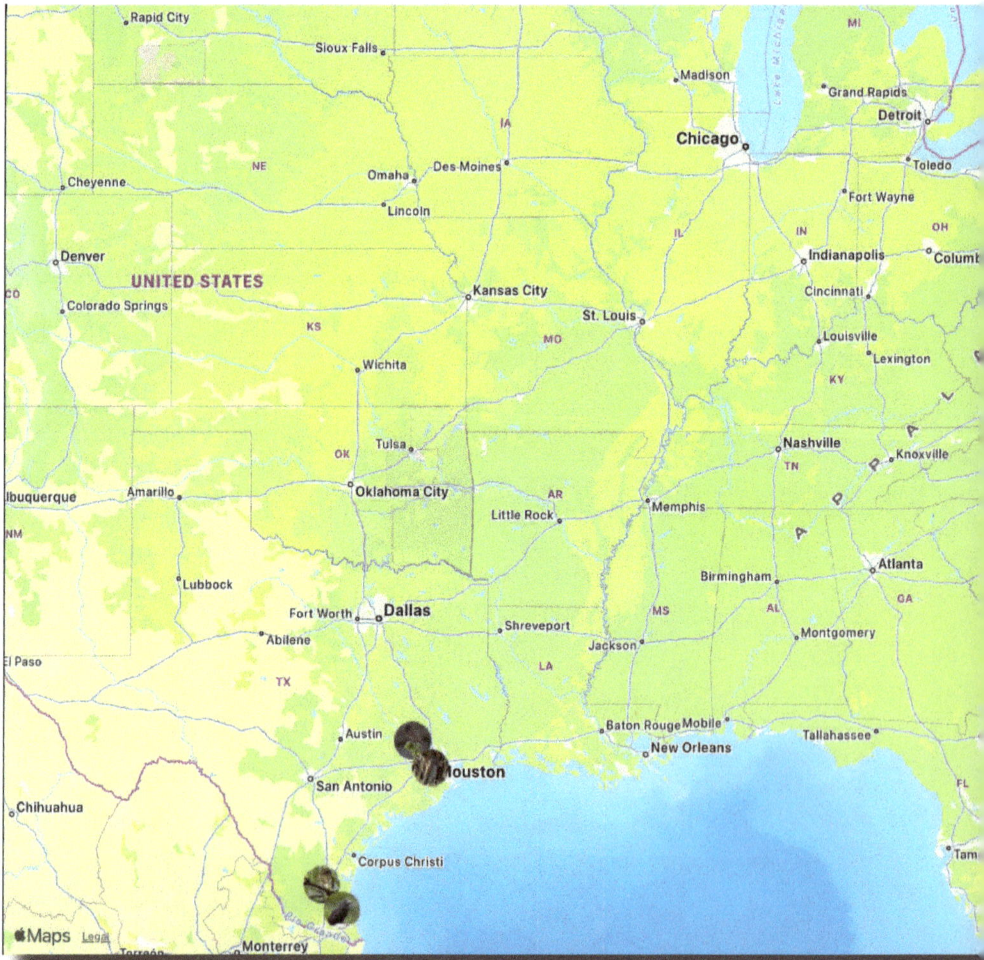

Common Gull

Once back home in Maine, we prepared for a minor construction project, babysat the world's most adorable grandson and planned for a final push into Texas and the Gulf Coast later in the month.

In the birding community, November is known as vagrant season as migrating birds occasionally show up in the darnedest places. We had overnight bags packed and sitting by the door as we waited for something chaseable to show up.

On Thursday, our phones started to buzz as a Common Gull had been found on a resort golf course in Rockport, Maine just an hour away. Vagrancy season had begun!!! Sadly, though, we already had a Common Gull for the year in a Connecticut Walmart parking lot back in January. So, we thanked each of our callers and went about our chores.

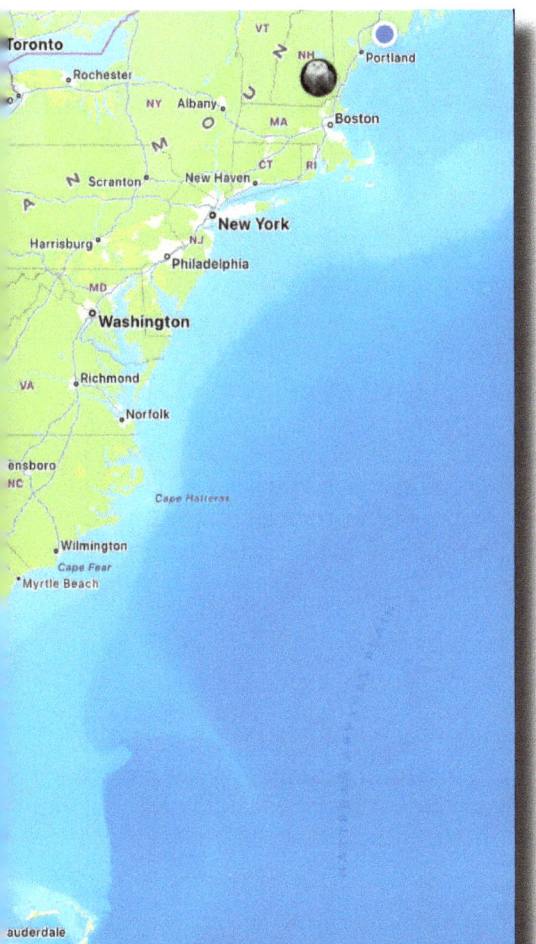

The Common Gull used to be called the "Mew Gull", with populations found in Europe, Siberia, Alaska and the North American West Coast. In 2021, the Mew Gull was split into the aforementioned "Common Gull" and the "Short-billed Gull".

Common Gull sightings in Maine are very rare, with confirmed sightings in 2000, 2022 and this past January. The latter was seen by our friend Rich Garrigus who had the foresight to photograph the bird before it disappeared.

Ingrid had plans to spend time with our grandson, and Ethan really wanted a Common Gull for his Maine list. So, for one of the rare times this year, we went in different directions. Ethan north and Ingrid south.

Ethan spent over an hour and a half walking the Samoset Resort's golf course, then closed for the season, which was covered with hundreds of gulls. He would approach a flock and go through the birds one at a time, quickly eliminating the larger Great Black-backed Gulls and American Herring Gulls and then going through

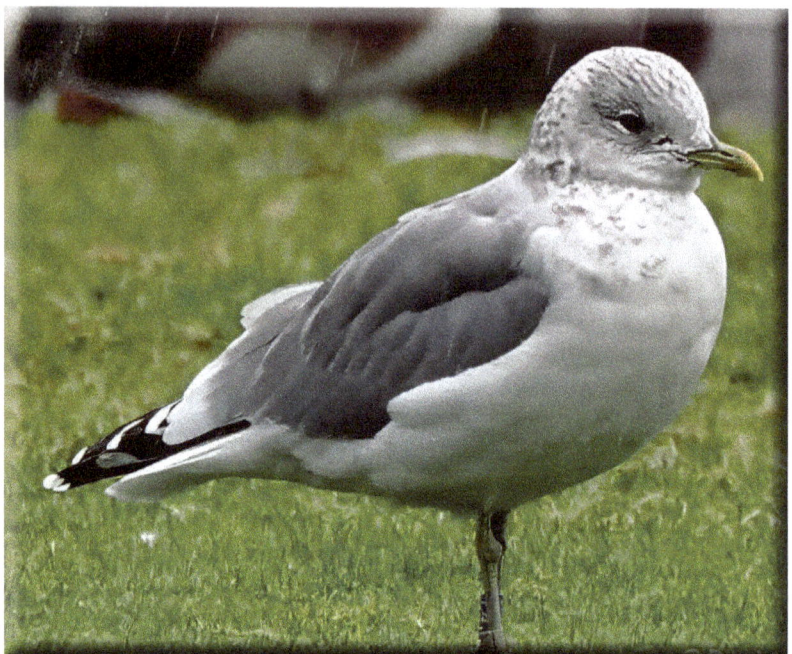
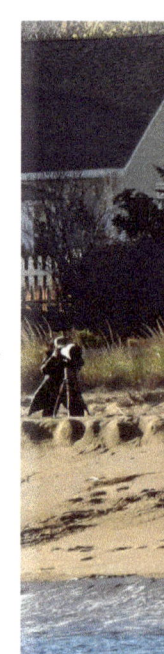

smaller Ring-billed Gulls, hoping to find a single bird with a distinctive bill and subtly darker mantle.

After failing miserably, he went back to the car, grabbed his spotting scope and planned to scan through a flock of Ring-bills hanging out by a large pond.

He set up the scope, casually pointed it at the flock, looked in the eye piece, and there was the Common Gull! Ethan snapped a bunch of photos, put them out on the Maine Rare Bird Alert and eBird, and within ten minutes other birders started to arrive.

Now here is where the story got really interesting. Doug Hitchcox, Maine Audubon's Staff Naturalist and an expert on birding in Maine, noticed something different between the photos of the bird taken on Thursday and the one Ethan (and others) took on Friday. The Friday bird had a blue ID band on it. Thursday's bird did not.

This was a second Common Gull … in the same location!

We all went to work trying to read the code on the leg from distant photos. Working with Doug and birding friend Magill Weber, we determined that the code was 74J, which means this bird was banded in Denmark. This same bird was sighted in Cohasset, Massachusetts in 2018. Had this bird been on this side of the Atlantic for six years?

Snowy Owl

November remained a quiet month. There were lots of vagrants moving around

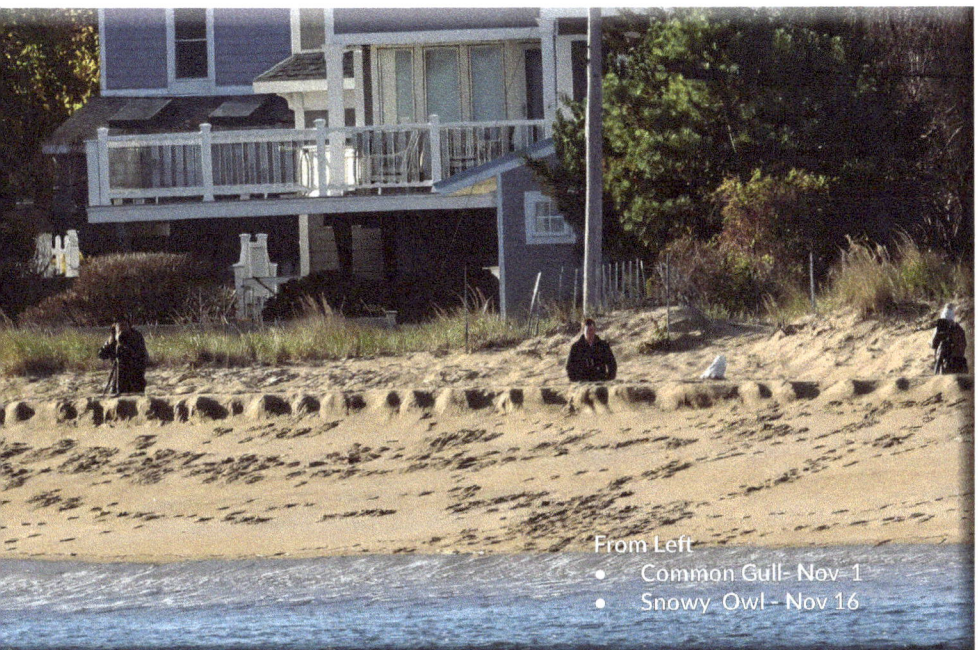

From Left
- Common Gull- Nov 1
- Snowy Owl - Nov 16

New England - a Rufous Hummingbird in Maine, a Scissor-tailed Flycatcher in Massachusetts and Cave Swallows all over the place - all rare birds for the Northeast but common birds in the south, and birds we had picked up long ago.

Late in the week, we began to notice an interesting trend. For the first time since early 2022, Snowy Owls started to appear in decent numbers in the Continental United States. Some New England winters we see lots of Snowy Owls - sometimes as many as three in a single morning. And then there are winters like the last two (2022-2023 and 2023-2024) when they are not seen at all.

On November 12, two Snowy Owls were seen, one in Wisconsin and the other in Michigan. The next day, three birds were seen, ranging from Ohio to Massachusetts. On the 14th, a new Snowy was reported in upstate NY. Then, on the 15th, nineteen birds were reported across the northern states, with several of the reports coming from Massachusetts.

The next morning we were in the car at dawn heading for Massachusetts hoping to add a Snowy Owl to our Big Year list. Our dear New Hampshire friends, Maura and Karen, met us, and we began to look for Snowy Owls.

What is the best way to find a Snowy Owl, you ask? The best tip is to look for a whole bunch of cars and folks with expensive optical gear all pointed in the same direction. In most cases, they will be looking at a Snowy Owl.

We found the Snowy Owl paparazzi staring at a sand berm about six hundred yards away. There sat a Snowy Owl, bird # 702 for the year.

And then we witnessed one of the problems associated with owling - people getting too close to the bird. As a rule of thumb, if an Owl is visibly reacting to your presence — fidgeting, staring at you, head-bobbing or changing position, you're too close, and need to back off immediately.

But as so often happens, some photographers were determined to get the perfect up close shot and eventually, thanks to their carelessness and inconsideration, the owl took off to the south. This was unfortunate both for the Owl and for the people who had just arrived at our distant location and missed seeing it.

Texas for the Third Time

By the end of October, we had spent 130 days away from home. This included thirty-six take offs and landings, nineteen rental cars and twelve boat trips.

Then in November, it kind of stopped. Short of the Snowy Owl, there wasn't much to be found in the Northeast. Therefore, when we headed to the Portland International Jetport on Sunday, we were giddy to be on the road again.

We landed in Houston mid-afternoon and traveled to the Houston Reservoir and its wooded trails surrounded by condominiums, apartment buildings and busy highways. We were looking for a bird from the Indian subcontinent, the Red-vented Bulbul. A popular caged bird kept as pets, enough have escaped in Houston to form a small breeding population in the wild, if you want to call downtown Houston "the wild."

Known for its song, we had hoped to hear the Red-vented Bulbuls, and we did. But it was so faint up against the traffic noise that it wasn't very helpful. Finally, we saw a couple of medium-sized birds fly from tree to tree with the highway as a backdrop. When they perched, we had our Bulbuls...Bird # 703 of the year.

The next morning we headed to Galveston Island State Park in search of a Black Rail, often considered the most elusive of North American Breeding Birds. The size of a small hen, this black bird with an exotic looking red eye is almost never seen, as it lives among reeds, rarely emerging. During breeding season, males can be heard at night doing their "ki-ki-krr" song quite aggressively, but we had missed the breeding season.

So, we spent Monday morning walking through the Galveston marshes, getting eaten by mosquitoes and hoping that we wouldn't run across any alligators. Periodically we would play a Black Rail call, and we got responses several times. Countable ... #704 but very unsatisfying.

Then as we were driving out of the park, on a narrow road with marshy reeds on both sides, a small dark bird popped up and flew in front of the car and dropped down into the reeds. It was a two-second glimpse at best and certainly too short to find our cameras, aim and focus, but we had just seen a Black Rail. Wow!

Thank You

Thanks to Alex Lamoreaux, Amy Segars, Andy Baker, Bradley Whitaker, Brandon Sullivan, Brian Patterson, Cameron Cox, Chuck Barnes, David Gersten, David McQuade, David Simpson, Doug Hitchcox, Eddy Edwards, Edward Abbey, Ezekiel Dobson, Ezra Cohen, Fred Hochstaedter, Glenn Hodgkins, Gordon Payne, Greg Miller, Hanyang Ye, Jake Molhmann, Jake Thompson, Janice Travis, John Yerger, Judd Brink, Kadynn Hatfield, Kate Sutherland, Kathie Brown, Kathy Rawdon, Killian Sullivan, JJ Furuno, Linda Gardrel, Lisa Bonato, Louis Bevier, Malcom Burson, Magil Weber, Marian Zimmerman, Mary Jo Ballator, Maya Furuno, Paula Aschim, Patrick Magee, Rob Spiers, Richard Garrigus, Robin Ohrt, Ryan Dibala, Sally Slick, Simon Kiacz, Sister Marty Dermody, Tammy McQuade, Tanner Whitaker, Tova Mellen and Zach Johnson.

And many others that helped us along the way

Tuesday was spent at the famous King Ranch. At 825,000 acres, it is the biggest ranch in the United States. This cattle ranch is larger than Rhode Island and the nation of Luxembourg. In addition to cattle and agriculture, King Ranch offers hunting and guided tours, including birding trips.

And King Ranch was our opportunity to get a rare Ferruginous-Pygmy Owl, the only Owl in the lower 48 states that we had yet to see or hear. We contacted the ranch and hired Janice Travis to help us find this rare species.

We met Janice at one of the electronic gates, and she escorted us to a cluster of ranch houses where we left our car and continued in her van. From there we were transported into a world we had only seen in the movies: fields of grazing cattle, deer with enormous racks, cowboys, narrow dirt roads through the Mesquite and gates that had to be opened and closed every five minutes or so.

The soil at that part of the ranch is very sandy and only Mesquite and grasses can grow there, but in the few areas where there is water, one finds Oak Islands, where Live Oaks thrive on the ranch. These 'islands' are where you find the Ferruginous-Pygmy Owls. Here the owls nest in holes excavated by Golden-fronted Woodpeckers.

Janice brought us to one of these Oak Islands, and we spent three hours looking for the tiny six-inch creatures. She crawled through thickets while we explored more accessible nooks. With a half hour left before we had to leave, we sat down for lunch and Janice told us that what we were experiencing with the Owl was unusual, not having at least heard one of the two to four Owls living in this Oak Island.

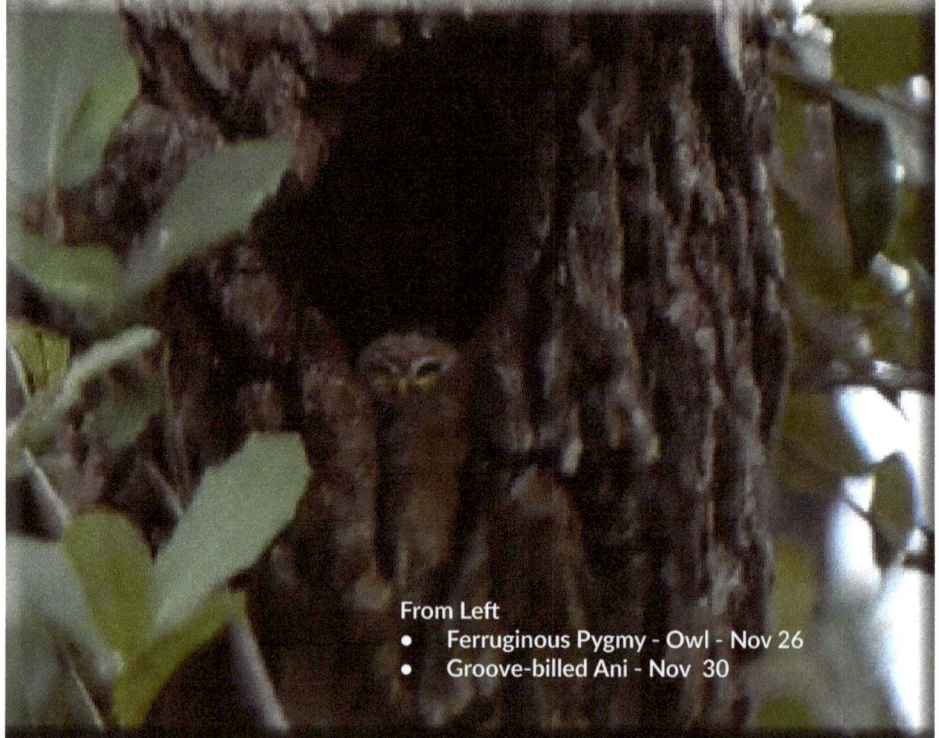

From Left
- Ferruginous Pygmy - Owl - Nov 26
- Groove-billed Ani - Nov 30

We had gone back to searching, the three of us going in different directions, when we heard it. The two of us made our way toward the sound. The bird was calling from deep in the tangles. Janice arrived, and we moved closer to the sound. And then it stopped.

The Ferruginous-Pygmy Owl had called loudly for about a minute, but we never got our eyes on the elusive creature. But identifying a bird by sound is countable in a Big Year, making it bird # 705 and our twentieth Owl.

A week later we were reviewing photos of the Ranch, when we noticed the Owl staring at us from the bottom of the nesting hole.

Groove-billed Ani

The Groove-billed Ani is a large, black bird with a long tail and a huge honker of a bill. Related to Cuckoos, it breeds in the summer in southern Texas. They were still being seen regularly two weeks before our trip, but we feared we may have gotten there too late to get one.

On our way to the Rio Grande Valley, we stopped at San Juan Wetlands Park where a pair had been seen a few days before. But no luck. However, we had never birded in this park before and discovered it to be a terrific spot. In just one hour, we observed thirty-four species there.

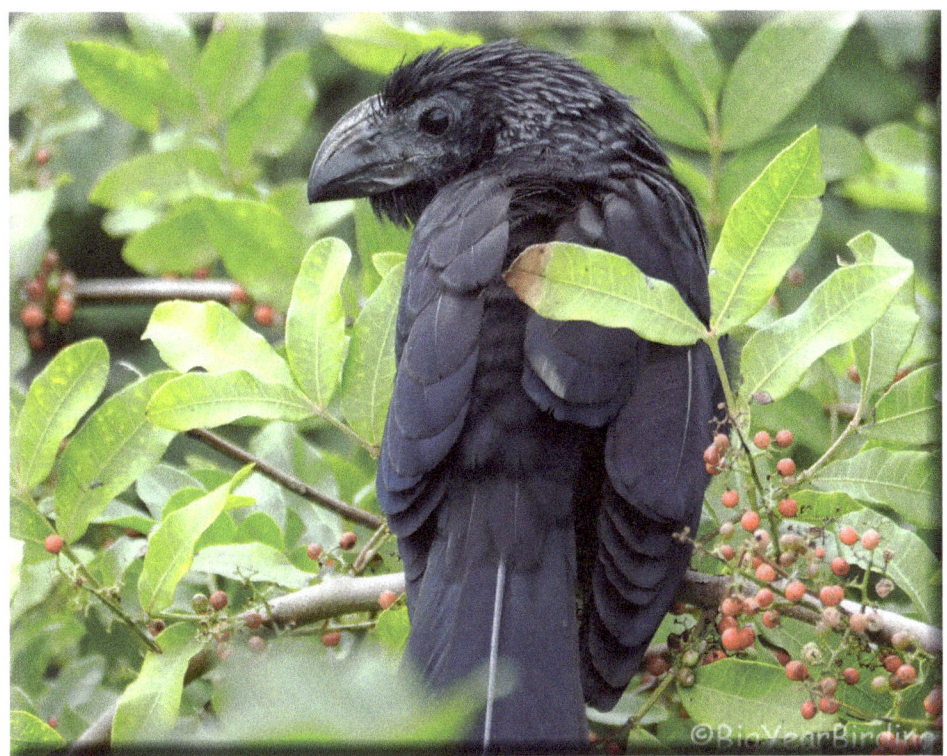

Another location we had heard a lot about from other birders but had not visited was Salineño Wildlife Preserve, which sits on the north side of the Rio Grande. There have been numerous times when a rarity reported at Santa Margarita Ranch, just half a mile away, has also been seen here. We had our fingers crossed that one of our target birds, the Hooked-billed Kite, might make an appearance.

As with many Texas wildlife preserves, Salineño has park hosts. Park hosts volunteer to maintain bird feeders and habitat and interact with the public in exchange for a site at which to park their RVs for the season. In this case, the park hosts were a couple from Maine, and, incredibly, three other birders who were there when we arrived at the feeding station were also from Maine. An invasion of Texas by Mainers!

Unfortunately, an hour of scoping from the river bank did not turn up any Hook-billed Kites. Not to worry, we were scheduled to visit the ranch in a couple of days.

The next morning was Thanksgiving, and we took a couple of days off from birding and headed north to Jourdanton, Texas, just south of San Antonio. Here we enjoyed two days with our son and daughter-in-law.

With full bellies, we returned to our number one mission, finding a Groove-billed Ani. This quest took us to South Padre Island where one had been reported that very morning along the boardwalk at the Convention Center. This sounded promising!

Texas was experiencing a drought at the time, attracting birds to any available source of freshwater. Our strategy when we arrived put Ethan on stake-out at the water feature while Ingrid walked up and down the boardwalk. After about an hour of searching, Ingrid's eyes fell upon the Ani tucked among the leaves of a Pepper bush where he was feasting on berries. After snapping a quick photo, she called Ethan and got him on the bird. Bird # 706!

In February we made a trip to Santa Margarita Ranch in Roma, Texas. We made a return trip with the hope of adding the Hook-billed Kite to our year and life lists. This Kite is a Mexican bird that feeds on terrestrial snails. It is rarely seen north of Mexico.

The ranch is located along the Rio Grande and is traversed by the border wall, which is about a mile from the river. Here, all birding is done between the wall and the river. You actually walk through a door in the wall to get to the birding spots. A truly unique experience.

We began our day on the bluff overlooking the Rio Grande, the location from which the Kites are most often seen. After a three hour wait, the Kites took pity on us, came in and flew around the area before perching for a VERY distant photo. Bird # 707.

We spent the rest of the afternoon at the ranch enjoying a return visit with many of the same birds we had seen in February, but got much more extensive looks and better photos. This was a real treat, as so many of these birds we will likely never see again. Add to this the joy of birding just for the sake of birding and not aggressively chasing one bird after another, and it was a fantastic day.

This marked the end of the last planned trip of our Big Year.

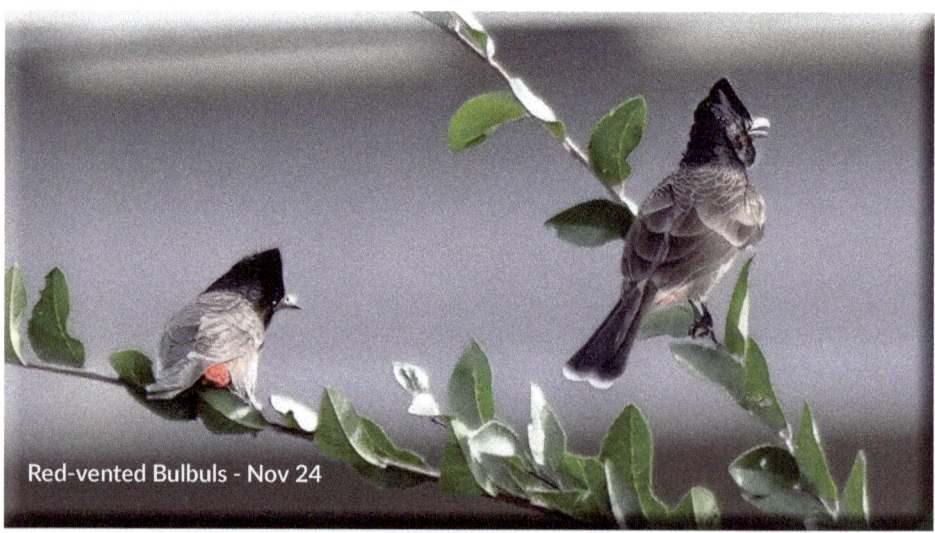

Red-vented Bulbuls - Nov 24

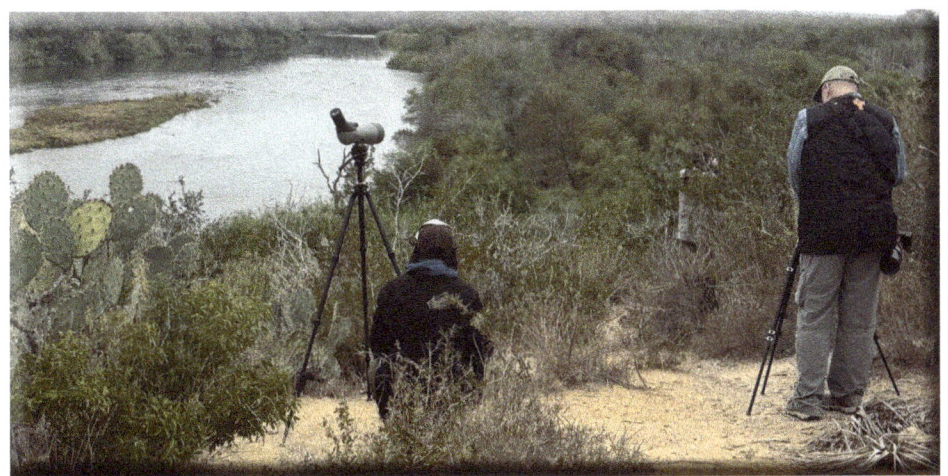

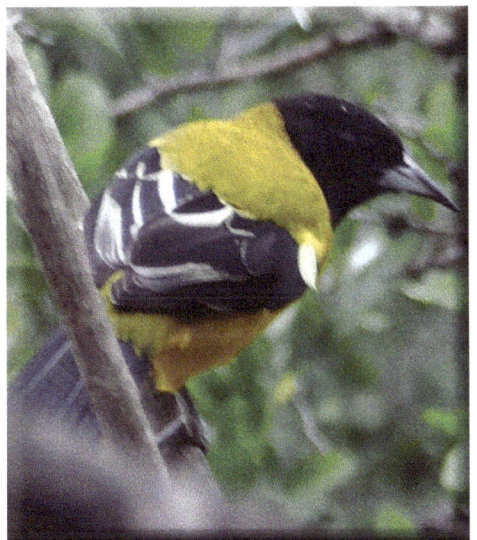
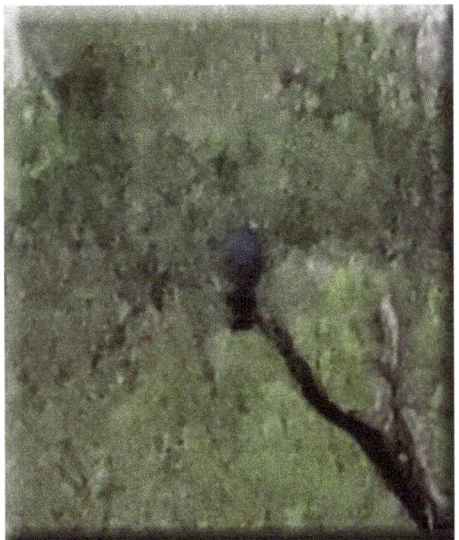

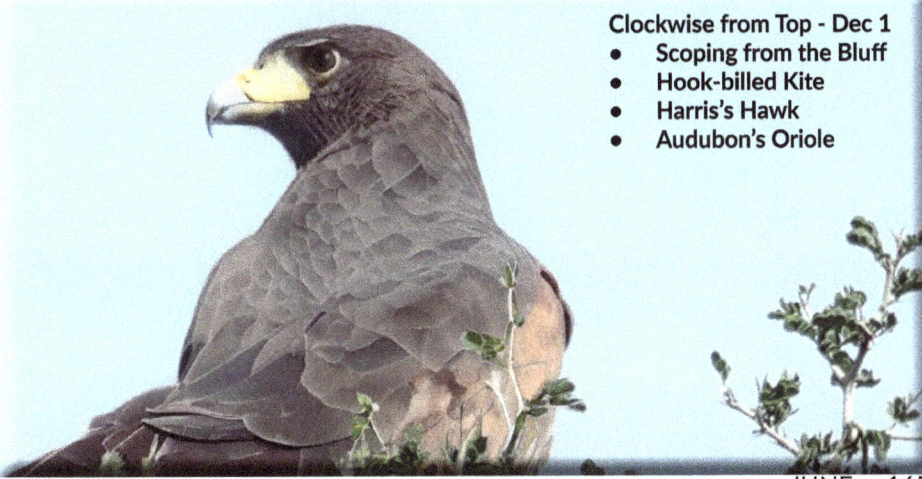

Clockwise from Top - Dec 1
- Scoping from the Bluff
- Hook-billed Kite
- Harris's Hawk
- Audubon's Oriole

December

Travel	#
Plane Flights	2
Rental Cars	1
Nights Away	3
Boat Trips	2

State	Year Birds
Massachusetts	1
Texas	1
Total	2

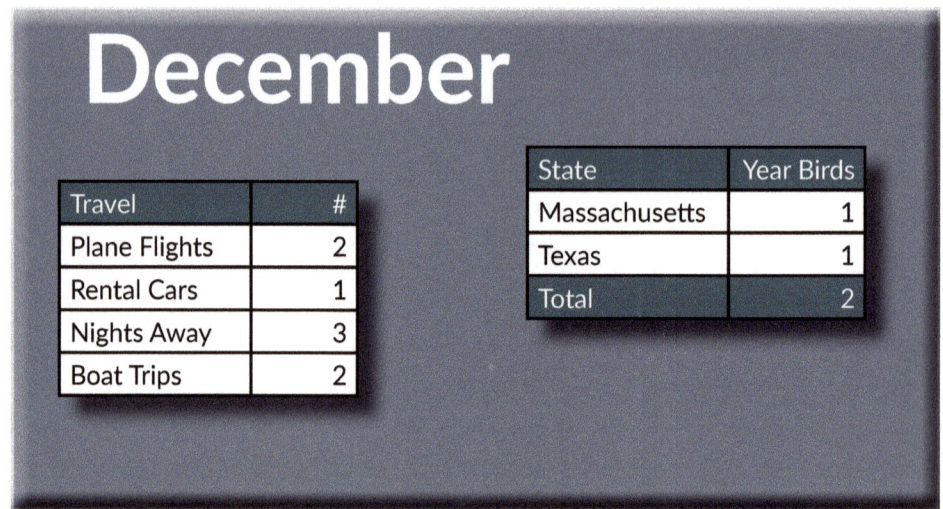

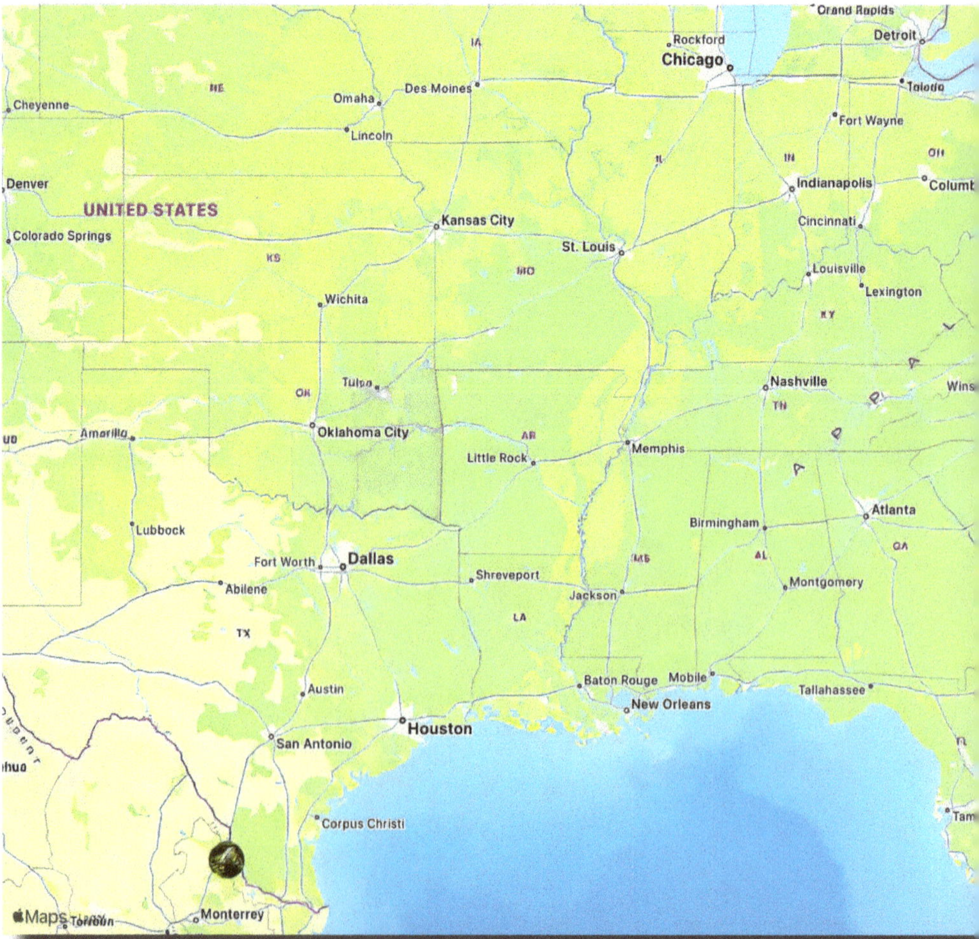

All Good Things ...

During a Big Year, there is a lot of time for reading ... long car rides, plane flights and insomnia caused by too much Tex-Mex.

During the year, Ingrid had enjoyed a series of books set on Nantucket Island written by author Elin Hilderbrand. These stories brought back memories of visits to Nantucket during her childhood.

While in Texas, we learned of a Northern Lapwing foraging on the farm fields of Nantucket. A Eurasian bird, it should have been in Southern Spain or Northern Africa by then, and we wanted one more bird for our Big Year.

Unfortunately, being in Texas and given that it was Thanksgiving weekend, the logistics (and expense) of getting to an island 30 miles off of Cape Cod from Houston were prohibitive.

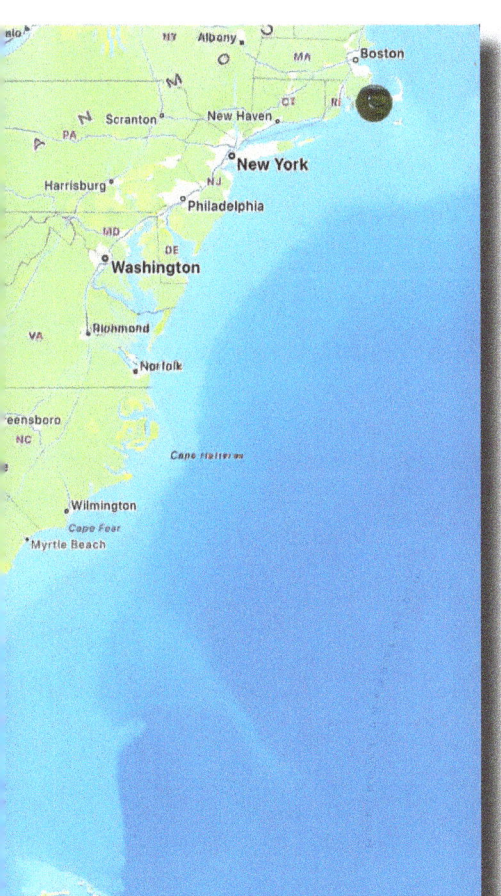

Once back at home in Maine, we began to look for a window to get to Nantucket. But New England storms, the multi-day Christmas Stroll festival on the island and appointments all made things difficult

And how long would the Northern Lapwing remain on Nantucket?

Finally, on Monday, December 9 we had an opening:
- Low winds on Nantucket Sound that would allow the ferries to run
- Mild weather on the Island
- The Christmas Festival was over
- And incredibly, the bird was still being reported

When we arrived at the Hyannis Ferry, we watched 350 Christmas Stroll festival-goers unload, while only a couple dozen riders joined us for the trip out to the island.

We sat up in the glassed-in bow of the high speed catamaran, which makes the journey to Nantucket in an hour.

We entertained (or annoyed) our fellow passengers by calling out the birds that we passed "Brant, Surf Scoter, Long-tail, Dovekie, Razorbill".

One of two large islands located off of Cape Cod - the other being Martha's Vineyard - Nantucket was once a major whaling port. Today, it is better known as a picturesque tourist destination.

Nantucket was just like Ingrid remembered it ... stately Sea Captain homes with weathered shakes, tasteful shops, a whaling museum, cobblestone roads and brick sidewalks. This was Ethan's first visit; he was impressed by the three bedroom houses for sale at 3.5 million dollars!

We rented a car to get to the agricultural areas outside of town and struggled a bit to find the solar fields and compost area, but when we did, we were able to get the Northern Lapwing in our spotting scope in less than a minute. Thankfully, it was still here.

We ended up with 708 birds for the year, which put us in second place. We had hoped for 600 and maybe the top fifteen.

Final Bird of the Year

Year Bird # 708

Northern Lapwing

December 9, 2:10 PM

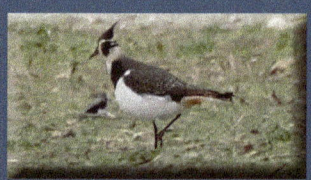

Ezekiel Dobson

The winner was Ezekiel Dobson, a 20 year old who crisscrossed the country in his car, often sleeping in it. He accumulated an incredible 757 birds breaking the 2022 record of 751. We communicated with Ezekiel off and on throughout the year and helped each other get on specific birds. Incredibly we only ran into him once ... on Long Island chasing the Northern Wheatear.

The previous Lower 48 State Record had been

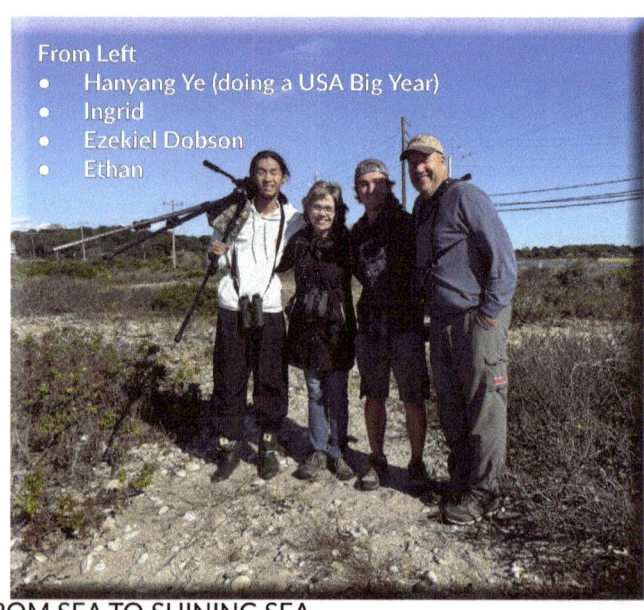

From Left
- Hanyang Ye (doing a USA Big Year)
- Ingrid
- Ezekiel Dobson
- Ethan

set in 2022 by two brothers from Tennessee, Victor and Rueben Stoll. While planning for our Big Year, Ethan announced confidently that the Stoll record was unbreakable. Ezekiel proved Ethan wrong.

Ezekiel's record breaking bird was a Fork-tailed Flycatcher in Florida, a rarity that stayed for two weeks but was gone by the time we were able to fly back to Florida.

All told, we spent 141 nights away from home to get our 708 species. We are sure Ezekiel spent at least twice as much time on the road as we did, and we salute his commitment, energy, ambition and youth!

Points of the Compass

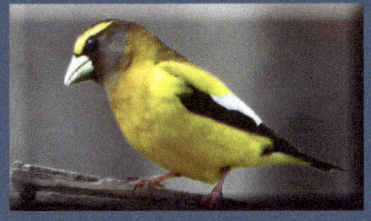

Our Northernmost bird of the year was an Evening Grosbeak in Minnesota.

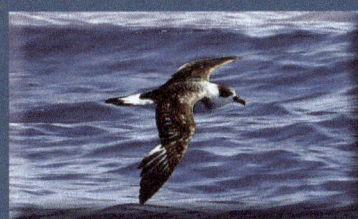

The Southernmost was a Black-capped Petrel that flew past our boat on the ride back to Key West from the Dry Tortugas,

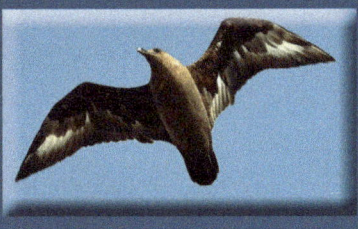

The Easternmost bird was the South Polar Skua on a Whale Watch out of Bar Harbor, Maine.

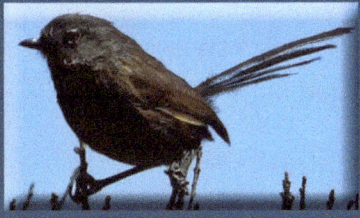

And the Western Most bird was the Wrentit in Newport, Oregon.

Woody Had It Right

We ended our Big Year very happy and grateful for all the birds that we saw, people we met, and the unforgettable experiences we shared together. Our stories will last us a lifetime!

We named this book *Every Bird from Sea to Shining Sea*, as a nod to Woody Guthrie's ode to America, "This Land is Your Land." While our twelve month adventure was an effort to see as many birds as possible, what will stick in our mind in the years ahead will be America itself.

We saw the towering skyscrapers of Manhattan Island and the six-toed cats of Ernest Hemingway's House in Key West.

We sweltered in the heat of Phoenix, AZ and two hours later drove through a snow storm in Flagstaff.

We crossed the floating bridges of Washington State and the 17.6 mile long Chesapeake Bay Bridge-Tunnel.

We passed NASA's launch facilities in Cape Canaveral, FL, SpaceX's in Brownsville, TX and Vandenberg Space Force Base in California.

We ate crab legs in Washington State and authentic Mexican food in Arizona.

We toured the magnificent natural monuments of Arches National Park and the Pueblo-style architecture of Santa Fe.

We fought off sea sickness on a boat in Monterey Bay and plucked skin piercing briers off of our clothes on a Texas Ranch.

We saw trains cars that went on for miles and Amish buggies sharing the road.

We saw the Redwood Forest and the Gulf Stream Waters ... this land was made for you and me.

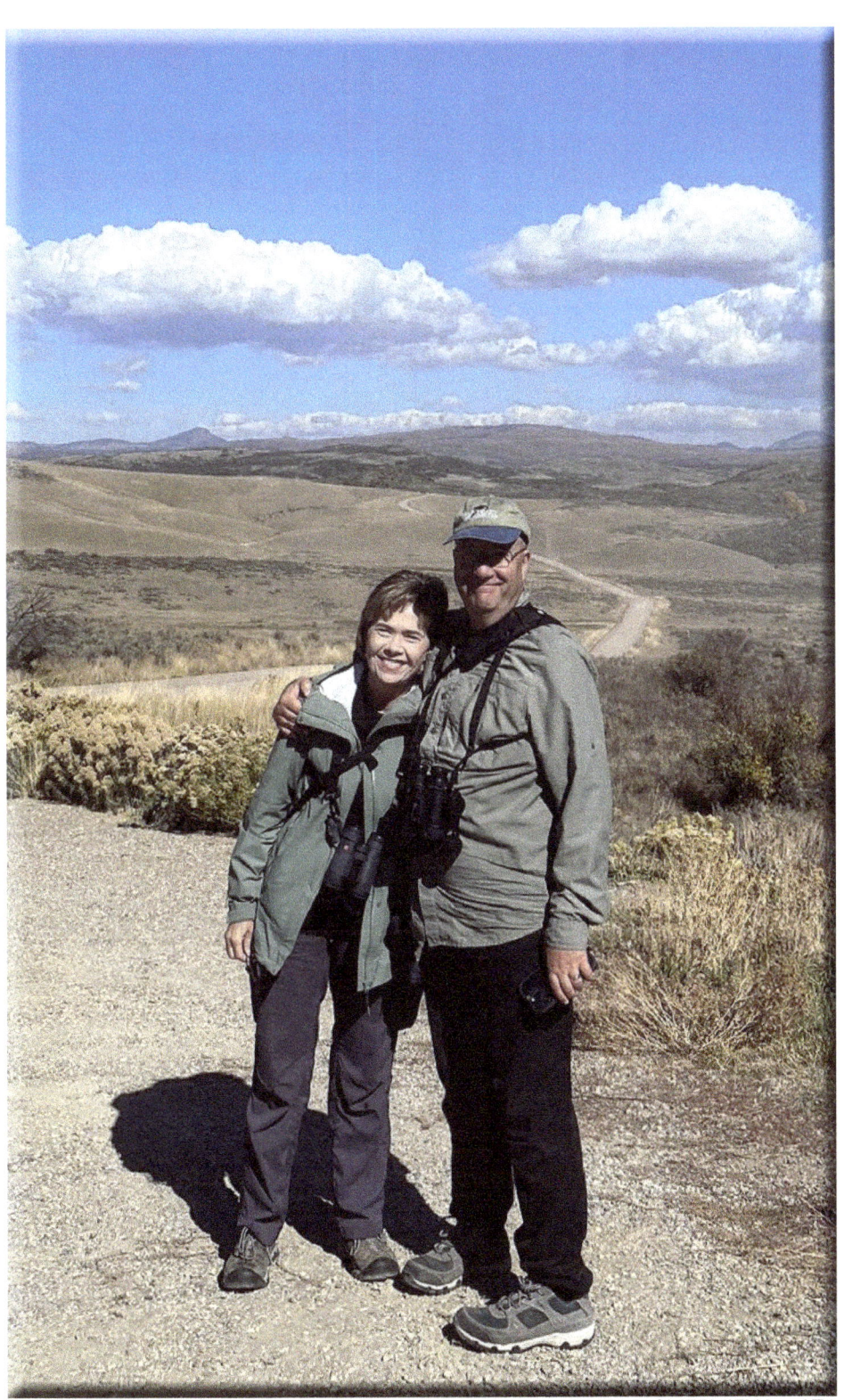

Big Year Overview

Travel	#
Plane Flights	40
Rental Cars	14
Nights Away	141
Boat Trips	14

Month	Year Birds
January	165
February	207
March	58
April	61
May	65
June	57
July	8
August	21
September	47
October	11
November	5
December	2
Total	708

State	Year Birds
Arizona	79
California	42
Colorado	8
Connecticut	8
Delaware	2
Florida	121
Illinois	4
Kansas	4
Louisiana	4
Massachusetts	68
Maryland	10
Maine	98
Michigan	3
Minnesota	13
Missouri	3
North Carolina	32
New Hampshire	7
New Jersey	13
New Mexico	18
New York	1
Oregon	3
South Carolina	8
Texas	117
Utah	5
Virginia	4
Vermont	1
Washington	31
Wyoming	1
Total	708

Superlatives

- Hottest Temperature: 118 degrees Salton Sea in September
- Coldest Temperature: -22 degrees Sax-Zim Bog in January
- Worst Road: Forest Service 42, AZ (Mexican Chickadees)
- Favorite Bird: Great Gray Owl (Ethan) & Elegant Trogon (Ingrid)
- Longest Stakeout: Yellow-headed Caracara (20 Hours over 3 Days)
- Heaviest Bird: Trumpeter Swan (26 lbs)
- Lightest Bird: Calliope Hummingbird (.1 Oz)
- Tallest Bird: Whooping Crane (5 ft)
- Shortest Bird: Calliope Hummingbird (3" Long)
- Largest Wingspan: California Condor (109")
- Shortest Wingspan: Calliope Hummingbird (4.2")
- Best Meal: Steiner Ranch at Lake Travis, TX
- Miles Driven: 29,340
- Miles Flown: 27,063
- Miles on a Boat: 724
- Friendliest People: Everyone in Utah
- Rudest Drivers: Miami
- Most Colorful Bird: Painted Bunting
- Rarest Bird: Mottled Owl
- Most Unique State: Utah
- Most year birds State: Florida (121)
- Favorite State (not Maine): Arizona (Ingrid) & Washington State (Ethan)
- Ugliest Bird: Turkey Vulture
- Meanest Bird: Rivoli's Hummingbird
- Prettiest Bird: Western Tanager
- Oddest Bird: Roseate Spoonbill
- Most Surprising Get: Yellow Rail
- Favorite Adventure: Dry Tortugas National Park
- We'd most like to Return to: Albuquerque (Ethan) & Florida Keys (Ingrid)
- Luckiest Get: Yellow Grosbeak & Rufous-backed Robin in the same tree
- Best Road Trip Bathrooms: McDonald's
- Favorite Road Snack: Blue Diamond Roasted Almonds
- Life Birds: Ethan (200), Ingrid (212)
- States Visited: 37
- Lowest Elevation Bird: -226 Feet - Salton Sea (Yellow-footed Gull)
- High Elevation Bird: 11,706 Feet - Rocky Mountains NP (White-tailed Ptarmigan)
- Biggest Strategic Mistake: Too Few Visits to California & Pacific Northwest

Year Bird Map

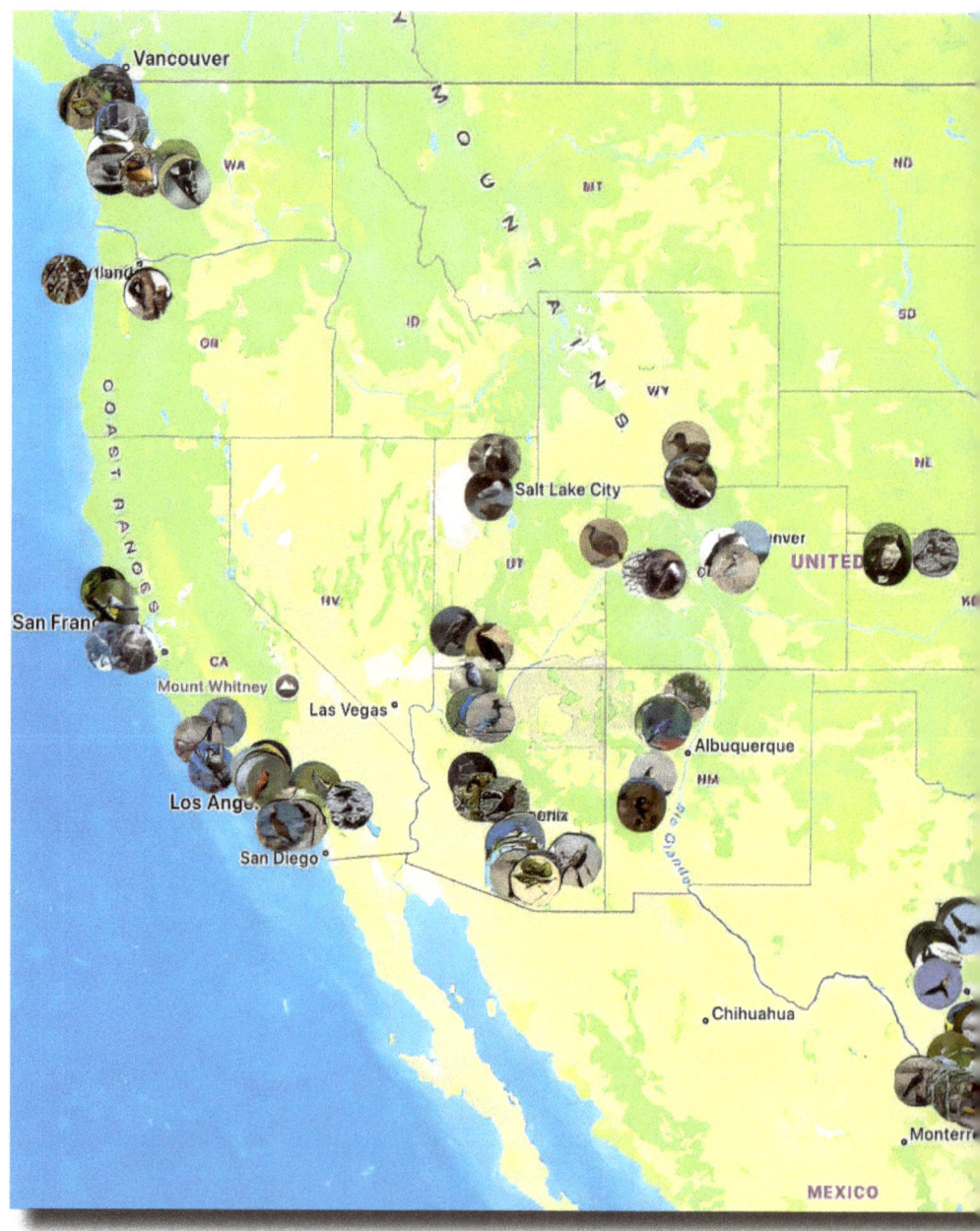

174 EVERY BIRD FROM SEA TO SHINING SEA

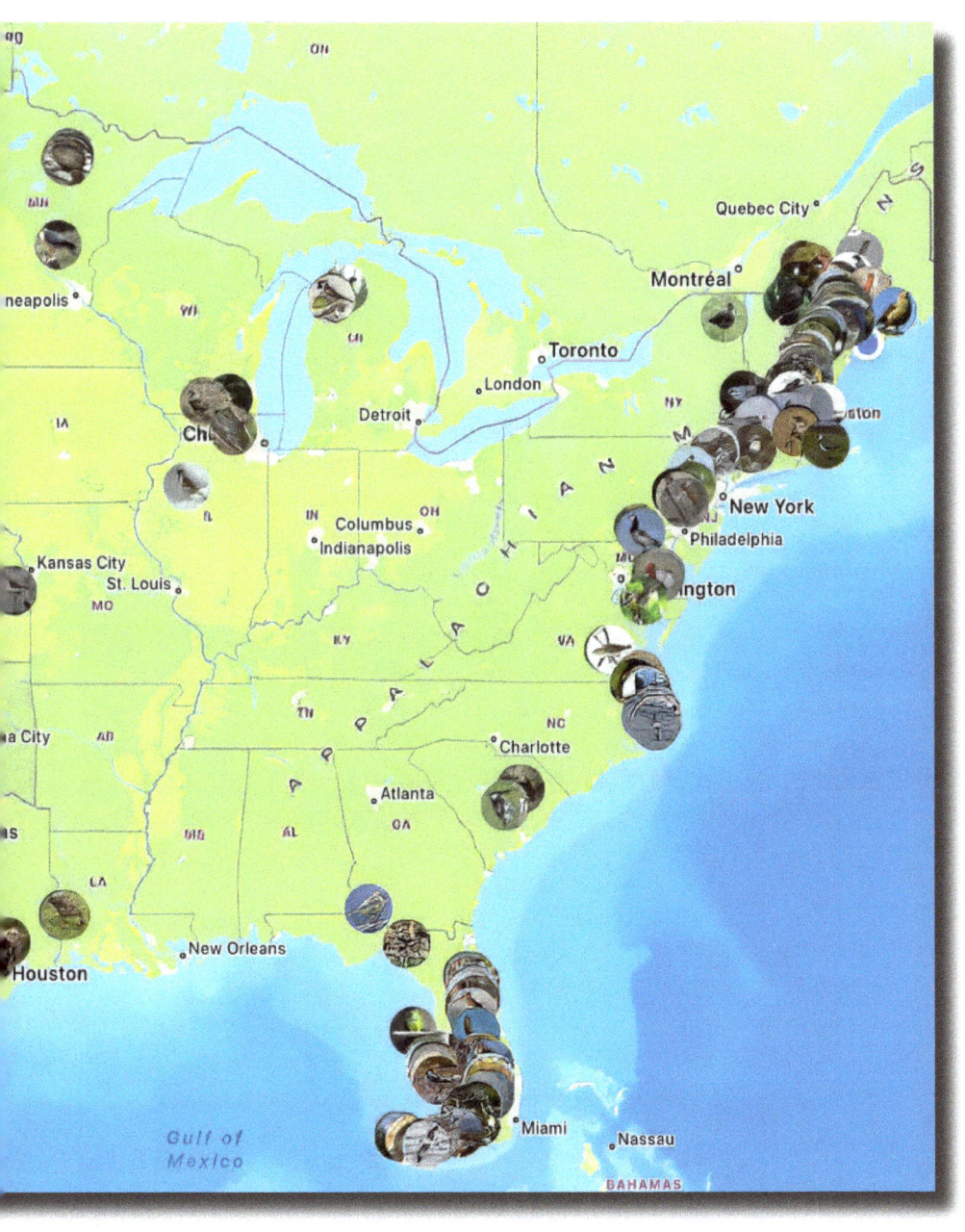

BIG YEAR OVERVIEW 175

Top 100 eBirders in USA Lower 48 by species, 2024 — 804 Species

		Complete checklists	Species (% of total)	Most recent addition
1.	Ezekiel Dobson	1,876	757 94.15%	Tundra Bean-Goose (Dec 31, 2024)
2.	Ethan Whitaker	511	708 88.06%	Northern Lapwing (Dec 9, 2024)
2.	Ingrid Whitaker	497	708 88.06%	Northern Lapwing (Dec 9, 2024)
4.	Tim Ryan	833	700 87.06%	Smooth-billed Ani (Dec 31, 2024)
5.	David McQuade	560	696 86.57%	Northern Lapwing (Dec 13, 2024)
5.	Tammy McQuade	488	696 86.57%	Northern Lapwing (Dec 13, 2024)
7.	larry nigro	493	692 86.07%	Common Gull (Dec 31, 2024)
8.	Hanyang Ye	439	687 85.45%	American Dipper (Dec 21, 2024)
9.	David Gersten	749	674 83.83%	Glaucous Gull (Dec 29, 2024)
10.	Molly Donahue	386	669 83.21%	Common Gull (Dec 31, 2024)
11.	Alex Lamoreaux	1,884	655 81.47%	Chestnut-collared Longspur (Nov 26, 2024)
12.	Kyle Rambo	2,228	653 81.22%	Eurasian Tree Sparrow (Dec 31, 2024)
13.	Chris Brown	821	626 77.86%	Northern Shrike (Dec 29, 2024)
14.	Beatriz Hernandez	651	620 77.11%	Snowy Owl (Dec 17, 2024)
15.	Connor Fox	444	619 76.99%	Sharp-tailed Grouse (Dec 29, 2024)
16.	Dan Shuber	314	613 76.24%	Groove-billed Ani (Dec 13, 2024)
17.	Kathryn Kay	461	592 73.63%	Rosy-faced Lovebird (Dec 22, 2024)
18.	Aaron Jackson	506	589 73.26%	Elegant Trogon (Dec 31, 2024)
19.	Kadynn Hatfield	1,426	588 73.13%	Nelson's Sparrow (Dec 30, 2024)
20.	Skye Haas	639	580 72.14%	Snow Bunting (Nov 9, 2024)
20.	Simon Kiacz	631	580 72.14%	Kelp Gull (Dec 31, 2024)
20.	Adrian Lakin	514	580 72.14%	Rosy-faced Lovebird (Dec 22, 2024)
23.	Quentin Reiser	213	579 72.01%	White Wagtail (Dec 31, 2024)
24.	Kevin Hayes	448	577 71.77%	American Tree Sparrow (Dec 28, 2024)
24.	Owen Reiser	193	577 71.77%	White Wagtail (Dec 31, 2024)
26.	Steve Glover	1,092	574 71.39%	Sagebrush Sparrow (Dec 31, 2024)
27.	Nick Glover	655	573 71.27%	Kelp Gull (Dec 31, 2024)
27.	Ron Clark	460	573 71.27%	Eurasian Wigeon (Dec 29, 2024)
29.	Gavin Awerbuch	525	571 71.02%	Eastern Whip-poor-will (Dec 30, 2024)
30.	Jim and Brenda Carpenter	489	570 70.9%	Razorbill (Dec 31, 2024)
31.	Angelo DelloMargio	1,007	567 70.52%	Rufous-capped Warbler (Dec 28, 2024)
31.	Troy Hibbitts	654	567 70.52%	White Wagtail (Dec 29, 2024)
31.	Stefan Schlick	626	567 70.52%	Arctic Loon (Dec 29, 2024)

Gallery

Albatrosses 191
Amazons (Parrots) 198
Anhingas 191
Anis 183
Auklets 187
Avocets 183
Becards 195
Bitterns 191
Blackbirds 212
Bluebirds 204
Boobies 188
Bulbuls 195
Buntings 205
Caracaras 195
Cardinals & Allies 206
Chachalacas 213
Chats 203
Chickadees 202
Coots 185
Cormorants 190
Cowbirds 212
Cranes 182
Creepers 201
Crossbills 206
Crows 198
Cuckoos 182
Curlews 185
Dippers 203
Doves 182
Dowitchers 184
Ducks (Dabbling) 178
Ducks (Diving) 178
Eagles 193
Egrets 192
Eiders 179
Eurasian Escapees 193
Exotics 198
Falcons 194
Finches 206
Flamingos 183
Flickers 195
Flycatchers 197
Flycatchers 200
Fowl 181
Frigatebirds 189
Fulmars 190
Gallinules 184
Gannets 189
Geese 178
Gnatcatchers 205
Godwits 185
Goldeneyes 178
Goldfinches 206
Grackles 213
Grebes 180
Grosbeaks 206

Grouse 181
Guillemots 187
Gulls 188
Harriers 195
Hawks (Accipiters) 193
Hawks (Buteos) 192
Herons 193
Hummingbirds 182
Ibises 193
Jaegers 187
Jays 198
Juncos 205
Kingbirds 196
Kingfishers 183
Kinglets 203
Kiskadees 197
Kites 192
Lapwings 184
Larks 201
Limpkin 181
Longspurs 204
Loons 189
Lovebirds 197
Macaws 199
Magpies 199
Meadowlarks 207
Mergansers 180
Mimics 202
Murrelets 187
Murres 186
New World Quail 181
Night-Herons 191
Nightjars 184
Noddies 189
Nutcrackers 199
Nuthatches 202
Old World Sparrows 207
Orioles 212
Ospreys 193
Other Auks 186
Owls (Barn) 194
Owls (Typical) 194
Oystercatchers 183
Parakeets 198
Parrotbills 199
Pelicans 191
Pewees 196
Phalaropes 187
Pheasants 180
Phoebes 197
Pigeons 180
Pintails 178
Pipits 204
Plovers 184
Prairie-Chickens 180
Ptarmigans 181

Puffins 186
Rails 184
Ravens 198
Roadrunners 182
Rosy-Finches 205
Sage-Grouse 181
Sandpipers 186
Sapsuckers 194
Scaups 179
Scoters 181
Scrub-Jays 201
Shearwaters 190
Shrikes 194
Silky 197
Skimmers 213
Skuas 187
Snipes 185
Sparrows 208
Spoonbills 203
Stilts 183
Storks 182
Storm-Petrels (Northern) 188
Storm-Petrels (Southern) 188
Swallows 204
Swans 178
Swifts 213
Tanagers 206
Teal 180
Terns 190
Thrushes 204
Titmice 202
Tits 199
Towhees 196
Trogons 207
Tropicbirds 190
Turkeys 180
Turnstones 185
Tyrants 196
Verdins 201
Vireos 200
Vultures 192
Wagtails 213
Waxwings 199
Wheatears 200
Whistling-Ducks 179
Wigeons 179
Wood Warblers 210
Woodcocks 185
Woodpeckers 196
Wrens 202
Yellowlegs 186

Geese

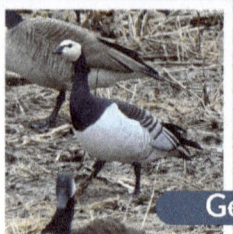
Barnacle Goose
May 19, 2024
New Hampshire

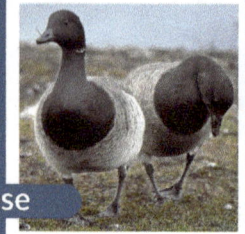
Brant
January 29, 2024
Maryland

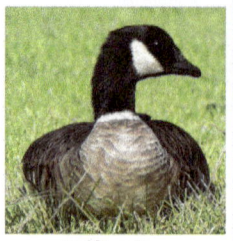
Cackling Goose
January 3, 2024
New Jersey

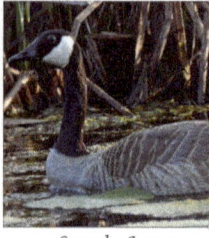
Canada Goose
January 1, 2024
Massachusetts

Swans

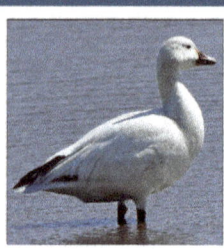
Snow Goose
January 1, 2024
Massachusetts

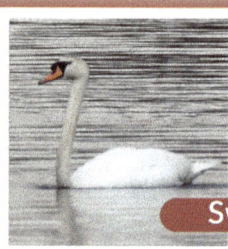
Mute Swan
January 1, 2024
Massachussetts

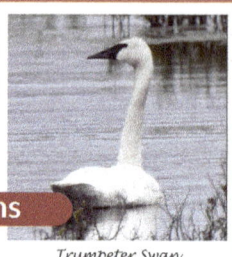
Trumpeter Swan
January 3, 2024
New Jersey

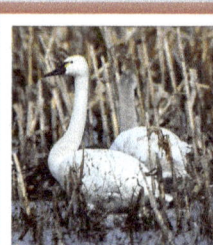
Tundra Swan
January 4, 2024
Connecticut

Ducks (Dabbling)

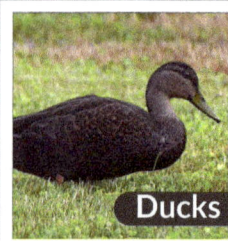
American Black Duck
January 1, 2024
Massachusetts

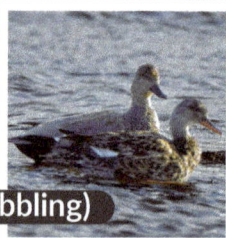
Gadwalls
January 1, 2024
Massachusetts

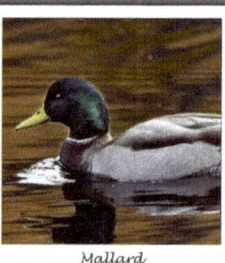
Mallard
January 1, 2024
Massachussets

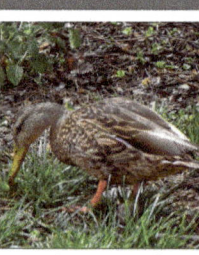
Mexican Duck
February 25, 2024
Texas

Ducks (Diving)

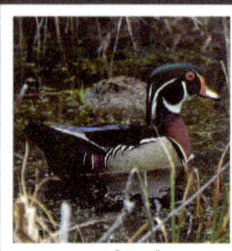
Wood Duck
February 6, 2024
Florida

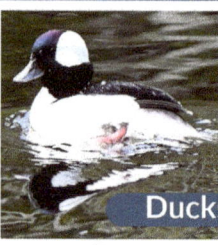
Bufflehead
January 1, 2024
Massachusetts

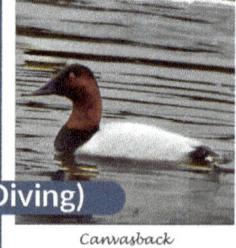
Canvasback
January 30, 2024
Maryland

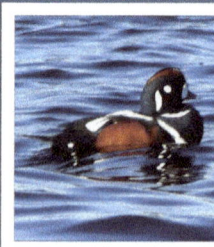
Harlequin Duck
January 1, 2024
Massachusetts

Pintails

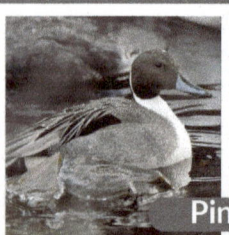
Northern Pintail
January 1, 2024
Massachussets

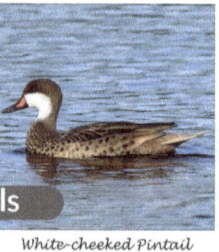
White-cheeked Pintail
May 6, 2024
Florida

Goldeneyes

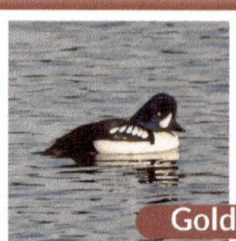
Barrow's Goldeneye
January 6, 2024
Maine

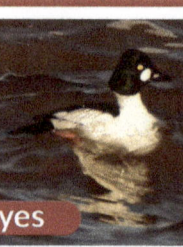
Common Goldeneye
January 1, 2024
Massachusetts

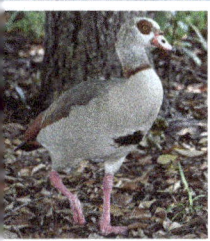
Egyptian Goose
February 8, 2024
Florida

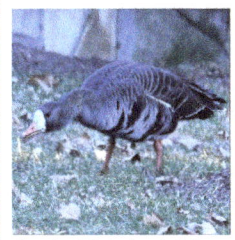
Greater White-fronted Goose
February 15, 2024
Louisiana

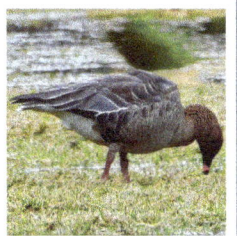
Pink-footed Goose
January 29, 2024
New Jersey

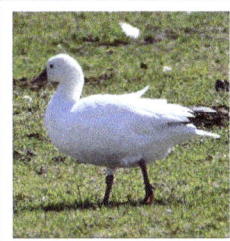
Ross's Goose
February 21, 2024
Texas

Whistling-Ducks

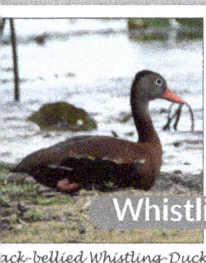
Black-bellied Whistling-Duck
February 4, 2024
Florida

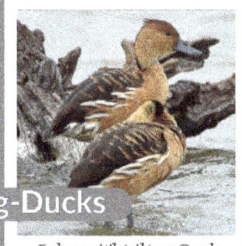
Fulvous Whistling-Duck
February 6, 2024
Florida

Wigeons

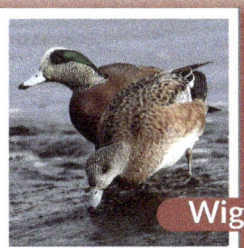
American Wigeon
January 1, 2024
Massachusetts

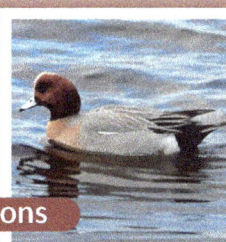
Eurasian Wigeon
January 4, 2024
Connecticut

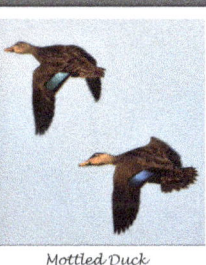
Mottled Duck
February 3, 2024
Florida

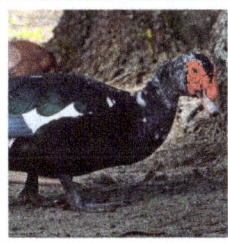
Muscovy Duck
February 4, 2024
Florida

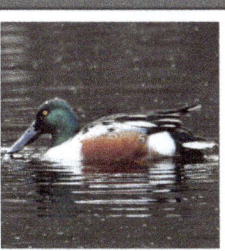
Northern Shoveler
January 1, 2024
Maine

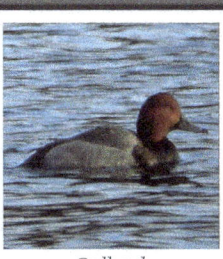
Redhead
January 30, 2024
Maryland

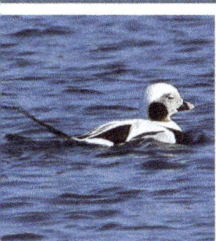
Long-tailed Duck
January 1, 2024
Massachussets

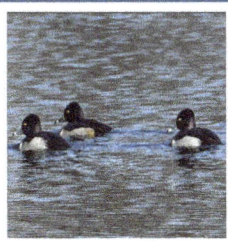
Ring-necked Duck
January 3, 2024
Connecticut

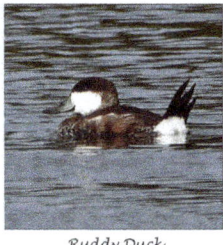
Ruddy Duck
January 2, 2024
Maine

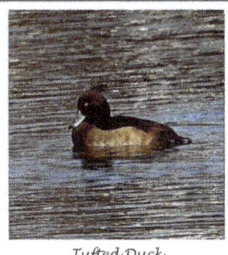
Tufted Duck
January 3, 2024
Connecticut

Scaups

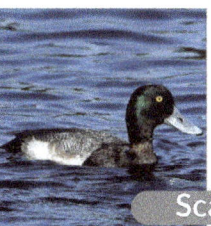
Greater Scaup
January 6, 2024
Maine

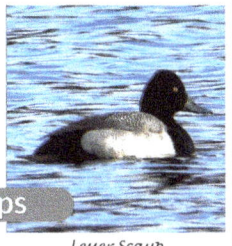
Lesser Scaup
January 2, 2024
Maine

Eiders / 179

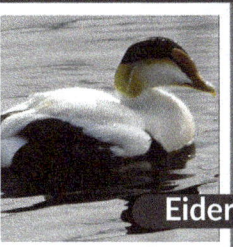
Common Eider
January 1, 2024
Massachusetts

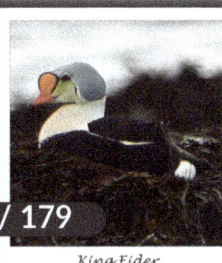
King Eider
January 20, 2024
Maine

Mergansers

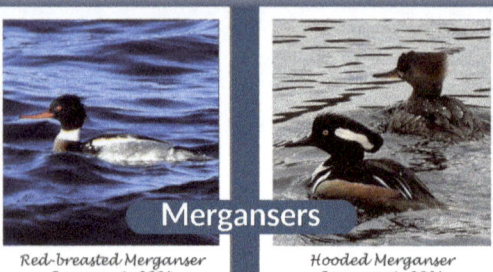

Red-breasted Merganser
January 1, 2024
Massachusetts

Hooded Merganser
January 1, 2024
Massachusetts

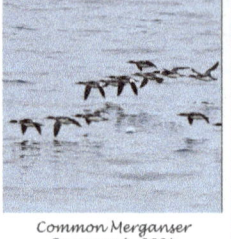

Common Merganser
January 4, 2024
New Jersey

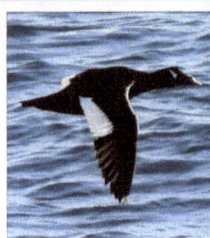

White-winged Scoter
January 2, 2024
Maine

Teal

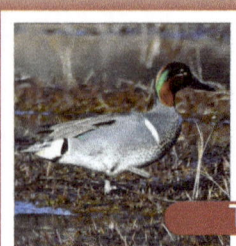

Green-winged Teal
January 1, 2024
Massachusetts

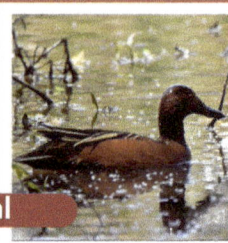

Cinnamon Teal
February 21, 2024
Texas

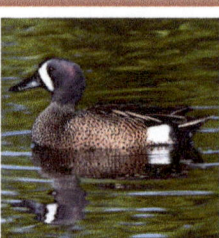

Blue-winged Teal
February 3, 2024
Florida

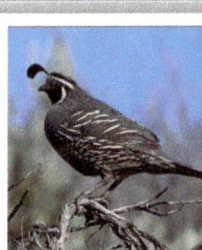

California Quail
September 16, 2024
California

Turkeys / Prairie-Chickens

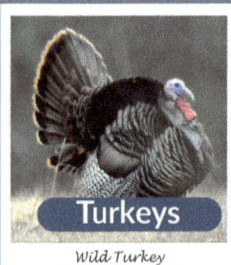

Wild Turkey
January 2, 2024
Maine

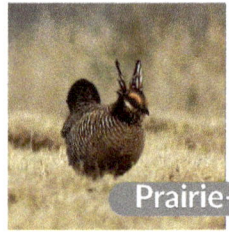

Lesser Prarie-Chicken
April 12, 2024
Kansas

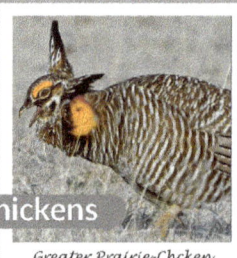

Greater Prairie-Chcken
April 12, 2024
Kansas

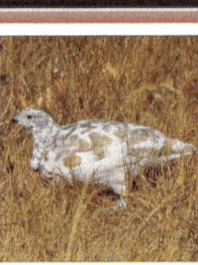

White-tailed Ptarmigan
October 16, 2024
Colorado

Pheasants / Pigeons

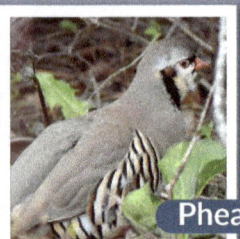

Chukar
October 15, 2024
Colorado

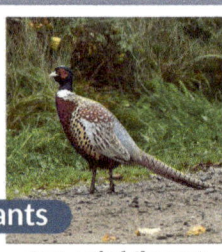

Ring-necked Pheasant
April 8, 2024
Utah

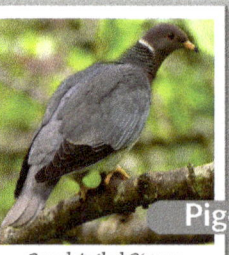

Band-tailed Pigeon
June 24, 2024
Washington State

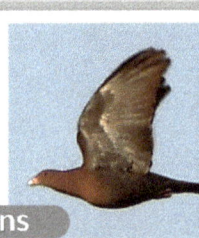

Red-billed Pigeon
February 25, 2024
Texas

Grebes

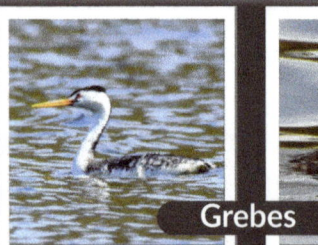

Clark's Grebe
March 28, 2024
New Mexico

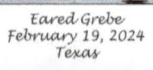

Eared Grebe
February 19, 2024
Texas

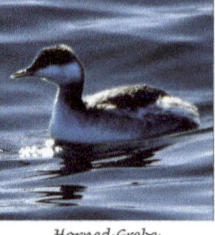

Horned Grebe
January 2, 2024
Maine

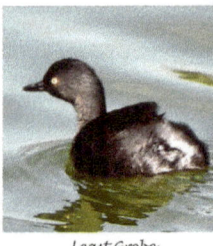

Least Grebe
February 19, 2024
Texas

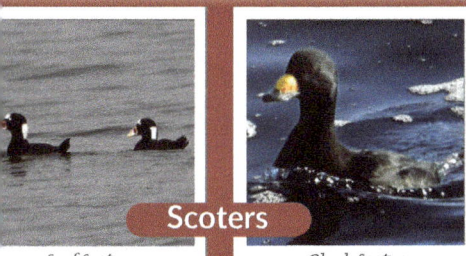
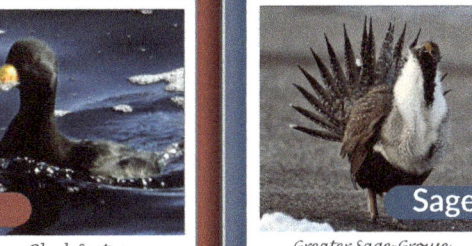
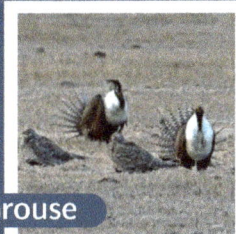

Scoters

Surf Scoter
January 6, 2024
Maine

Black Scoter
January 2, 2024
Maine

Sage-Grouse

Greater Sage-Grouse
April 8, 2024
Utah

Gunnison Sage-Grouse
April 10, 2024
Colorado

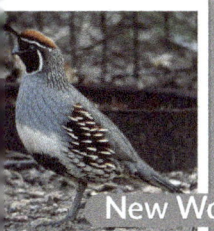
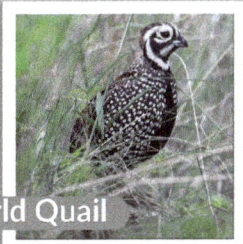
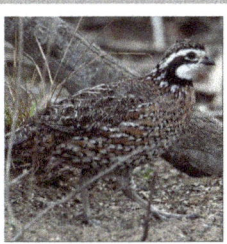
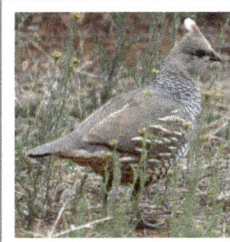

New World Quail

Gambel's Quail
March 28, 2024
Arizona

Montezuma Quail
August 12, 2024
Arizona

Northern Bobwhite
February 13, 2024
Florida

Scaled Quail
March 28, 2024
Arizona

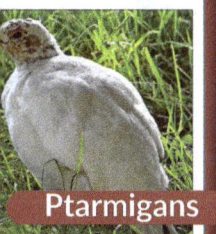
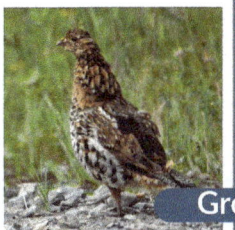
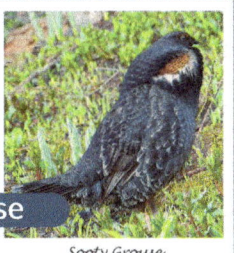
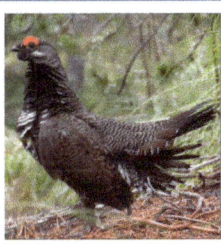

Ptarmigans

Grouse

Willow Ptarmigan
May 29, 2024
Maine

Ruffed Grouse
January 16, 2024
Minnesota

Sooty Grouse
June 23, 2024
Washington State

Spruce Grouse
June 13, 2024
Maine

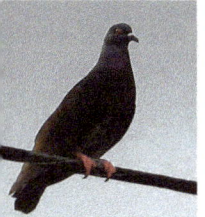
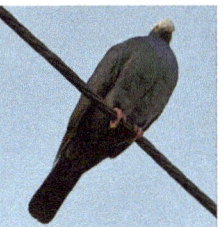
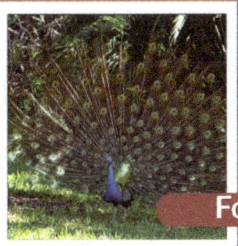
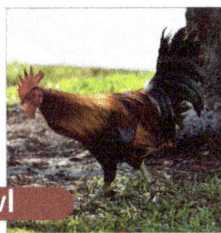

Fowl

Rock Pigeon
January 1, 2024
Massachusetts

White-crowned Pigeon
May 7, 2024
Florida

Indian Peafowl
May 5, 2024
Florida

Red Junglefowl
May 7, 2024
Florida

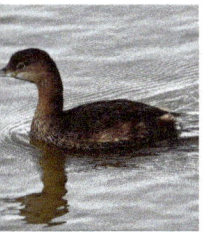
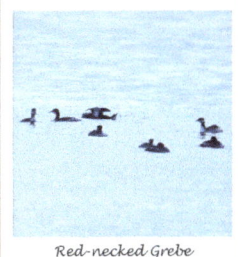
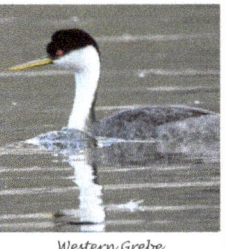
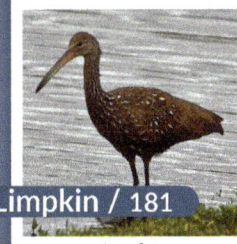

Limpkin / 181

Pied-billed Grebe
January 14, 2024
Maine

Red-necked Grebe
January 2, 2024
Maine

Western Grebe
March 28, 2024
New Mexico

Limpkin
February 4, 2024
Florida

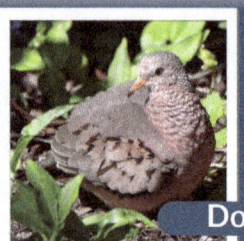
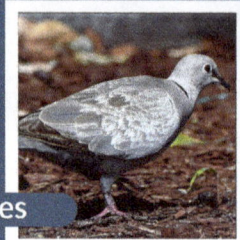
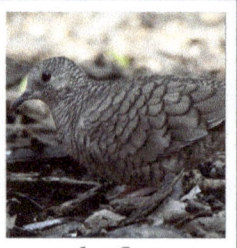
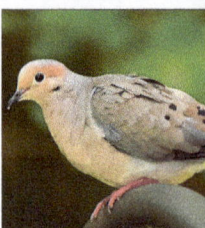

Doves

Common Ground Dove
February 3, 2024
Florida

Eurasian Collared-Dove
January 31, 2024
North Carolina

Inca Dove
February 17, 2024
Texas

Mourning Dove
January 1, 2024
Massachusetts

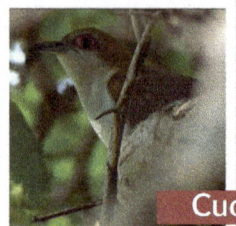
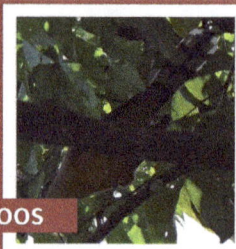
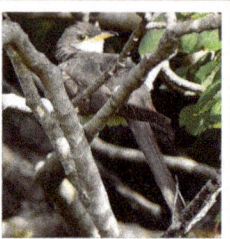
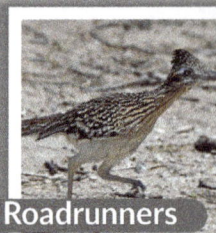

Cuckoos

Roadrunners

Black-billed Cuckoo
May 12, 2024
Maine

Mangrove Cuckoo
February 7, 2024
Florida

Yellow-billed Cuckoo
May 24, 2024
Maine

Greater Roadrunner
February 21, 2024
Texas

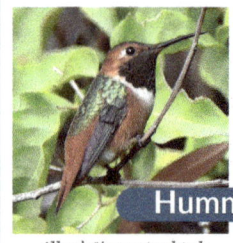
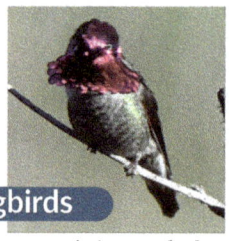
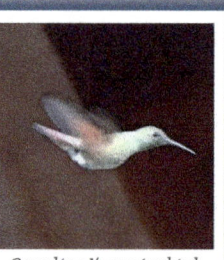
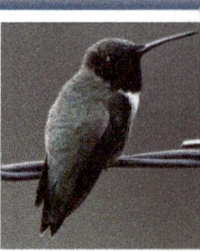

Hummingbirds

Allen's Hummingbird
September 4, 2024
California

Anna's Hummingbird
March 30, 2024
Arizona

Berryline Hummingbird
April 1, 2024
Arizona

Black-chinned Hummingbird
February 19, 2024
Texas

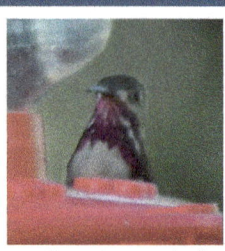
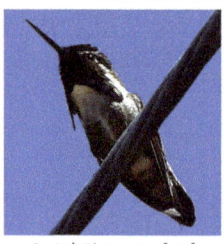
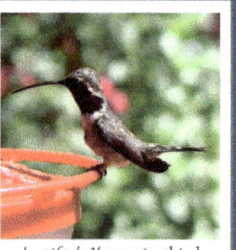
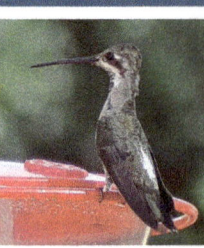

Calliope Hummingbird
June 28, 2024
Oregon

Costa's Hummingbird
April 3, 2024
Arizona

Lucifer's Hummingbird
August 5, 2024
Arizona

Plain-capped Starthroat
October 18, 2024
Arizona

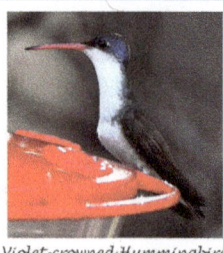
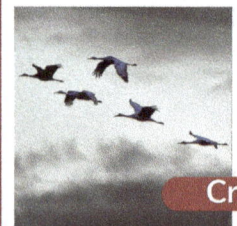
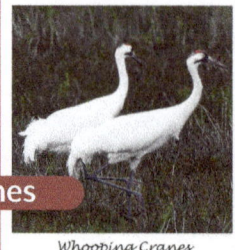
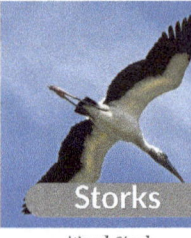

Cranes

Storks

Violet-crowned Hummingbird
March 30, 2024
Arizona

Sandhill Cranes
February 5, 2024
Florida

Whooping Cranes
February 16, 2024
Texas

Wood Stork
February 3, 2024
Florida

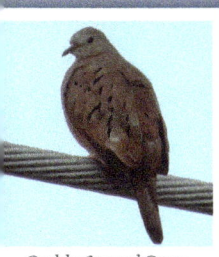
Ruddy Ground Dove
October 18, 2024
Arizona

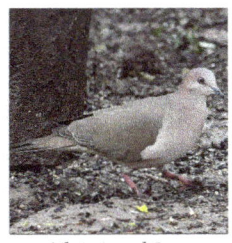
White-tipped Dove
February 17, 2024
Texas

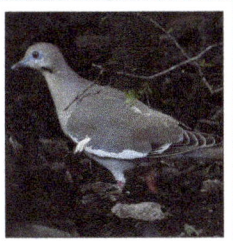
White-winged Dove
February 7, 2024
Florida

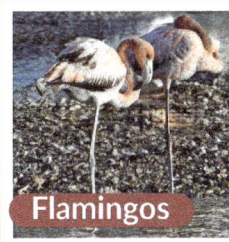
Flamingos
American Flamingo
February 3, 2024
Florida

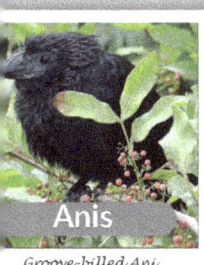
Anis
Groove-billed Ani
November 30, 2024
Texas

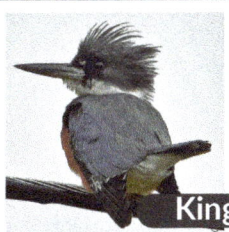
Kingfishers
Belted Kingfisher
January 3, 2024
Connecticut

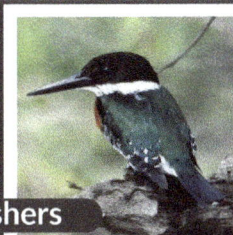
Green Kingfisher
February 19, 2024
Texas

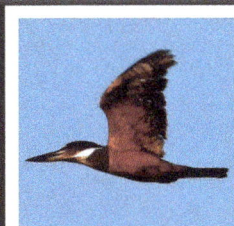
Ringed Kingfisher
February 25, 2024
Texas

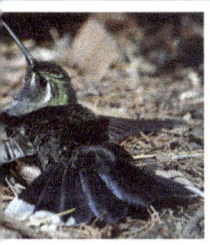
Blue-throated Mountain-gem
March 29, 2024
Arizona

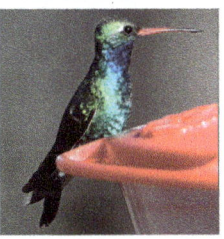
Broad-billed Hummingbird
March 29, 2024
Arizona

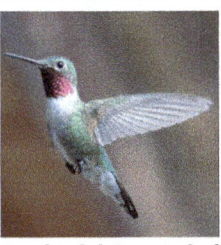
Broad-tailed Hummingbird
April 5, 2024
Arizona

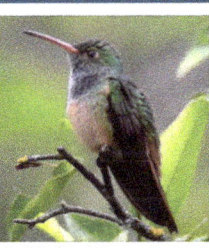
Buff-bellied Hummingbird
February 19, 2024
Texas

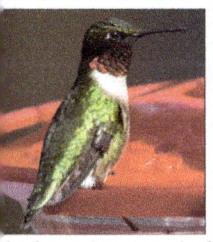
Ruby-throated Hummingbird
January 31, 2024
North Carolina

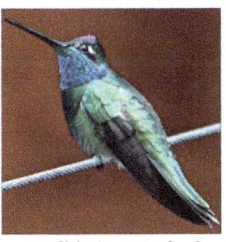
Rivoli's Hummingbird
March 31, 2024
Arizona

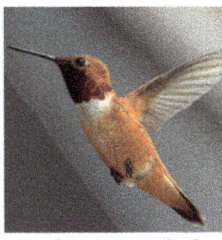
Rufous Hummingbird
February 23, 2024
Texas

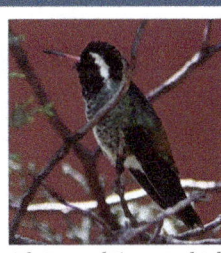
White-eared Hummingbird
August 12, 2024
Arizona

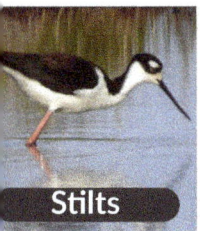
Stilts
Black-necked Stilt
January 31, 2024
North Carolina

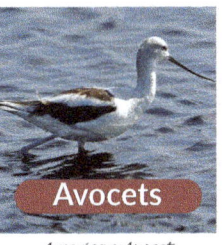
Avocets
American Avocet
January 31, 2024
North Carolina

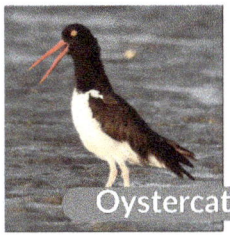
Oystercatchers / 183
American Oystercatcher
January 29, 2024
Maryland

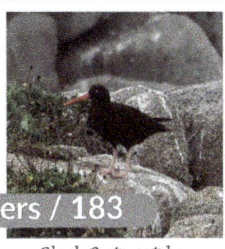
Black Oystercatcher
September 5, 2024
California

Nightjars

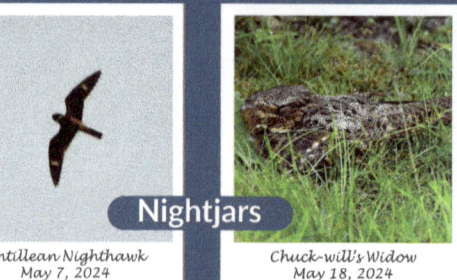

Antillean Nighthawk
May 7, 2024
Florida

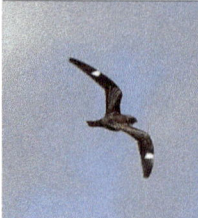

Chuck-will's Widow
May 18, 2024
Boston

Common Nighthawk
May 5, 2024
Florida

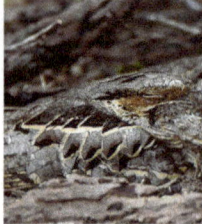

Common Pauraque
February 18, 2024
Texas

Rails

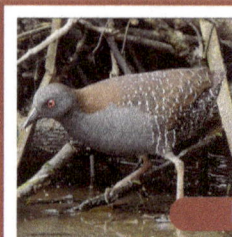

Black Rail
November 25, 2024
Texas

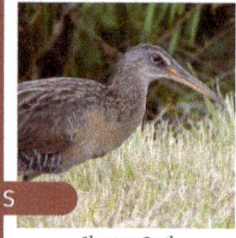

Clapper Rail
February 21, 2024
Texas

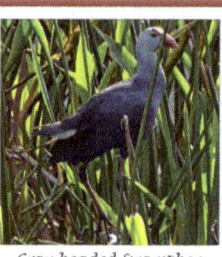

Gray-headed Swamphen
February 6, 2024
Florida

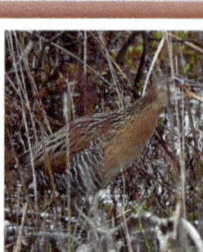

King Rail
April 30, 2024
Massachusetts

Gallinules

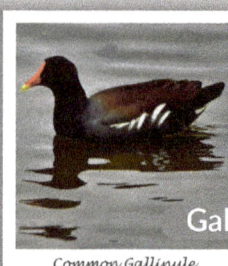

Common Gallinule
February 2, 2024
Florida

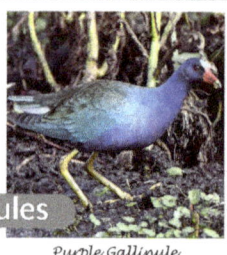

Purple Gallinule
February 4, 2024
Florida

Dowitchers

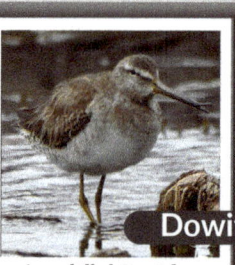

Long-billed Dowitcher
January 31, 2024
North Carolina

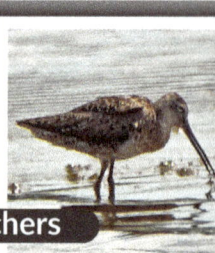

Short-billed Dowitcher
January 31, 2024
North Carolina

Plovers

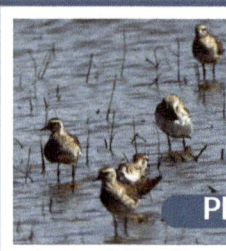

American Golden-Plover
April 13, 2024
Missouri

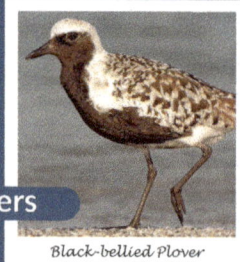

Black-bellied Plover
January 31, 2024
North Carolina

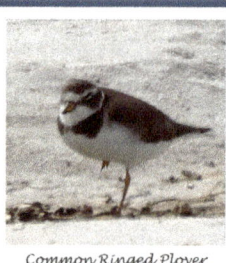

Common Ringed Plover
September 18, 2024
Massachusetts

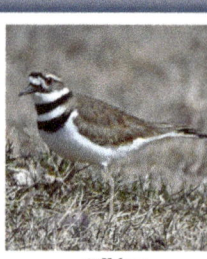

Killdeer
June 4, 2024
Connecticut

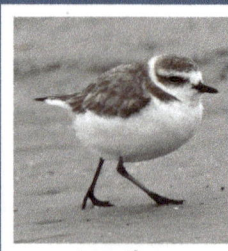

Snowy Plover
February 20, 2024
Texas

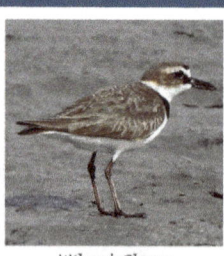

Wilson's Plover
February 8, 2024
Florida

Lapwings

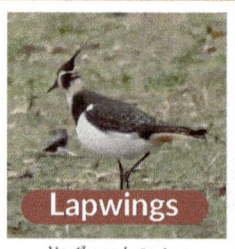

Northern Lapwing
December 9, 2024
Massachusetts

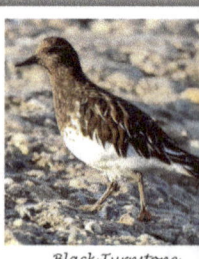

Black Turnstone
September 4, 2024
California

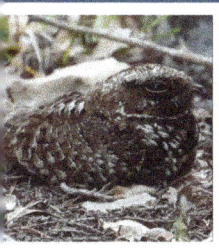
Common Poorwill
February 24, 2024
Texas

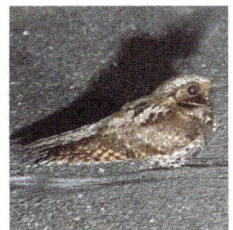
Eastern Whip-poor-will
May 13, 2024
Massachusetts

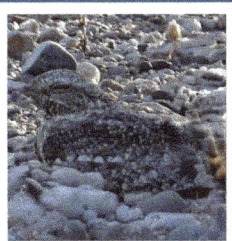
Lesser Nighthawk
August 5, 2024
Arizona

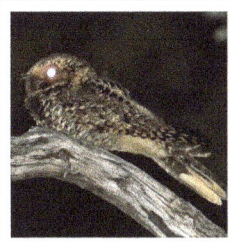
Mexican Whip-poor-will
August 4, 2024
Arizona

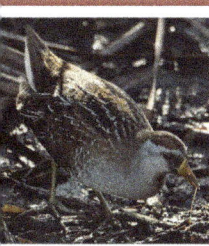
Sora
February 5, 2024
Florida

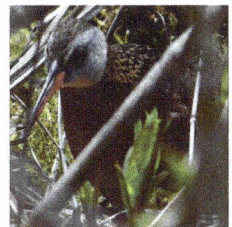
Virginia Rail
February 5, 2024
Florida

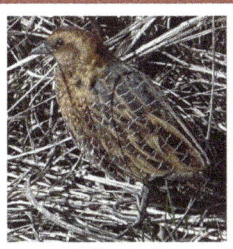
Yellow Rail
June 7, 2024
Michigan

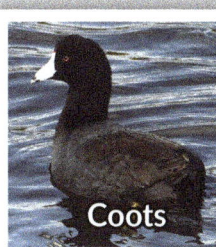
Coots
American Coot
January 2, 2024
Maine

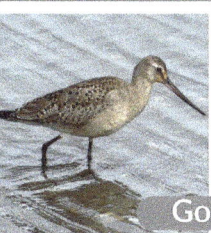
Godwits
Hudsonian Godwit
August 14, 2024
Maine

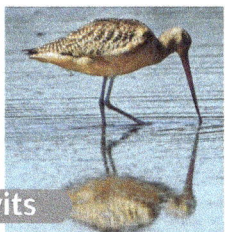
Marbled Godwit
February 6, 2024
Florida

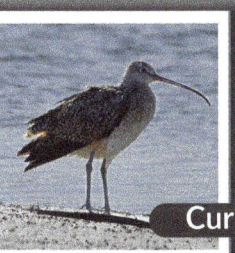
Curlews
Long-billed Curlew
February 19, 2024
Texas

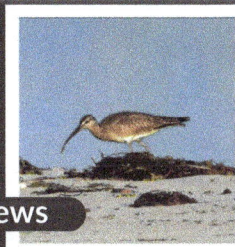
Whimbrel
February 20, 2024
Texas

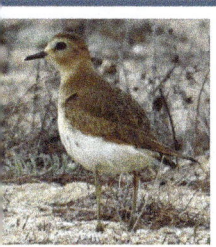
Mountain Plover
April 10, 2024
Colorado

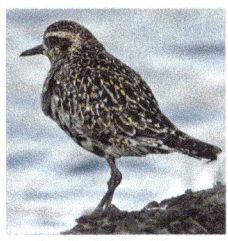
Pacific Golden-Plover
September 10, 2024
California

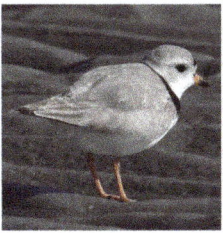
Piping Plover
February 18, 2024
Texas

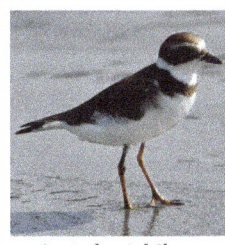
Semipalmated Plover
January 31, 2024
North Carolina

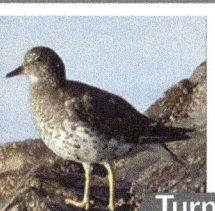
Turnstones
Surfbird
September 5, 2024
California

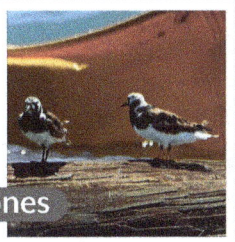
Ruddy Turnstone
January 29, 2024
Maryland

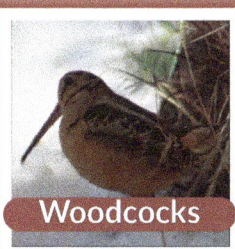
Woodcocks
American Woodcock
February 1, 2024
South Carolina

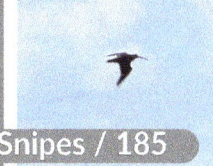
Snipes / 185
Wilson's Snipe
February 5, 2024
Florida

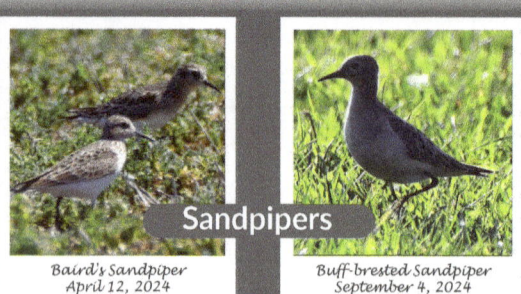
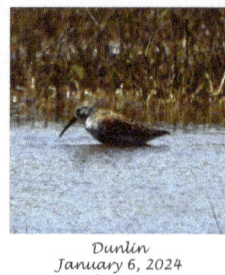
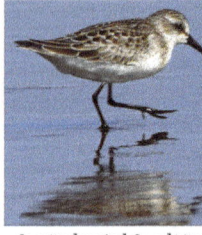

Sandpipers

Baird's Sandpiper
April 12, 2024
Kansas

Buff-brested Sandpiper
September 4, 2024
New Hampshire

Dunlin
January 6, 2024
Maine

Semipalmated Sandpiper
April 13, 2024
Missouri

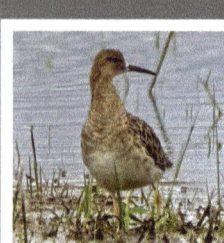
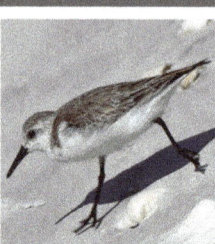
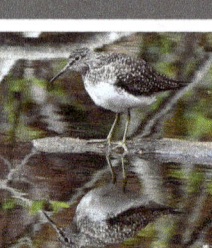
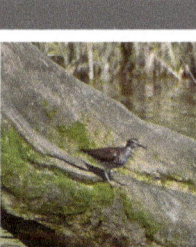

Ruff
April 20, 2024
Vermont

Sanderling
January 29, 2024
Maryland

Solitary Sandpiper
May 10, 2024
Maine

Spotted Sandpiper
February 6, 2024
Florida

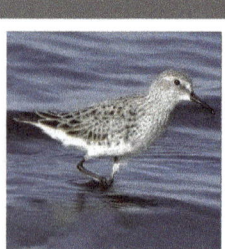
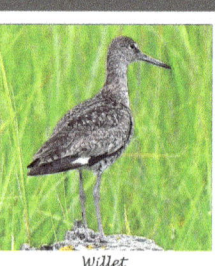
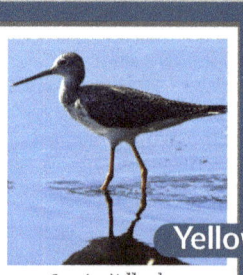
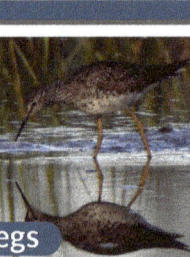

White-rumped Sandpiper
May 6, 2024
Florida

Willet
February 3, 2024
Florida

Yellowlegs

Greater Yellowlegs
February 3, 2024
Florida

Lesser Yellowlegs
February 3, 2024
Florida

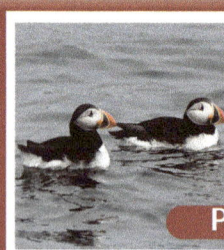
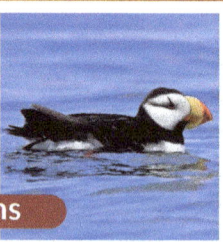
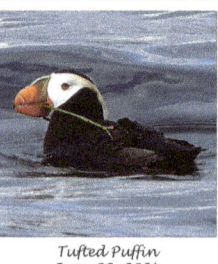
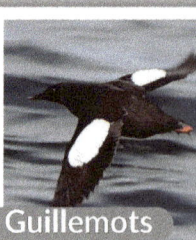

Puffins

Atlantic Puffin
May 22, 2024
Maine

Horned Puffin
June 22, 2024
Washington State

Tufted Puffin
June 22, 2024
Washington State

Guillemots

Black Guillemot
January 2, 2024
Maine

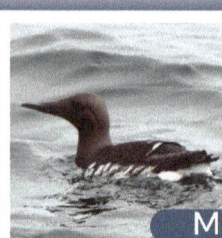
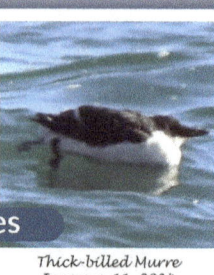
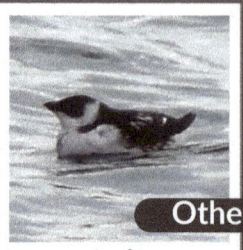
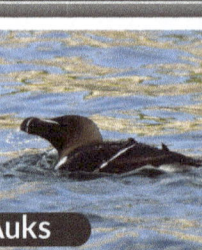

Murres

Common Murre
June 22, 2024
Washington State

Thick-billed Murre
January 11, 2024
Maine

Other Auks

Dovekie
January 10, 2024
Maine

Razorbill
January 10, 2024
Maine

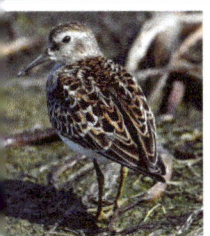
Least Sandpiper
February 6, 2024
Florida

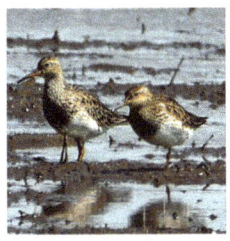
Pectoral Sandpiper
April 13, 2024
Missouri

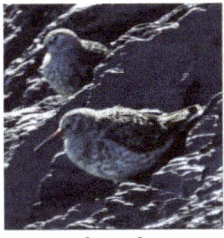
Purple Sandpiper
January 2, 2024
Maine

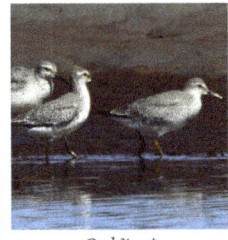
Red Knot
February 6, 2024
Florida

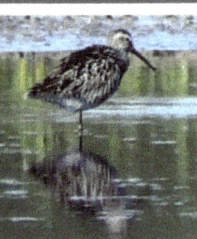
Stilt Sandpiper
February 6, 2024
Florida

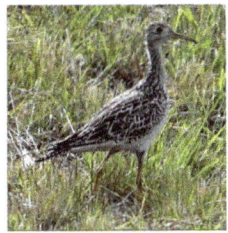
Upland Sandpiper
April 29, 2024
New Hampshire

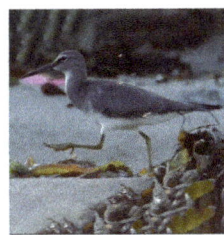
Wandering Tattler
September 5, 2024
California

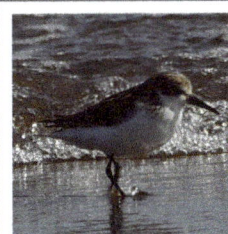
Western Sandpiper
February 6, 2024
Florida

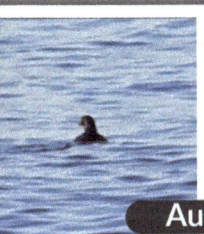
Auklets
Cassin's Auklet
September 7, 2024
California

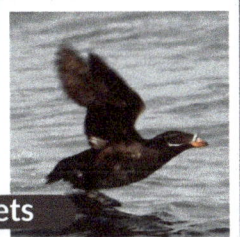
Rhinoceros Auklet
June 22, 2024
Washington State

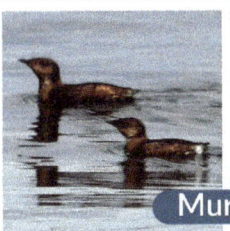
Murrelets
Marbled Murrelet
June 22, 2024
Washington State

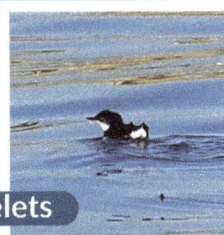
Scripp's Murrelet
Septmber 5, 2024
California

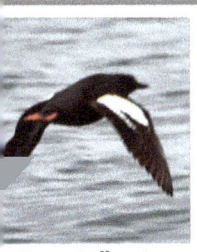
Pigeon Guillemot
June 21, 2024
Washington State

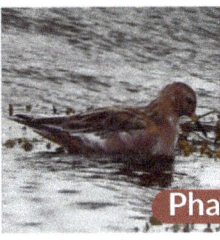
Phalaropes
Red Phalarope
July 16, 2024
Maine

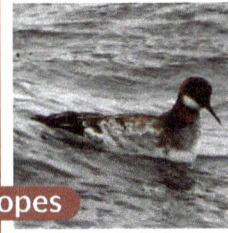
Red-necked Phalarope
June 3, 2024
North Carolina

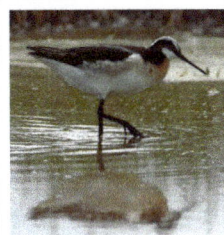
Wilson's Phalarope
May 2, 2024
Maine

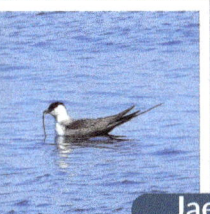
Jaegers
Long-tailed Jaeger
August 19, 2024
Massachusetts

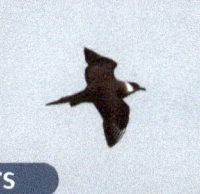
Parasitic Jaeger
June 3, 2024
North Carolina

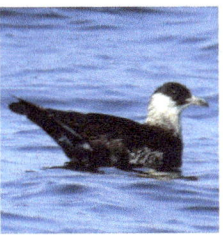
Pomarine Jaeger
June 3, 2024
North Carolina

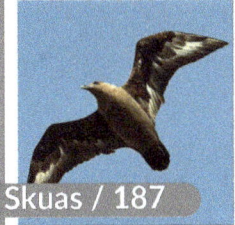
Skuas / 187
South Polar Skua
July 27, 2024
Maine

Gulls

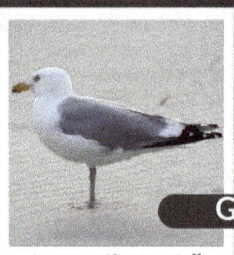
American Herring Gull
January 1, 2024
Massachusetts

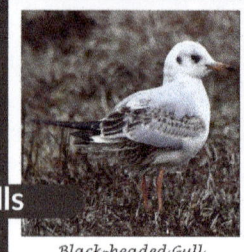
Black-headed Gull
January 4, 2024
New Jersey

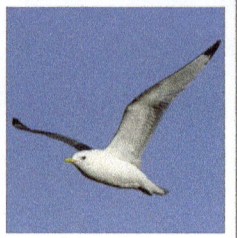
Black-legged Kittiwake
January 10, 2024
Maine

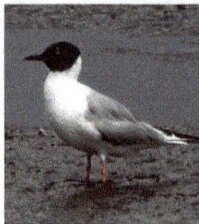
Bonaparte's Gull
January 13, 2024
Maine

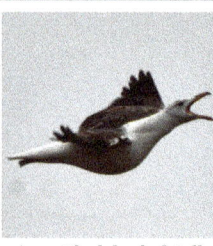
Lesser Black-backed Gull
February 21, 2024
Texas

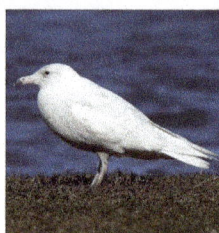
Glaucous Gull
June 6, 2024
Maine

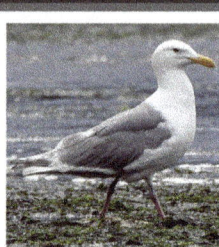
Glaucous-winged Gull
June 21, 2024
Washington State

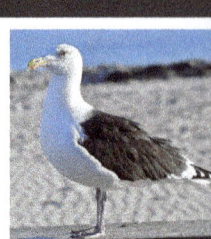
Great Black-backed Gull
January 1, 2024
Massachusetts

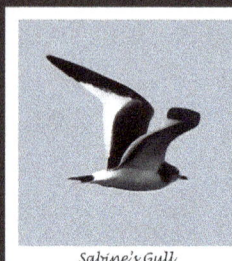
Sabine's Gull
September 7, 2024
California

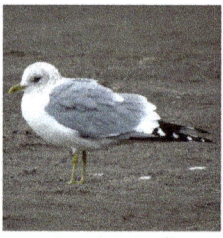
Short-billed Gull
April 7, 2024
Utah

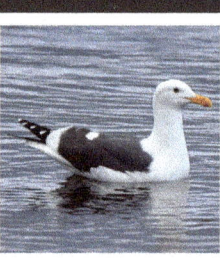
Western Gull
June 22, 2024
Washington State

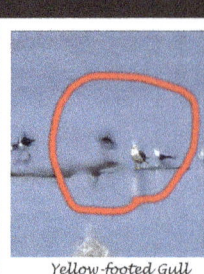
Yellow-footed Gull
September 8, 2024
California

Storm-Petrels (Northern)

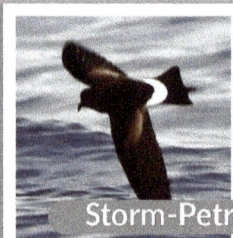
Band-rumped Storm-Petrel
June 3, 2024
North Carolina

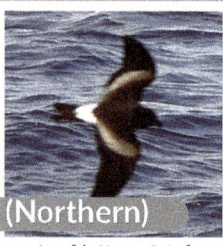
Leach's Storm-Petrel
June 3, 2024
North Carolina

Storm-Petrels (Southern)

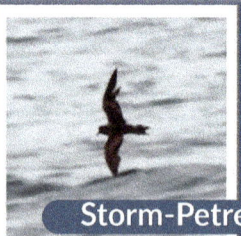
Ashy Storm-Petrel
September 15, 2024
California

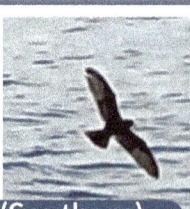
Black Storm-Petrel
September 15, 2024
California

Boobies

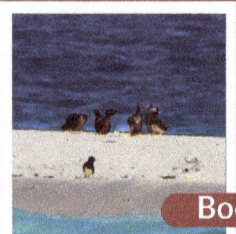
Brown Booby
May 8, 2024
Florida

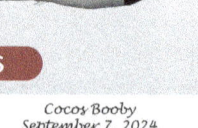
Cocos Booby
September 7, 2024
California

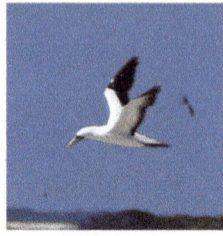
Masked Booby
May 8, 2024
Florida

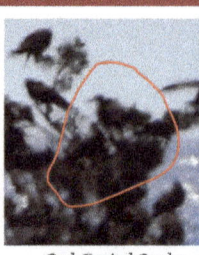
Red-Footed Booby
May 8, 2024
Florida

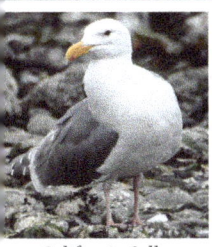
California Gull
April 7, 2024
Utah

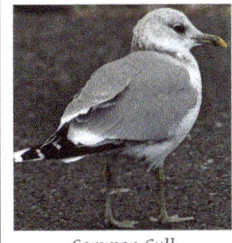
Common Gull
January 4, 2024
Connecticut

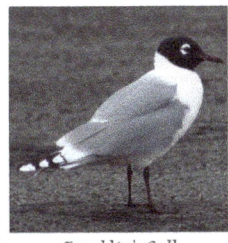
Franklin's Gull
February 23, 2024
Texas

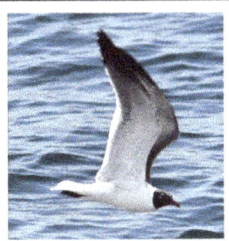
Laughing Gull
February 2, 2024
Florida

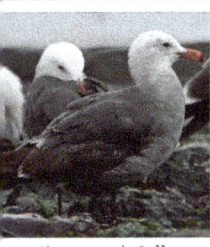
Heermann's Gull
June 22, 2024
Washington State

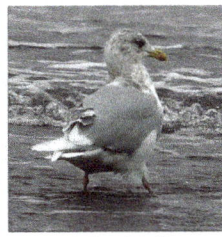
Iceland Gull
January 6, 2024
Maine

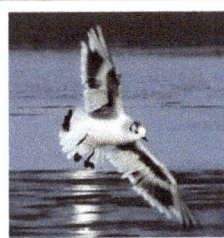
Little Gull
July 22, 2024
Maine

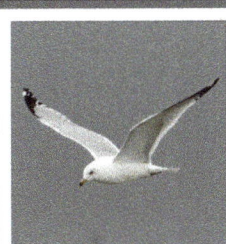
Ring-billed Gull
January 1, 2024
Massachusetts

Loons

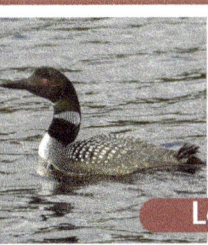
Common Loon
January 1, 2024
Massachusetts

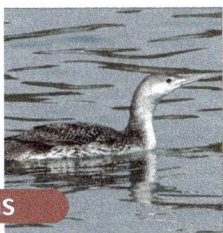
Red-throated Loon
January 8, 2024
Maine

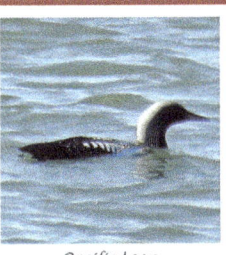
Pacific Loon
June 22, 2024
Washington State

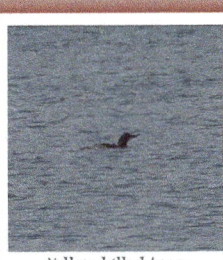
Yellow-billed Loon
October 13, 2024
Wyoming

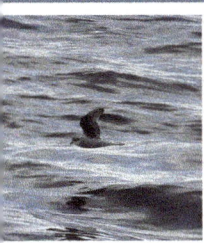
Fork-tailed Storm-Petrel
September 15, 2024
California

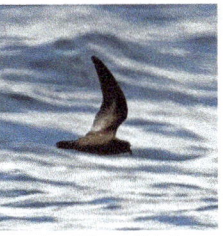
Least Storm-Petrel
September 7, 2024
California

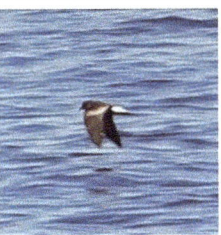
Townsend's Storm-Petrel
September 7, 2024
California

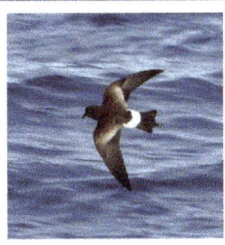
Wilson's Storm-Petrel
May 22, 2024
Maine

Gannets

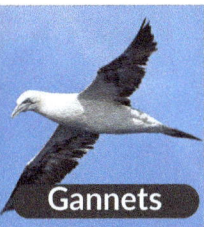
Northern Gannet
January 10, 2024
Maine

Noddies

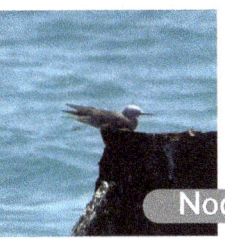
Black Noddy
May 8, 2024
Florida

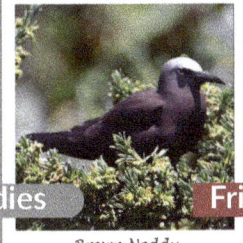
Brown Noddy
May 8, 2024
Florida

Frigatebirds

Magnificent Frigatebird
February 4, 2024
Florida

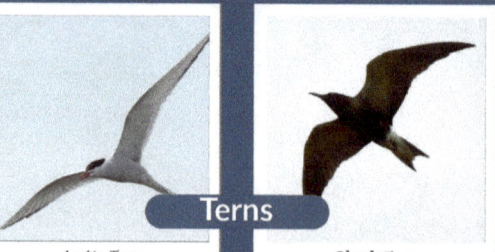
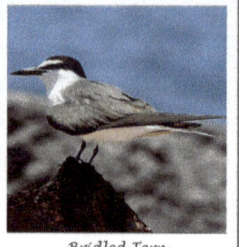
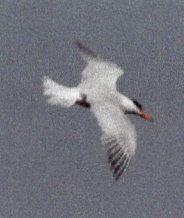

Terns

Arctic Tern
May 22, 2024
Maine

Black Tern
May 21, 2024
Maine

Bridled Tern
May 8, 2024
Florida

Caspian Tern
February 3, 2024
Florida

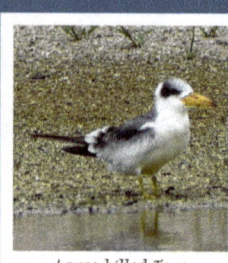
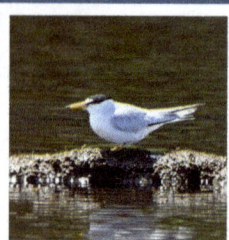
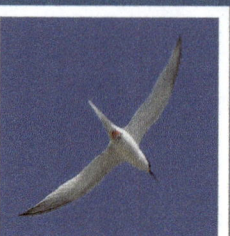
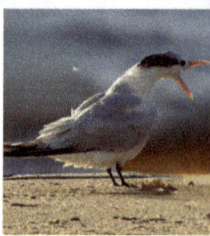

Large-billed Tern
July 10, 2024
Florida

Least Tern
May 6, 2024
Florida

Roseate Tern
May 7, 2024
Florida

Royal Tern
February 2, 2024
Florida

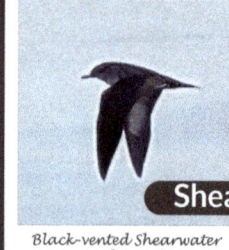
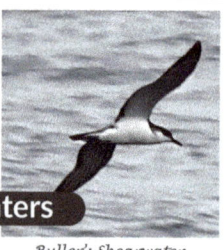
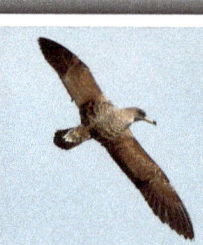
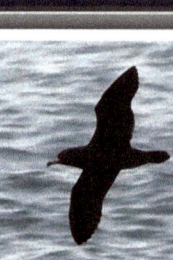

Shearwaters

Black-vented Shearwater
September 7, 2024
California

Buller's Shearwater
September 15, 2024
California

Cory's Shearwater
June 3, 2024
North Carolina

Flesh-footed Shearwater
September 15, 2024
California

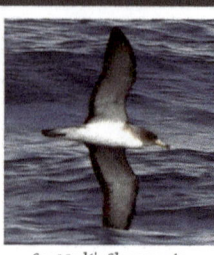
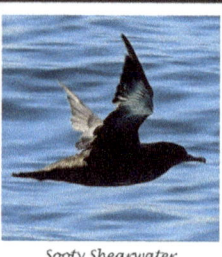
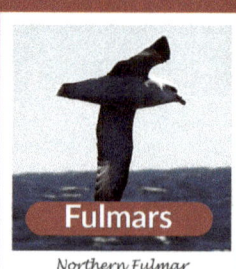
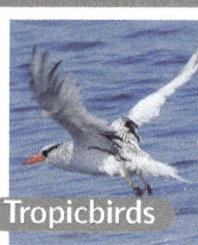

Scappoli's Shearwater
June 3, 2024
North Carolina

Sooty Shearwater
June 3, 2024
North Carolina

Fulmars

Northern Fulmar
July 16, 2024
Maine

Tropicbirds

Red-billed Tropicbird
September 7, 2024
California

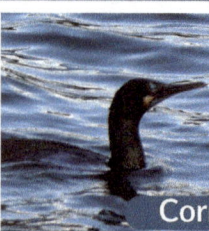
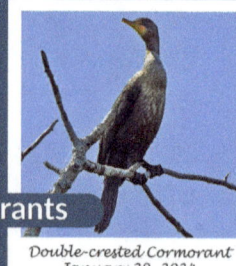
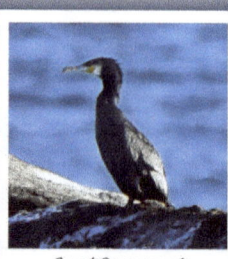
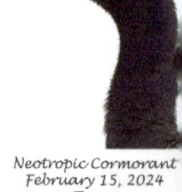

Cormorants

Brandt's Cormorant
June 21, 2024
Washington State

Double-crested Cormorant
January 29, 2024
Maryland

Great Cormorant
January 2, 2024
Maine

Neotropic Cormorant
February 15, 2024
Texas

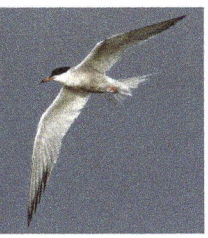
Common Tern
April 29, 2024
Massachusetts

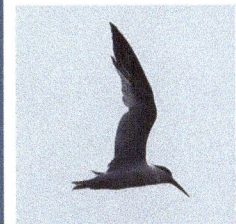
Elegant Tern
September 4, 2024
California

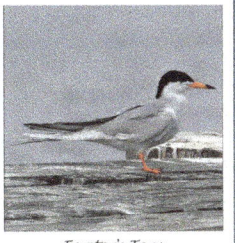
Forster's Tern
January 30, 2024
Maryland

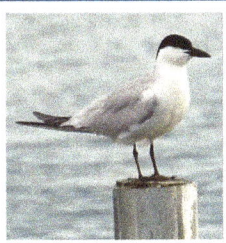
Gull-billed Tern
February 22, 2024
Texas

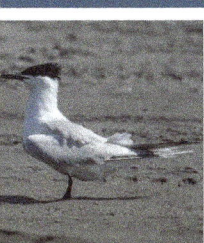
Sandwich Tern
February 5, 2024
Florida

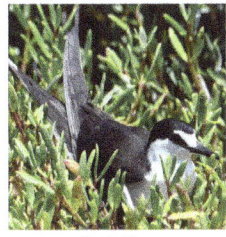
Sooty Tern
May 8, 2024
Florida

Petrels

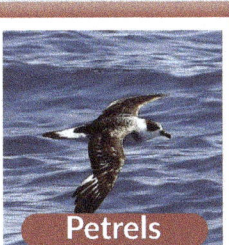
Black-capped Petrel
May 8, 2024
Florida

Albatrosses

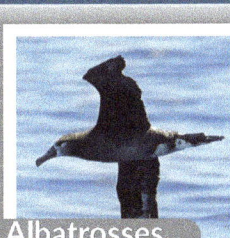
Black-footed Albatross
September 7, 2024
California

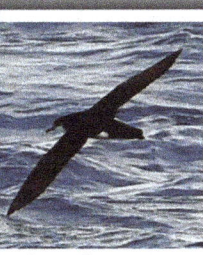
Manx Shearwater
June 3, 2024
North Carolina

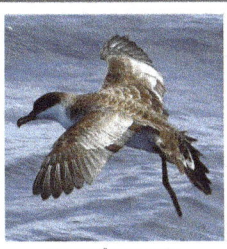
Great Shearwater
June 3, 2024
North Carolina

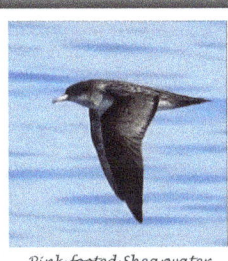
Pink-footed Shearwater
September 7, 2024
California

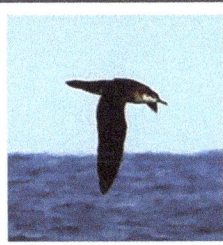
Sargasso Shearwater
May 8, 2024
Florida

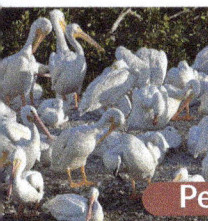
American White Pelican
January 31, 2024
North Carolina

Pelicans

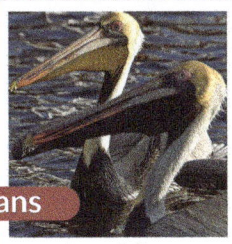
Brown Pelican
January 31, 2024
North Carolina

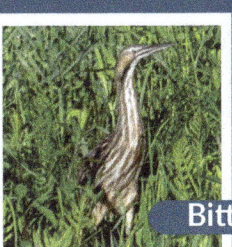
American Bittern
January 31, 2024
North Carolina

Bitterns

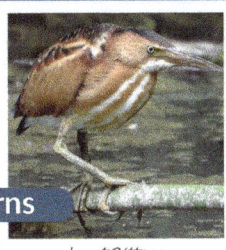
Least Bittern
February 6, 2024
Florida

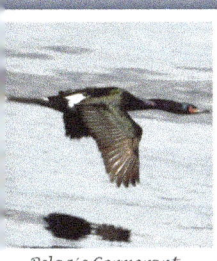
Pelagic Cormorant
June 21, 2024
Washington State

Anhingas

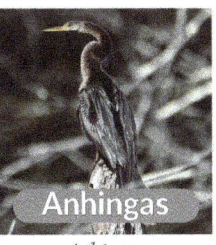
Anhinga
February 3, 2024
Florida

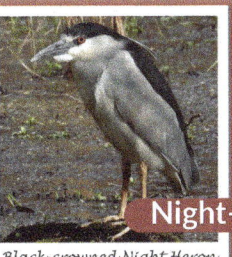
Black-crowned Night Heron
February 9, 2024
Florida

Night-Herons / 191

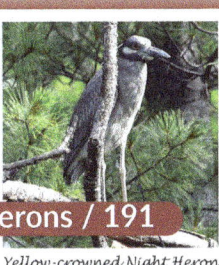
Yellow-crowned Night Heron
February 9, 2024
Florida

Vultures

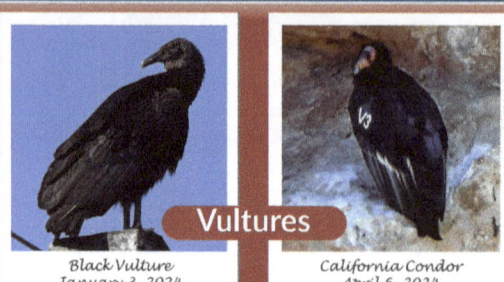
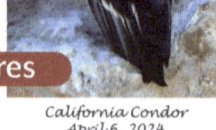
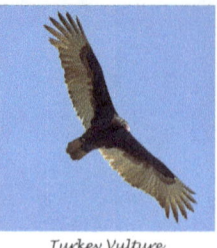
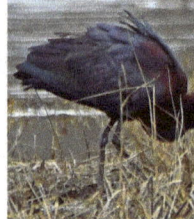

Black Vulture
January 3, 2024
New Jersey

California Condor
April 6, 2024
Arizona

Turkey Vulture
January 3, 2024
New Jersey

Glossy Ibis
February 3, 2024
Florida

Egrets

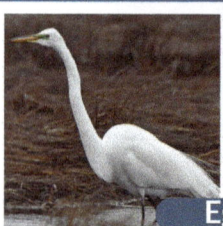
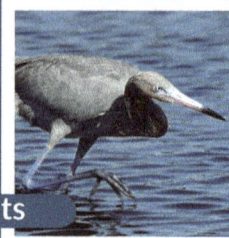
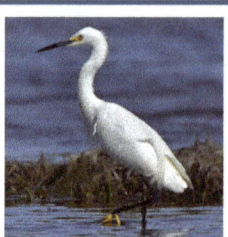
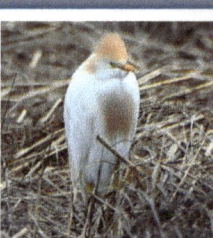

Great Egret
January 31, 2024
North Carolina

Reddish Egret
February 3, 2024
Florida

Snowy Egret
January 31, 2024
North Carolina

Western Cattle-Egret
February 3, 2024
Florida

Kites

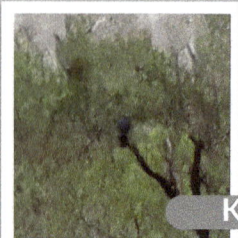
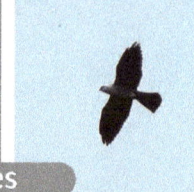
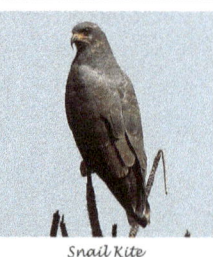
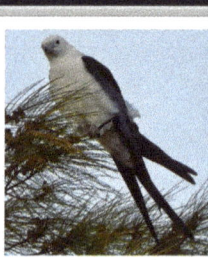

Hook-billed Kite
December 1, 2024
Texas

Mississippi Kite
May 31, 2024
New Jersey

Snail Kite
February 5, 2024
Florida

Swallow-tailed Kite
April 30, 2024
Massachusetts

Hawks (Buteos)

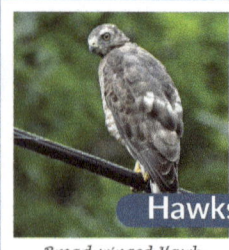
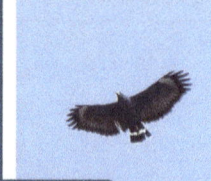
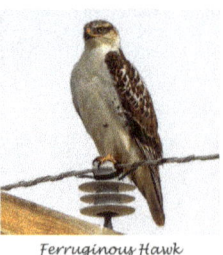
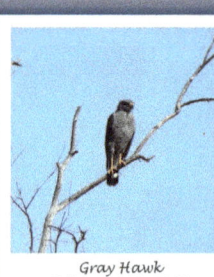

Broad-winged Hawk
February 6, 2024
Florida

Common Black Hawk
April 2, 2024
Arizona

Ferruginous Hawk
April 12, 2024
Kansas

Gray Hawk
February 24, 2024
Texas

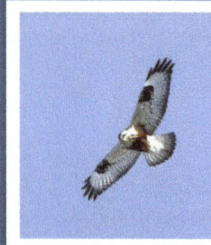
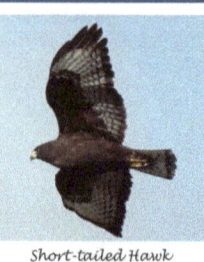
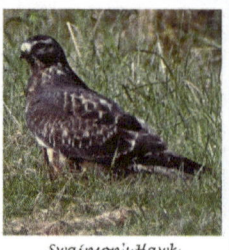
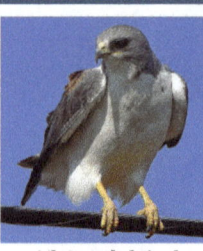

Rough-legged Hawk
January 15, 2024
Illinois

Short-tailed Hawk
February 5, 2024
Florida

Swainson's Hawk
February 25, 2024
Texas

White-tailed Hawk
February 19, 2024
Texas

Ibises

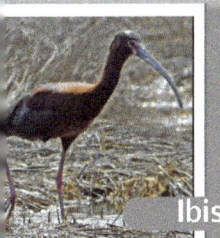
White-faced Ibis
February 15, 2024
Louisiana

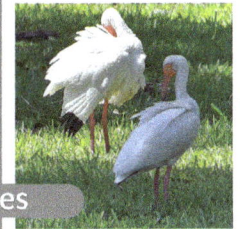
White Ibis
January 31, 2024
North Carolina

Eurasian Escapees

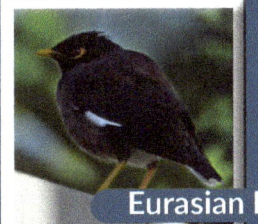
Common Myna
February 7, 2024
Florida

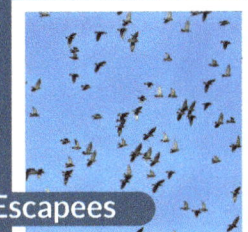
European Starlings
January 1, 2024
Massachusetts

Herons

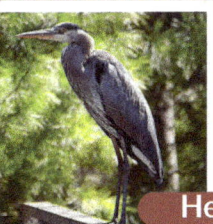
Great Blue Heron
January 3, 2024
New Jersey

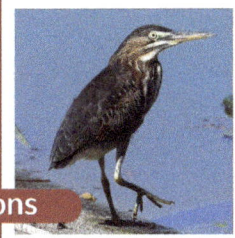
Green Heron
February 4, 2024
Florida

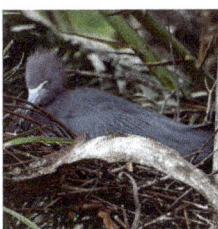
Little Blue Heron
February 3, 2024
Florida

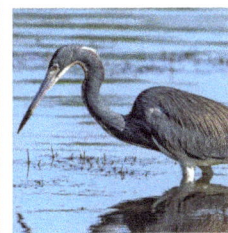
Tricolored Heron
January 31, 2024
North Carolina

Hawks (Accipiters)

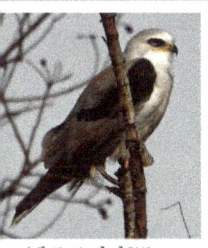
White-tailed Kite
February 15, 2024
Texas

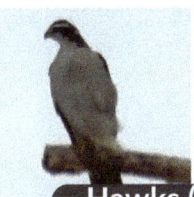
American Goshawk
January 8, 2024
Maine

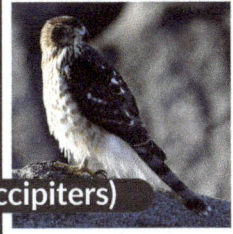
Cooper's Hawk
January 16, 2024
Minnesota

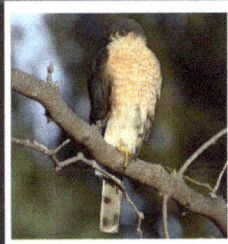
Sharp-shinned Hawk
January 4, 2024
New Jersey

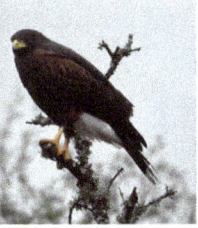
Harris's Hawk
February 16, 2024
Texas

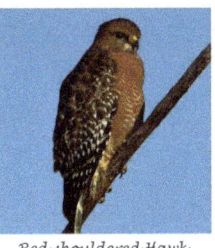
Red-shouldered Hawk
January 2, 2024
Maine

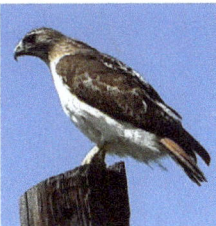
Red-tailed Hawk
January 1, 2024
Massachusetts

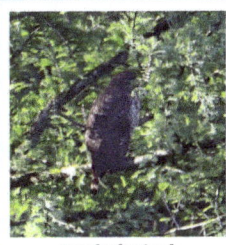
Roadside Hawk
February 18, 2024
Texas

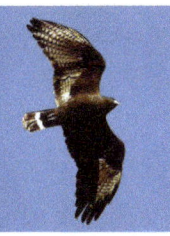
Zone-tailed Hawk
February 25, 2024
Texas

Eagles

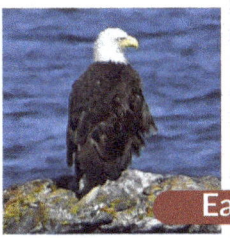
Bald Eagle
January 1, 2024
Massachusetts

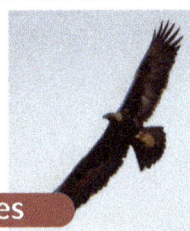
Golden Eagle
March 31, 2024
Arizona

Ospreys / 193

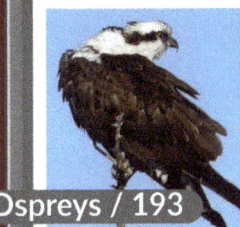
Osprey
February 2, 2024
Florida

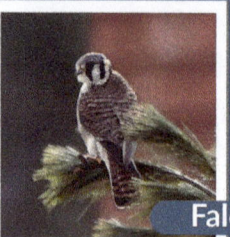
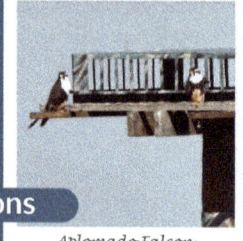
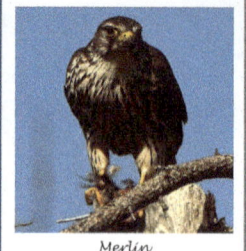
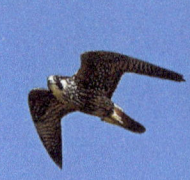

Falcons

American Kestrel
January 29, 2024
Maryland

Aplomado Falcon
February 20, 2024
Texas

Merlin
January 18, 2024
Minnesota

Peregrine Falcon
January 11, 2024
Maine

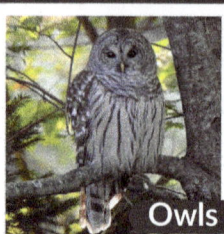
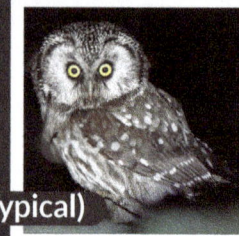
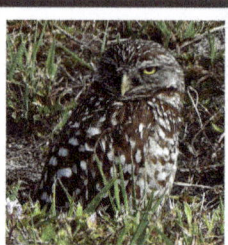
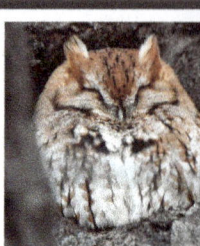

Owls (Typical)

Barred Owl
January 8, 2024
Maine

Boreal Owl
October 10, 2024
Coloardo

Burrowing Owl
February 9, 2024
Florida

Eastern Screech-Owl
January 1, 2024
Massachusetts

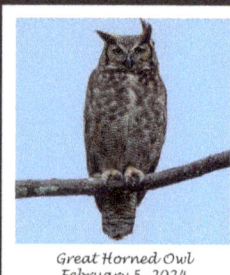
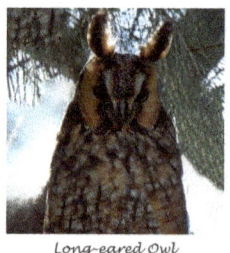
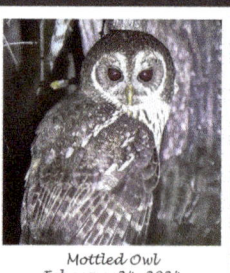
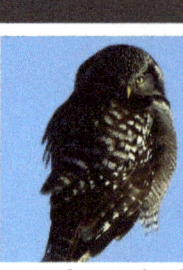

Great Horned Owl
February 5, 2024
Florida

Long-eared Owl
January 1, 2024
Massachusetts

Mottled Owl
February 24, 2024
Texas

Northern Hawk Owl
January 16, 2024
Minnesota

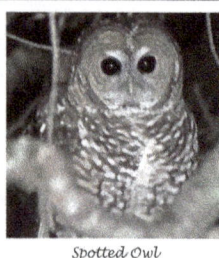
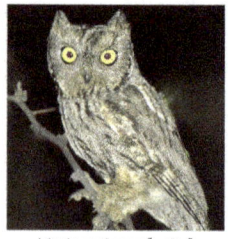
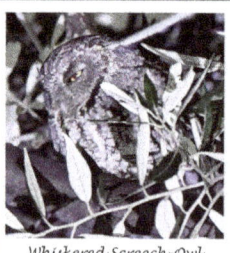
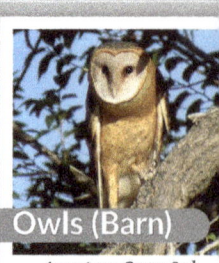

Owls (Barn)

Spotted Owl
October 12, 2024
Arizona

Western Screech-Owl
March 29, 2024
Arizona

Whiskered Screech-Owl
April 2, 2024
Arizona

American Barn Owl
February 24, 2024
Texas

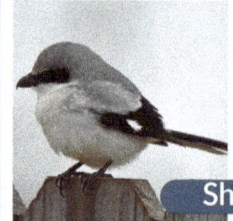
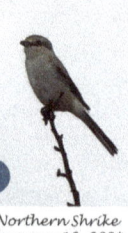
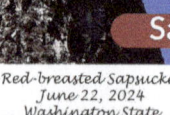

Shrikes

Sapsuckers

Loggerhead Shrike
February 4, 2024
Florida

Northern Shrike
January 16, 2024
Minnesote

Red-breasted Sapsucker
June 22, 2024
Washington State

Red-naped Sapsucker
June 24, 2024
Washington State

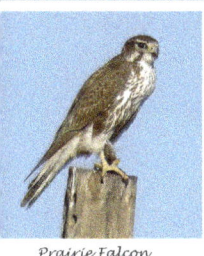
Prairie Falcon
February 18, 2024
Texas

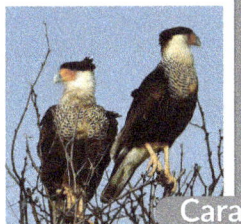
Crested Caracara
February 6, 2024
Florida

Caracaras

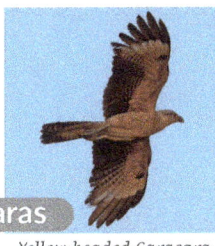
Yellow-headed Caracara
July 13, 2024
Florida

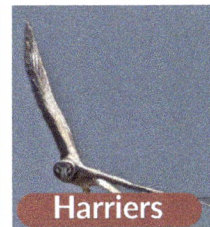
Harriers

Northern Harrier
January 1, 2024
Massachusetts

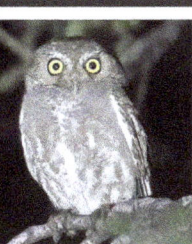
Elf Owl
March 29, 2024
Arizona

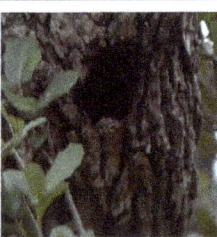
Ferruginous Pygmy-Owl
November 26, 2024
Texas

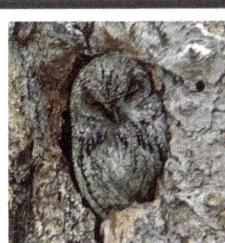
Flammulated Owl
June 26, 2024
Washington State

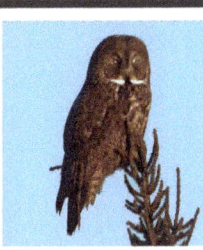
Great Gray Owl
January 17, 2024
Minnesota

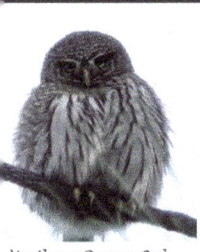
Northern Pygmy-Owl
April 2, 2024
Arizona

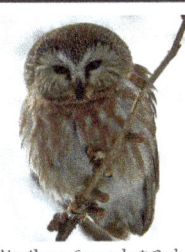
Northern Saw-whet Owl
March 9, 2024
Maine

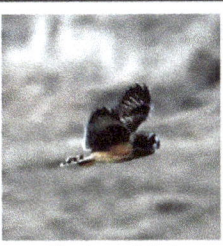
Short-eared Owl
January 12, 2024
Maine

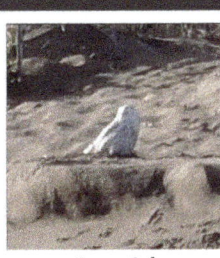
Snowy Owl
November 16, 2024
Massachusetts

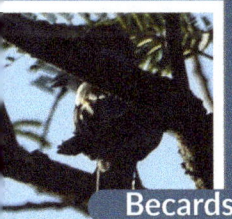
Becards

Gray-collared Becard
February 20, 2024
Texas

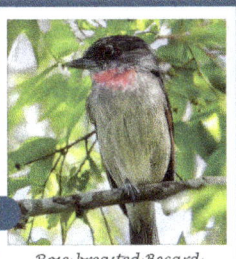
Rose-breasted Becard
February 25, 2024
Texas

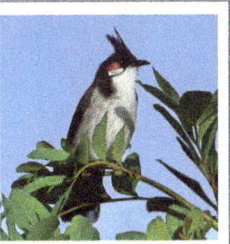
Red-whiskered Bulbul
February 11, 2024
Florida

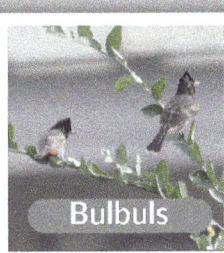
Bulbuls

Red-vented Bulbul
November 24, 2024
Texas

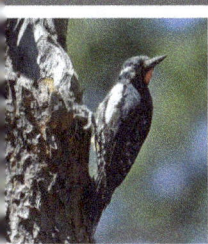
Williamson's Sapsucker
June 27, 2024
Oregon

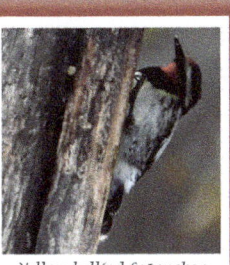
Yellow-bellied Sapsucker
January 3, 2024
New Jersey

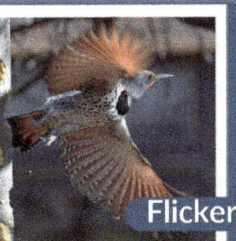
Flickers / 195

Gilded Flicker
April 4, 2024
Arizona

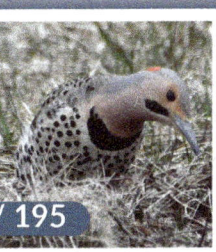
Northern Flicker
January 28, 2024
Maine

Woodpeckers

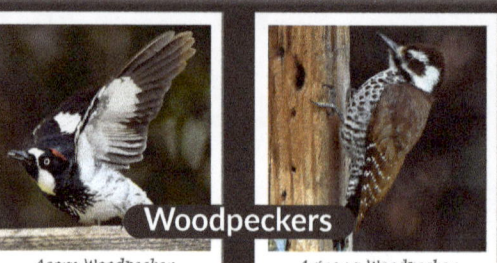
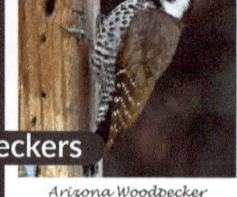
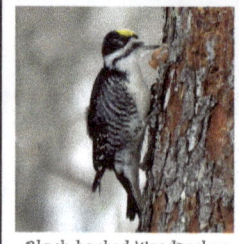
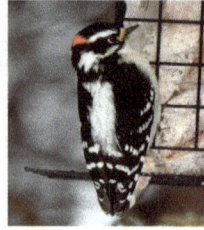

Acorn Woodpecker
March 29, 2024
Arizona

Arizona Woodpecker
March 29, 2024
Arizona

Black-backed Woodpecker
June 13, 2024
Maine

Downy Woodpecker
January 1, 2024
Maine

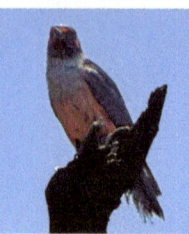
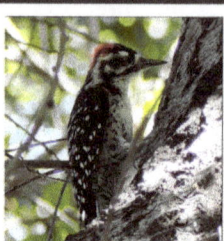
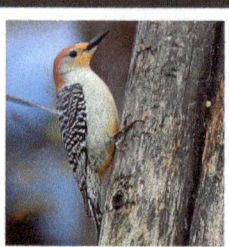
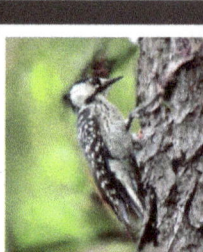

Lewis's Woodpecker
June 25, 2024
Washington State

Nuttall's Woodpecker
September 6, 2024
California

Red-bellied Woodpecker
January 2, 2024
Maine

Red-cockaded Woodpecker
February 2, 2024
South Carolina

Kingbirds

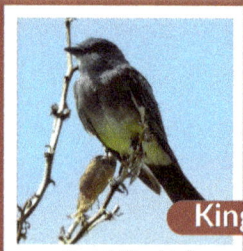
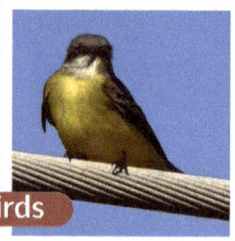
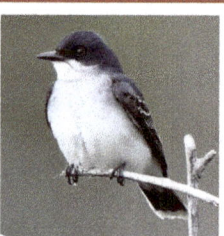
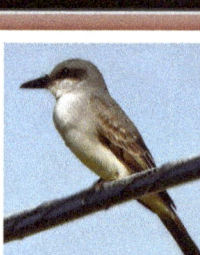

Cassin's Kingbird
April 2, 2024
Arizona

Couch's Kingbird
February 21, 2024
Texas

Eastern Kingbird
April 30, 2024
Massachusetts

Gray Kingbird
May 5, 2024
Florida

Pewees / Tyrants

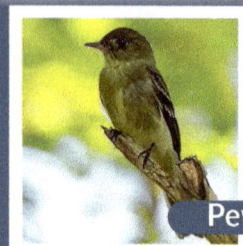
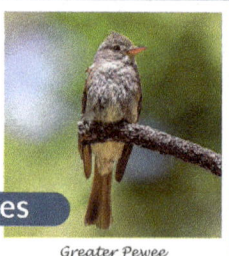
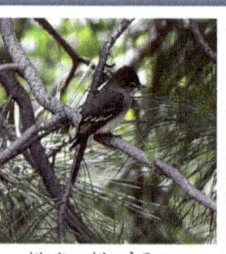
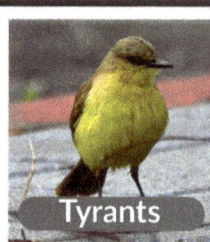

Eastern Wood-Pewee
May 30, 2024
Maine

Greater Pewee
August 10, 2024
Arizona

Western Wood-Pewee
June 22, 2024
Washington State

Cattle Tyrant
February 16, 2024
Texas

Towhees

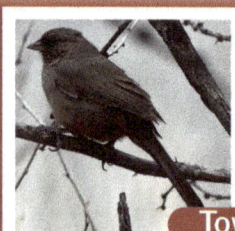
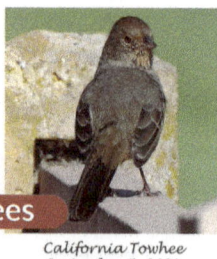
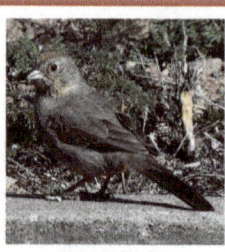
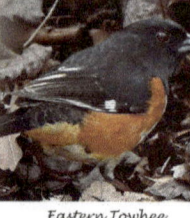

Abert's Towhee
March 30, 2024
Arizona

California Towhee
September 5, 2024
California

Canyon Towhee
March 27, 2024
New Mexico

Eastern Towhee
February 4, 2024
Florida

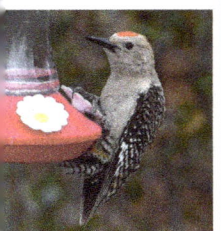
Gila Woodpecker
March 13, 2024
Texas

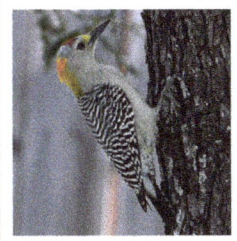
Golden-fronted Woodpecker
February 16, 2024
Texas

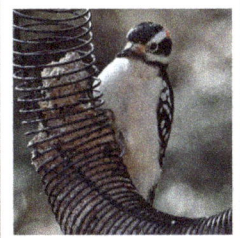
Hairy Woodpecker
January 2, 2024
Maine

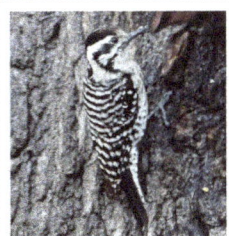
Ladder-backed Woodpecker
February 16, 2024
Texas

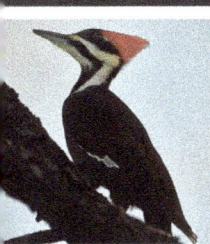
Pileated Woodpecker
January 1, 2024
Massachusetts

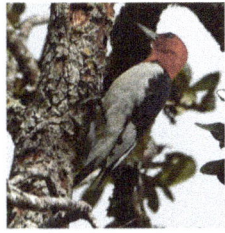
Red-headed Woodpecker
February 9, 2024
Florida

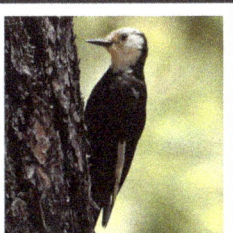
White-headed Woodpecker
June 25, 2024
Washington State

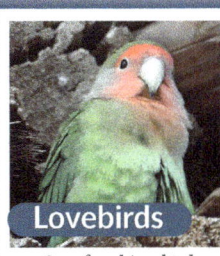

Lovebirds

Rosy-faced Lovebird
April 5, 2024
Arizona

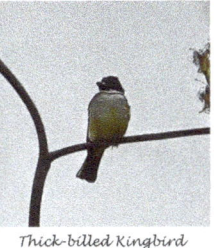
Thick-billed Kingbird
August 11, 2024
Arizona

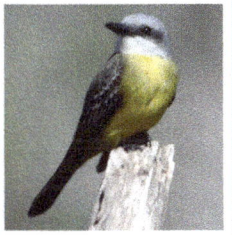
Tropical Kingbird
February 7, 2024
Florida

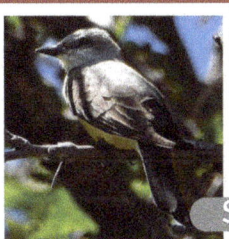
Western Kingbird
April 4, 2024
Arizona

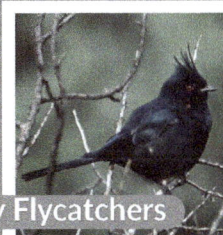

Silky Flycatchers

Phainopepla
March 29, 2024
Arizona

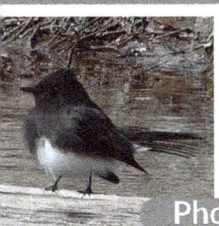
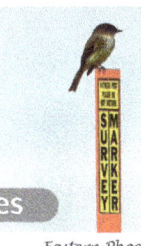

Phoebes

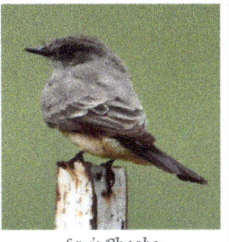
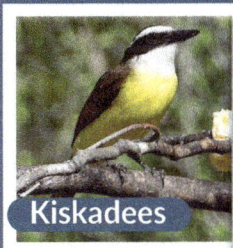

Kiskadees

Black Phoebe
February 18, 2024
Texas

Eastern Phoebe
January 31, 2024
North Carolina

Say's Phoebe
February 19, 2024
Texas

Great Kiskadee
February 17, 2024
Texas

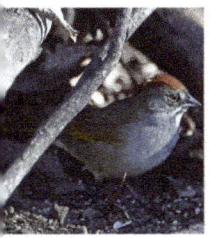
Green-tailed Towhee
March 30, 2024
Arizona

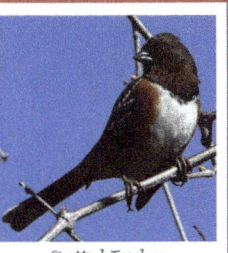
Spotted Towhee
February 29, 2024
Texas

Amazons (Parrots)

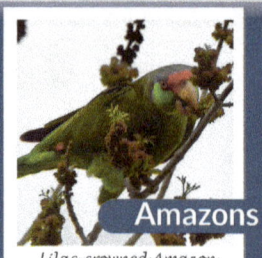
Lilac-crowned Amazon
February 26, 2024
Texas

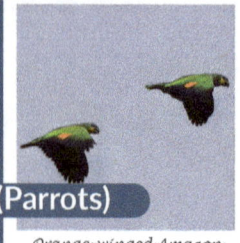
Orange-winged Amazon
May 5, 2024
Florida

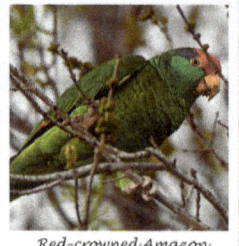
Red-crowned Amazon
February 19, 2024
Texas

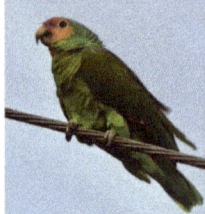
Red-lored Amazon
February 19, 2024
Texas

Parakeets

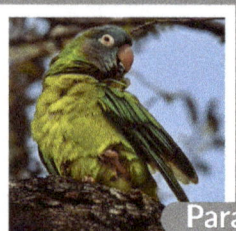
Blue-crowned Parakeet
February 11, 2024
Florida

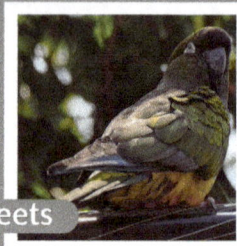
Burrowing Parakeet
September 9, 2024
California

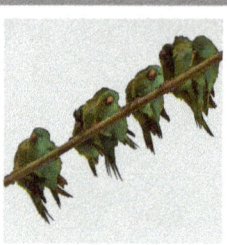
Green Parakeet
February 26, 2024
Texas

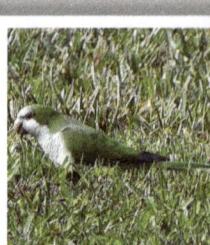
Monk Parakeet
February 9, 2024
Florida

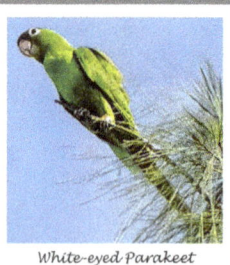
White-eyed Parakeet
May 5, 2024
Florida

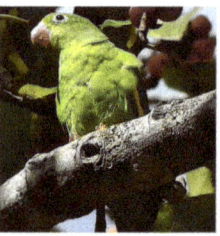
Yellow-chevroned Parakeet
May 5, 2024
Florida

Exotics

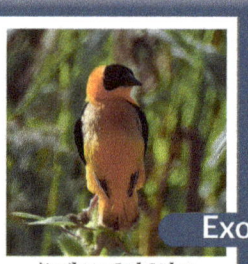
Northern Red Bishop
September 6, 2024
California

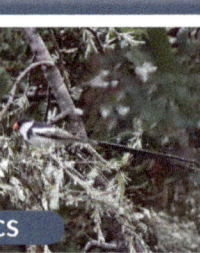
Pin-tailed Whydah
September 6, 2024
California

Jays

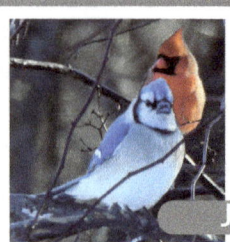
Blue Jay
January 1, 2024
Massachusetts

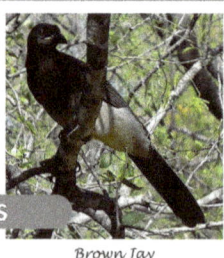
Brown Jay
February 25, 2024
Texas

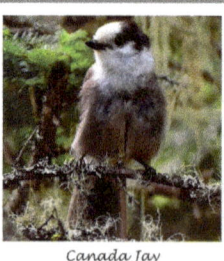
Canada Jay
January 16, 2024
Texas

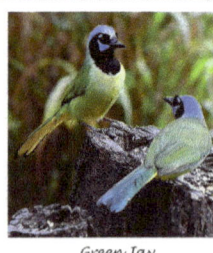
Green Jay
February 16, 2024
Texas

Crows

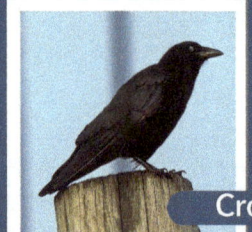
American Crow
January 1, 2024
Massachusetts

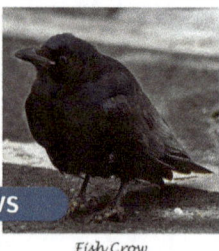
Fish Crow
January 20, 2024
Maine

Ravens

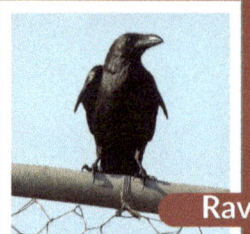
Chihuahuan Raven
February 25, 2024
Texas

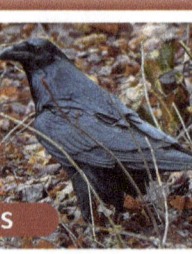
Common Raven
January 1, 2024
Massachusetts

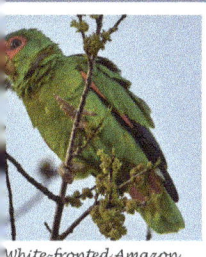
White-fronted Amazon
February 19, 2024
Texas

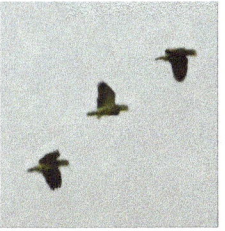
Yellow-headed Amazons
September 9, 2024
California

Macaws

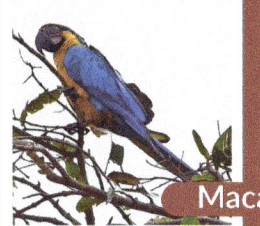
Blue-and-yellow Macaw
February 11, 2024
Florida

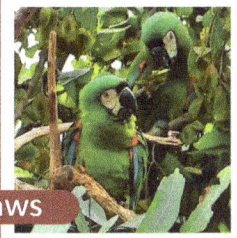
Chestnut-fronted Macaw
February 11, 2024
Florida

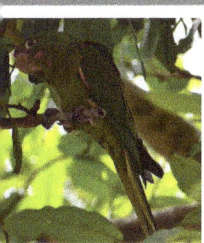
Mitred Parakeet
February 11, 2024
Florida

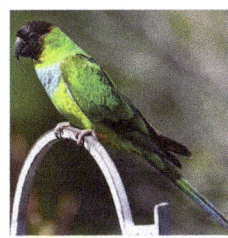
Nanday Parakeet
February 12, 2024
Florida

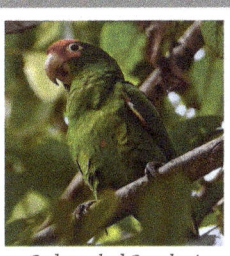
Red-masked Parakeet
February 11, 2024
Florida

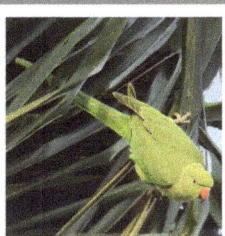
Rose-ringed Parakeet
July 10, 2024
Florida

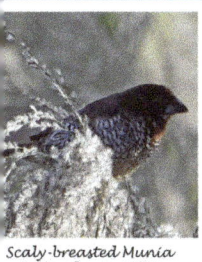
Scaly-breasted Munia
September 6, 2024
California

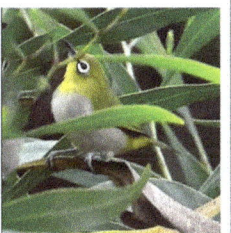
Swinhoe's White-ey
September 5, 2024
California

Waxwings

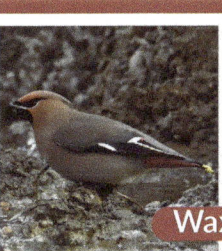
Bohemian Waxwing
January 21, 2024
Maine

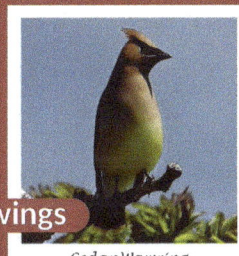
Cedar Waxwing
January 21, 2024
Maine

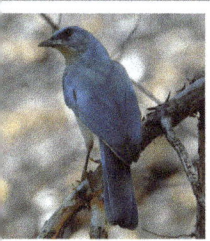
Mexican Jay
March 29, 2024
Arizona

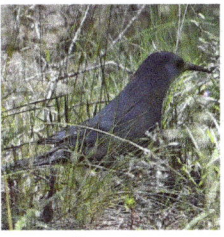
Pinyon Jay
April 6, 2024
Arizona

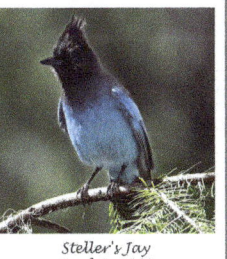
Steller's Jay
April 5, 2024
Arizona

Nutcrackers

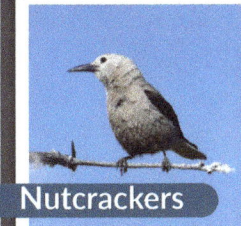
Clark's Nutcracker
April 6, 2024
Arizona

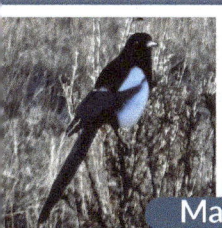
Black-billed Magpie
January 16, 2024
Minnesota

Magpies

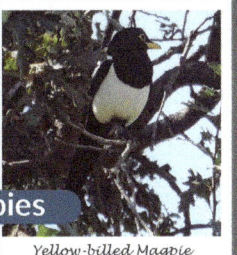
Yellow-billed Magpie
September 12, 2024
California

Parrotbills

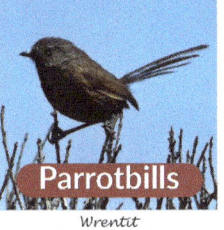
Wrentit
June 28, 2024
Oregon

Tits / 199

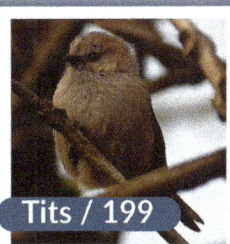
Bushtit
March 26, 2024
New Mexico

Flycatchers

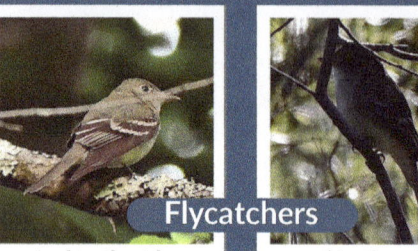
Acadian Flycatcher
June 1, 2024
Virginia

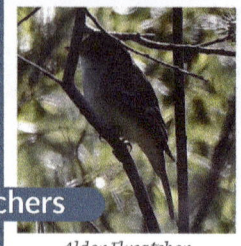
Alder Flycatcher
May 16, 2024
Maine

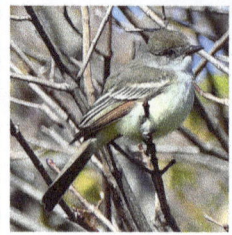
Ash-throated Flycatcher
March 24, 2024
Texas

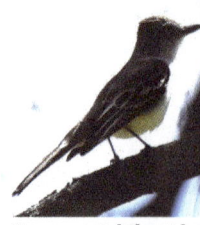
Brown-crested Flycatcher
August 7, 2024
New Mexico

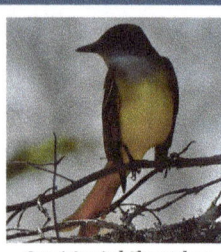
Great Crested Flycatcher
April 29, 2024
Massachusetts

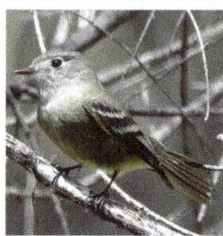
Hammond's Flycatcher
February 18, 2024
Texas

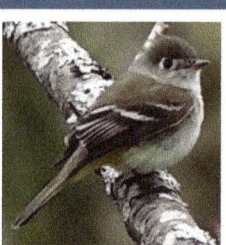
Least Flycatcher
February 7, 2024
Florida

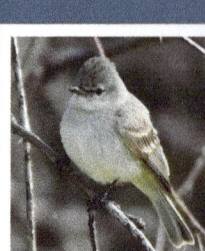
Northern Beardless-Tyrannulet
February 27, 2024
Texas

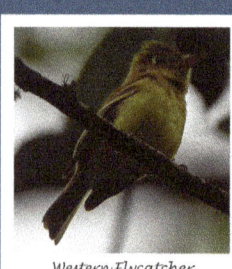
Western Flycatcher
June 22, 2024
Washington State

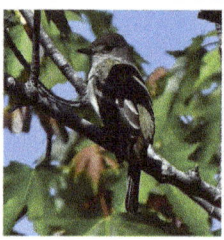
Willow Flycatcher
May 17, 2024
Maine

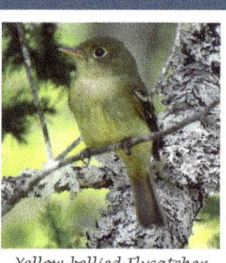
Yellow-bellied Flycatcher
May 14, 2024
Massachusetts

Wheatears

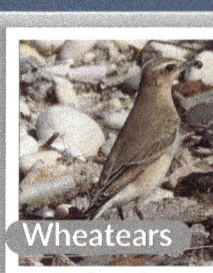
Northern Wheatear
October 10, 2024
New York

Vireos

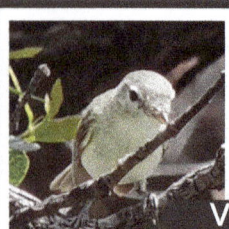
Bell's Vireo
April 2, 2024
Arizona

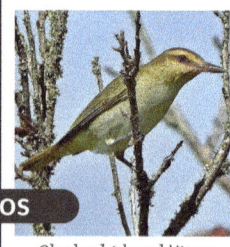
Black-whiskered Vireo
May 7, 2024
Florida

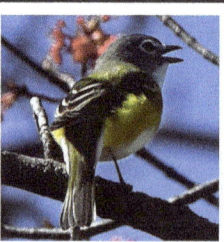
Blue-headed Vireo
February 2, 2024
South Carolina

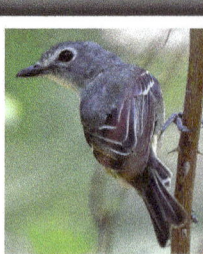
Cassin's Vireo
June 4, 2024
Washington State

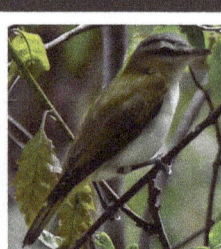
Red-eyed Vireo
May 10, 2024
Maine

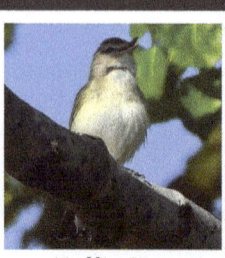
Warbling Vireo
May 2, 2024
Maine

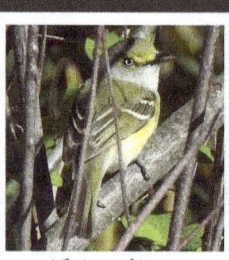
White-eyed Vireo
February 7, 2024
Florida

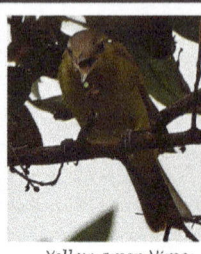
Yellow-green Vireo
July 11, 2024
Florida

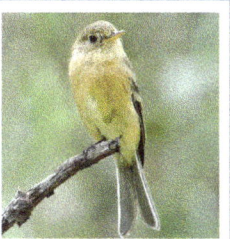
Buff-breasted Flycatcher
August 5, 2024
Arizona

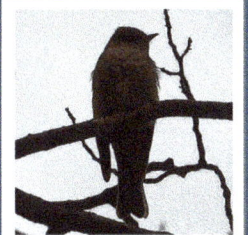
Dusky Flycatcher
June 26, 2024
Washington State

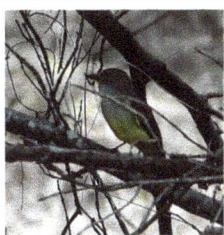
Dusky-capped Flycatcher
February 17, 2024
Texas

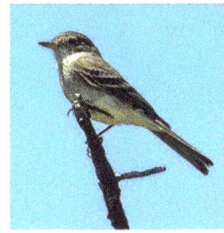
Gray Flycatcher
April 5, 2024
Arizona

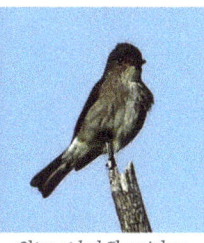
Olive-sided Flycatcher
June 13, 2024
Maine

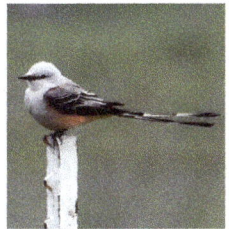
Scissor-tailed Flycatcher
March 24, 2024
Texas

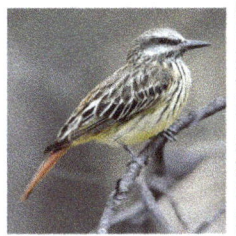
Sulphur-bellied Flycatcher
August 5, 2024
Arizona

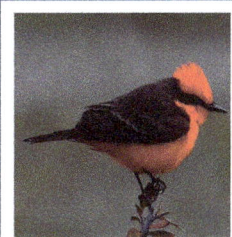
Vermilion Flycatcher
February 5, 2024
Florida

Scrub-Jays

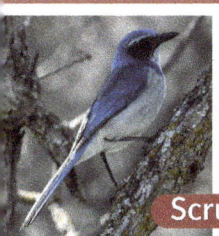
California Scrub-Jay
June 26, 2024
California

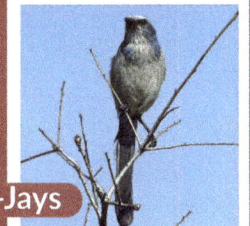
Florida Scrub-Jay
February 3, 2024
Massachusetts

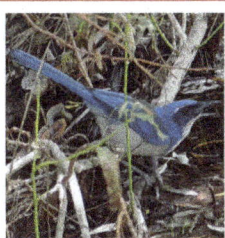
Island Scrub-Jay
September 11, 2024
California

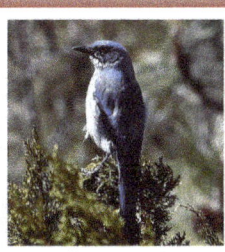
Woodhouse's Scrub-Jay
March 26, 2024
New Mexico

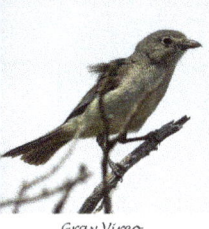
Gray Vireo
August 12, 2024
Arizona

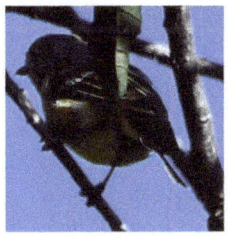
Hutton's Vireo
March 31, 2024
Arizona

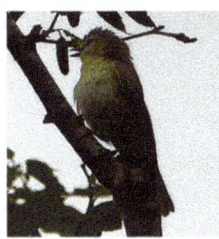
Philadelphia Vireo
May 27, 2024
Maine

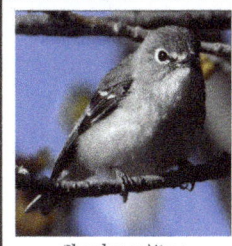
Plumbeous Vireo
April 2, 2024
Arizona

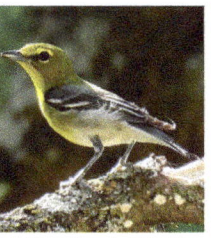
Yellow-throated Vireo
May 18, 2024
Massachusetts

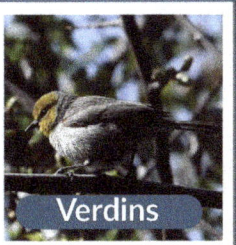
Verdins
Verdin
February 19, 2024
Texas

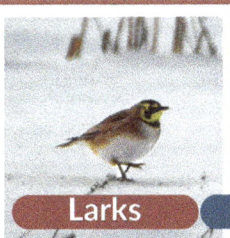
Larks
Horned Lark
January 8, 2024
Maine

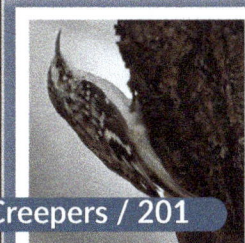
Creepers / 201
Brown Creeper
January 2, 2024
Maine

Chickadees

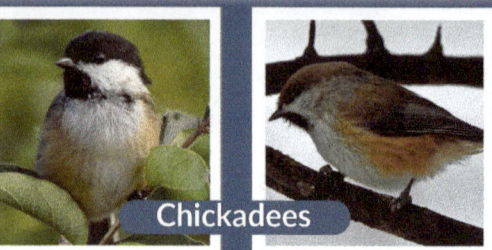

Black-capped Chickadee
January 1, 2024
Maine

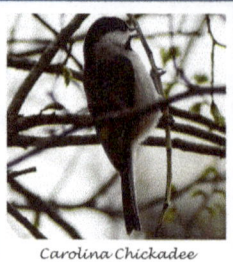

Boreal Chickadee
January 16, 2024
Minnesota

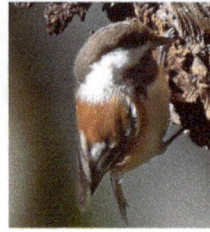

Carolina Chickadee
January 3, 2024
New Jersey

Chestnut-backed Chickadee
June 22, 2024
Washington State

Wrens

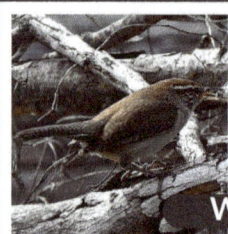

Bewick's Wren
February 19, 2024
Texas

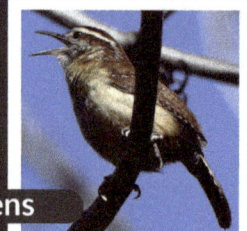

Carolina Wren
January 12, 2024
Maine

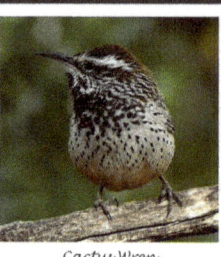

Cactus Wren
February 25, 2024
Texas

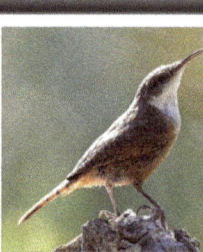

Canyon Wren
April 2, 2024
Arizona

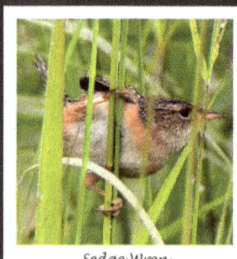

Sedge Wren
February 22, 2024
Texas

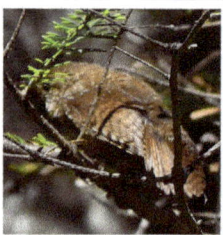

Winter Wren
February 25, 2024
Texas

Titmice

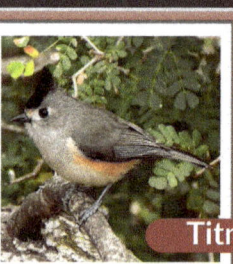

Black-crested Titmouse
February 16, 2024
Texas

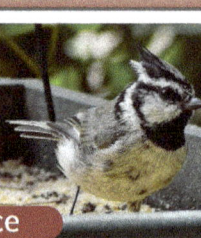

Bridled Titmouse
March 29, 2024
Arizona

Mimics

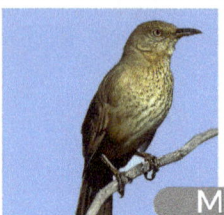

Bendire's Thrasher
August 7, 2024
Arizona

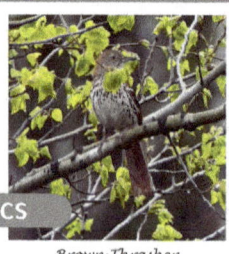

Brown Thrasher
February 4, 2024
Florida

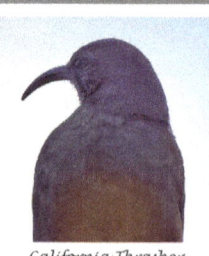

California Thrasher
September 6, 2024
California

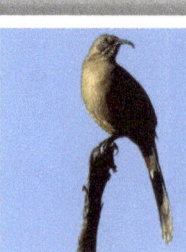

Crissal Thrasher
March 29, 2024
Arizona

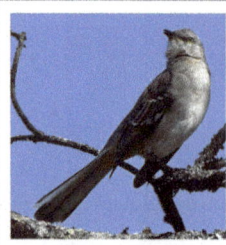

Northern Mockingbird
January 1, 2024
Massachusetts

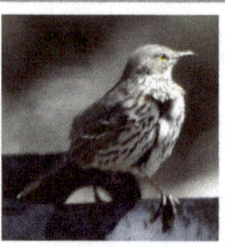

Sage Thrasher
April 9, 2024
Colorado

Nuthatches

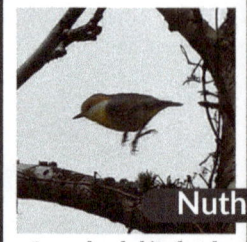

Brown-headed Nuthatch
January 31, 2024
North Carolina

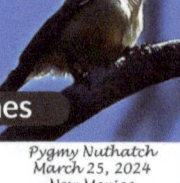

Pygmy Nuthatch
March 25, 2024
New Mexico

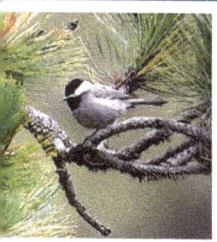
Mexican Chickadee
March 29, 2024
Arizona

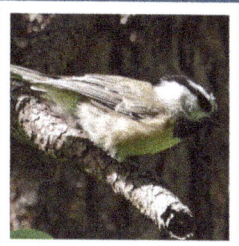
Mountain Chickadee
March 25, 2024
New Mexico

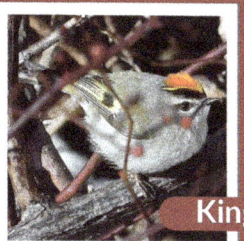
Golden-crowned Kinglet
January 12, 2024
Maine

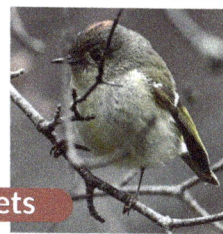
Ruby-crowned Kinglet
January 21, 2024
Maine

Kinglets

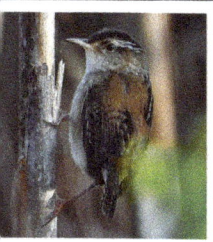
Marsh Wren
March 26, 2024
New Mexico

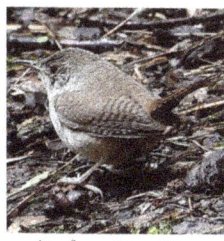
Northern House Wren
February 2, 2024
South Carolina

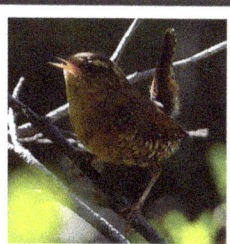
Pacific Wren
June 23, 2024
Washington State

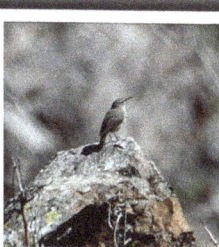
Rock Wren
February 25, 2024
Texas

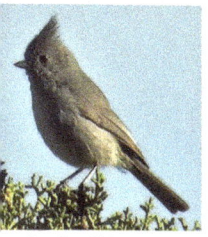
Juniper Titmouse
March 28, 2024
Arizona

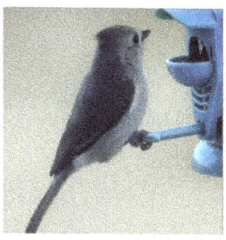
Oak Titmouse
September 9, 2024
California

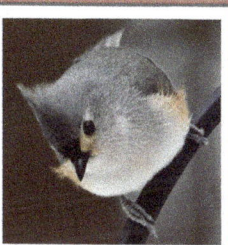
Tufted Titmouse
January 2, 2024
Maine

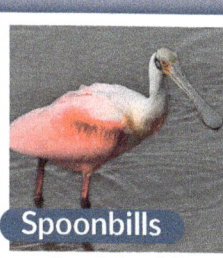
Roseate Spoonbill
February 3, 2024
Florida

Spoonbills

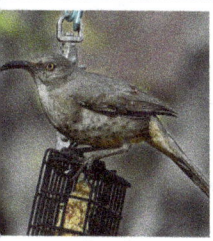
Curve-billed Thrasher
February 16, 2024
Texas

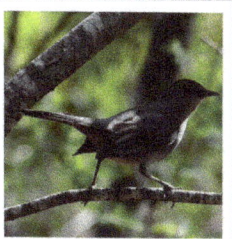
Gray Catbird
February 2, 2024
South Carolina

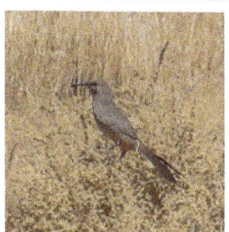
LeConte's Thrasher
September 17, 2024
California

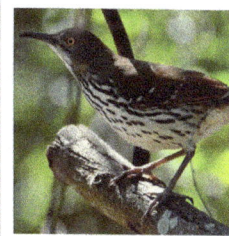
Long-billed Thrasher
February 17, 2024
Texas

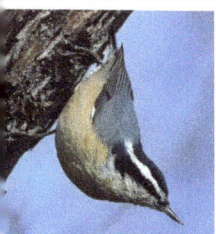
Red-breasted Nuthatch
January 2, 2024
Maine

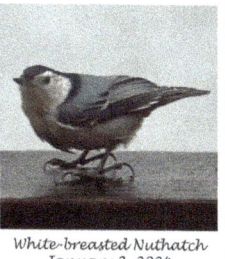
White-breasted Nuthatch
January 2, 2024
Maine

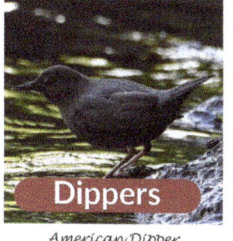
American Dipper
June 24, 2024
Washington State

Dippers

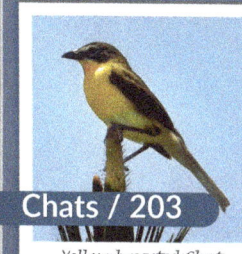
Yellow-breasted Chat
June 4, 2024
Virginia

Chats / 203

Swallows

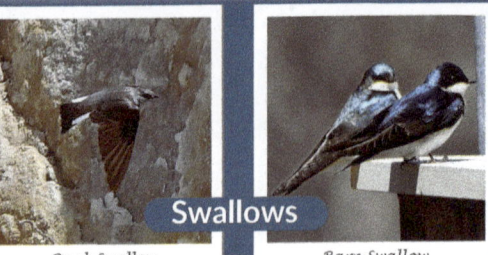
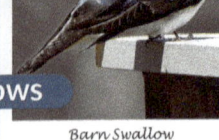
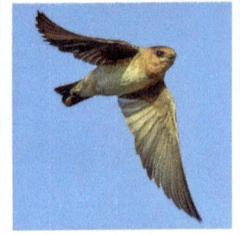
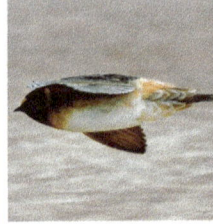

Bank Swallow
April 1, 2024
Arizona

Barn Swallow
January 29, 2024
Texas

Cave Swallow
February 21, 2024
Texas

Cliff Swallow
February 29, 2024
Texas

Thrushes

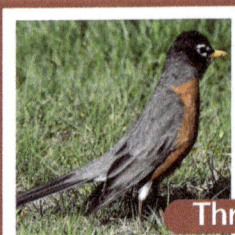
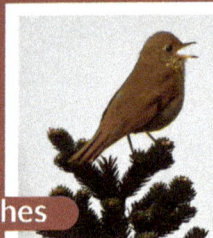
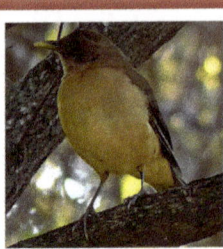
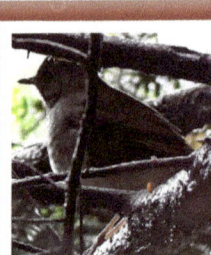

American Robin
January 1, 2024
Massachusetts

Bicknell's Thrush
May 28, 2024
New Hampshire

Clay-colored Thrush
February 18, 2024
Texas

Gray-cheeked Thrush
May 30, 2024
Massachusetts

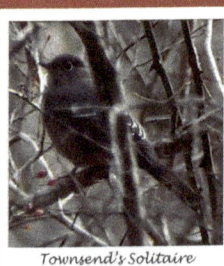
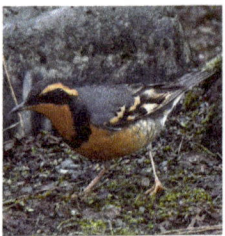
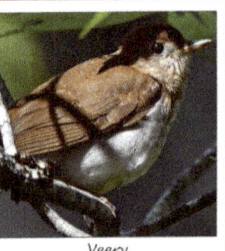
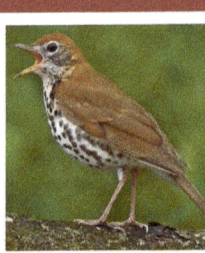

Townsend's Solitaire
April 10, 2024
Colorado

Varied Thrush
June 25, 2024
Washington State

Veery
April 23, 2024
Maine

Wood Thrush
April 30, 2024
Massachusetts

Bluebirds

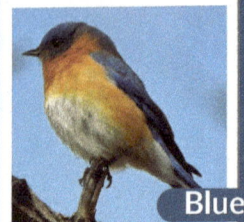
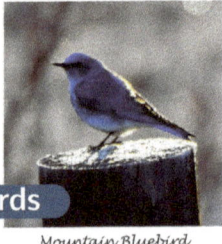
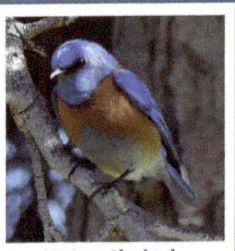
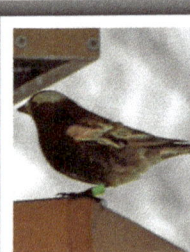

Eastern Bluebird
January 5, 2024
Maine

Mountain Bluebird
April 6, 2024
Arizona

Western Bluebird
May 26, 2024
New Mexico

Black Rosy-Finch
March 25, 2024
New Mexico

Pipits · Longspurs

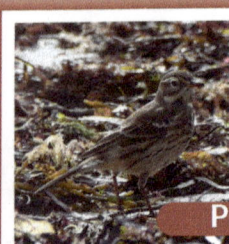
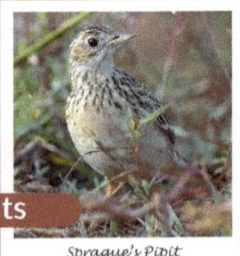
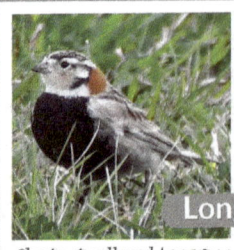
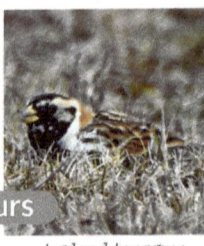

American Pipit
February 15, 2024
Louisiana

Sprague's Pipit
February 29, 2024
Texas

Chestnut-collared Longspur
February 29, 2024
Texas

Lapland Longspur
March 19, 2024
New Hampshire

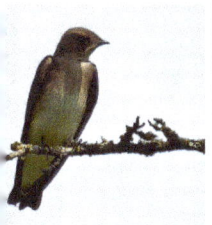
Northern Rough-winged Swallow
February 5, 2024
Florida

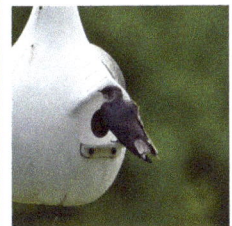
Purple Martin
February 5, 2024
Florida

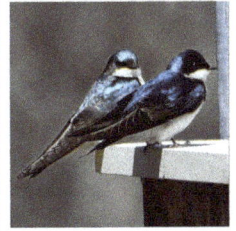
Tree Swallow
February 1, 2024
South Carolina

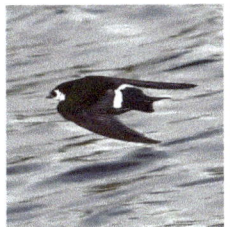
Violet-green Swallow
March 26, 2024
New Mexico

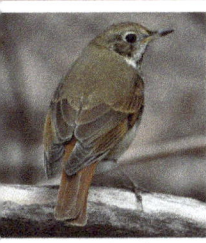
Hermit Thrush
January 3, 2024
New Jersey

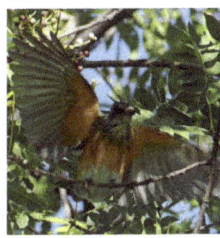
Rufous-backed Robin
October 17, 2024
Arizona

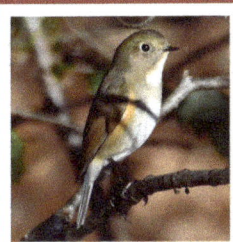
Red-flanked Bluetail
January 3, 2024
New Jersey

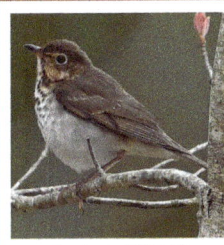
Swainson's Thrush
May 11, 2024
Maine

Buntings

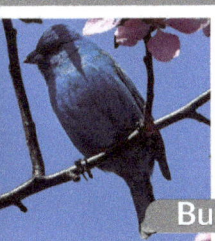
Indigo Bunting
February 9, 2024
Florida

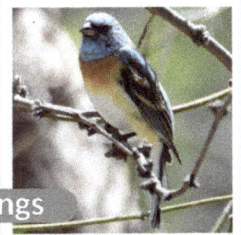
Lazuli Bunting
February 9, 2024
Florida

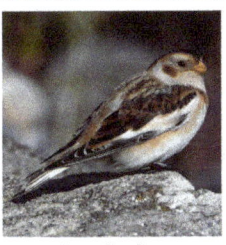
Snow Bunting
January 19, 2024
Maine

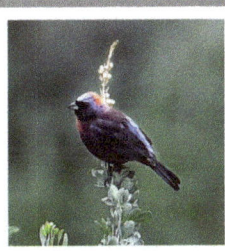
Varied Bunting
August 8, 2024
Arizona

Rosy-Finches

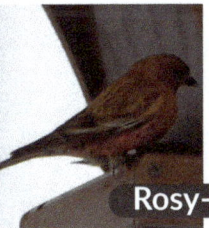
Brown-capped Rosy-Finch
March 25, 2024
New Mexico

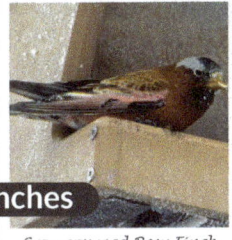
Gray-crowned Rosy-Finch
March 25, 2024
New Mexico

Juncos

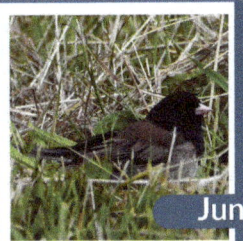
Dark-eyed Junco
January 1, 2024
Massachusetts

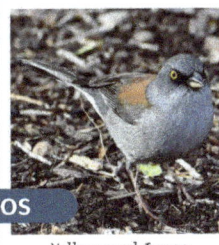
Yellow-eyed Junco
March 29, 2024
Arizona

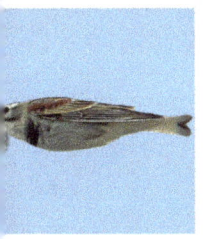
Thick-billed Longspur
April 11, 2024
Colorado

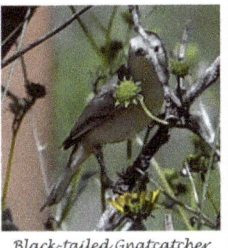
Black-tailed Gnatcatcher
April 4, 2024
Arizona

Gnatcatchers / 205

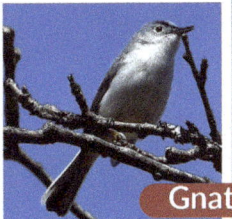
Blue-gray Gnatcatcher
February 4, 2024
Florida

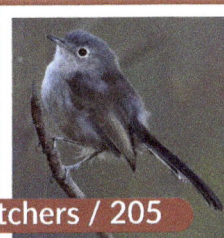
California Gnatcatcher
September 6, 2024
California

Grosbeaks

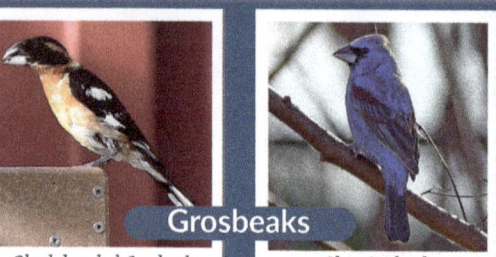

Black-headed Grosbeak
February 19, 2024
Texas

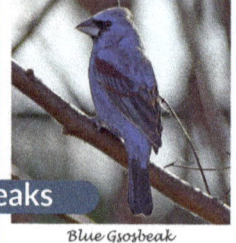

Blue Grosbeak
April 16, 2024
Massachusetts

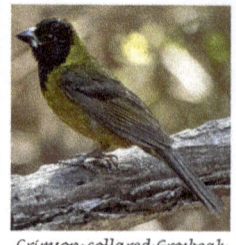

Crimson-collared Grosbeak
February 27, 2024
Texas

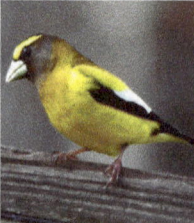

Evening Grosbeak
January 16, 2024
Minnesota

Crossbills

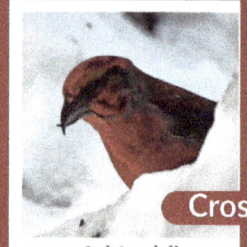

Red Crossbill
January 16, 2024
Minnesota

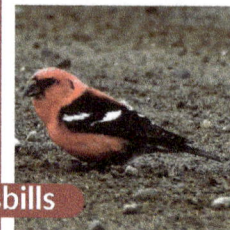

White-winged Crossbill
March 20, 2024
Maine

Goldfinches

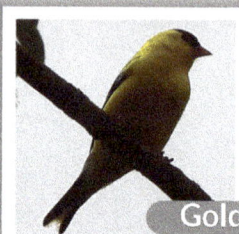

American Goldfinch
January 1, 2024
Massachusetts

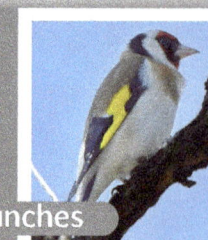

European Goldfinch
April 14, 2024
Illinois

Finches

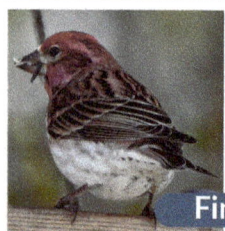

Cassin's Finch
March 26, 2024
New Mexico

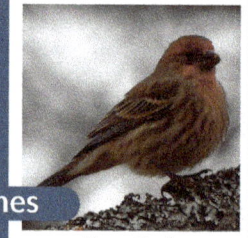

House Finch
March 2, 2024
Texas

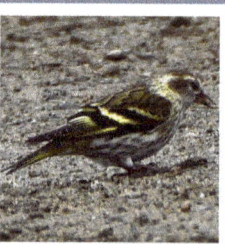

Pine Siskin
January 6, 2024
New Hampshire

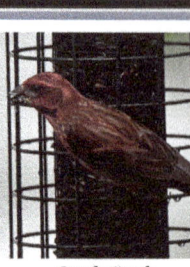

Purple Finch
March 12, 2024
Maine

Tanagers

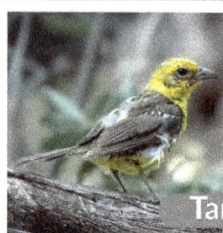

Flame-colored Tanager
August 5, 2024
Arizona

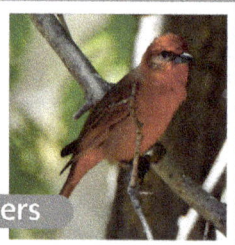

Heptatic Tanager
January 8, 2024
Maine

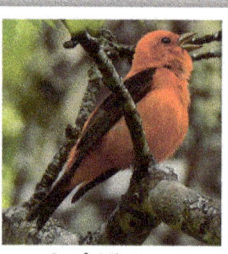

Scarlet Tanager
April 17, 2024
Massachusetts

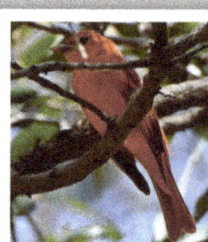

Summer Tanager
February 11, 2024
Florida

Cardinals & Allies

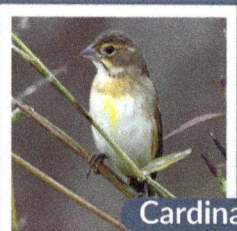

Dickcissel
June 5, 2024
Delaware

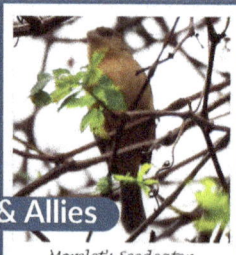

Morelet's Seedeater
February 25, 2024
Texas

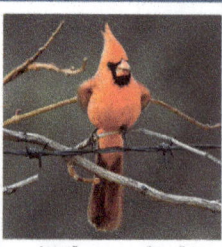

Northern Cardinal
January 1, 2024
Massachusetts

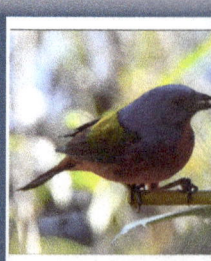

Painted Bunting
February 2, 2024
Florida

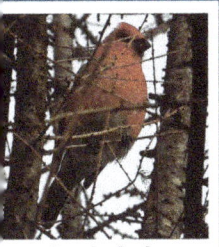
Pine Grosbeak
January 16, 2024
Minnesota

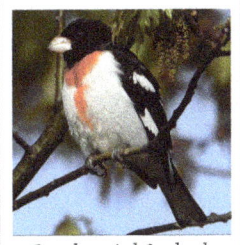
Rose-breasted Grosbeak
May 10, 2024
Maine

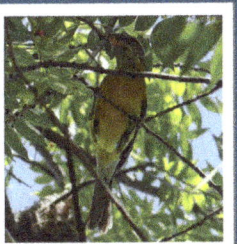
Yellow Grosbeak
October 17, 2024
Arizona

Trogons

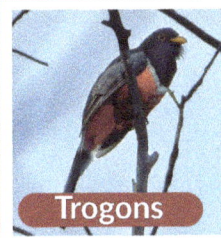
Elegant Trogon
March 29, 2024
Arizona

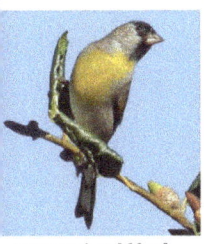
Lawrence's Goldfinch
September 9, 2024
California

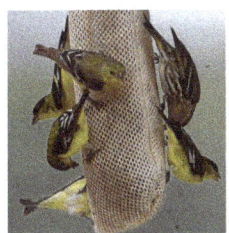
Lesser Goldfinch
February 18, 2024
Texas

Old World Sparrows

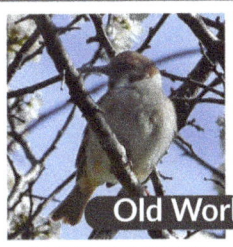
Eurasian Tree-Sparrow
April 14, 2024
Illinois

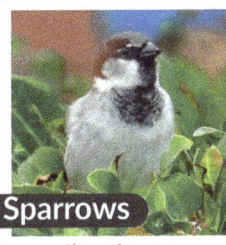
House Sparrow
January 1, 2024
Massachusetts

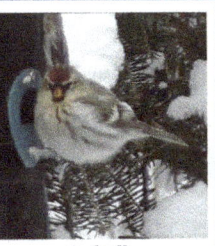
Redpoll
January 16, 2024
Minnesota

Meadowlarks

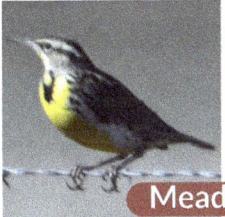
Chihuahuan Meadowlark
March 28, 2024
New Mexico

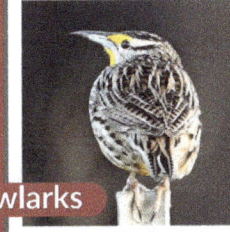
Eastern Meadowlark
January 31, 2024
North Carolina

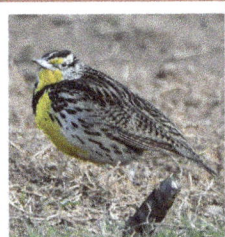
Western Meadowlark
February 22, 2024
Texas

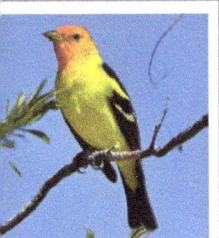
Western Tanager
January 9, 2024
Maine

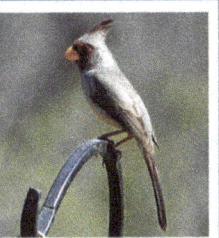
Pyrrhuloxia
February 25, 2024
Texas

207

Sparrows

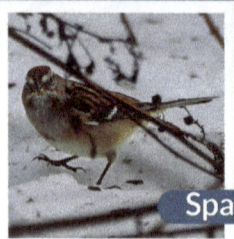
American Tree Sparrow
January 1, 2024
Massachusetts

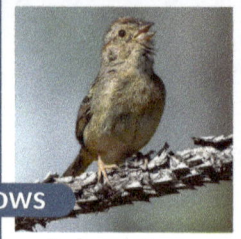
Bachman's Sparrow
February 13, 2024
Florida

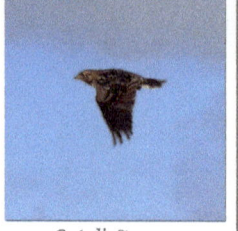
Baird's Sparrow
October 19, 2024
Arizona

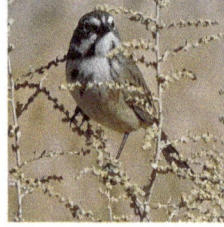
Bell's Sparrow
September 9, 2024
California

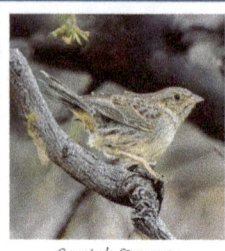
Cassin's Sparrow
February 18, 2024
Texas

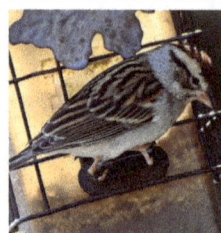
Chipping Sparrow
February 1, 2024
South Carolina

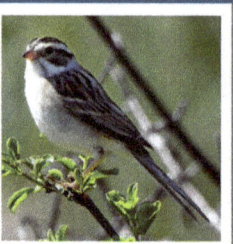
Clay-colored Sparrow
February 18, 2024
Texas

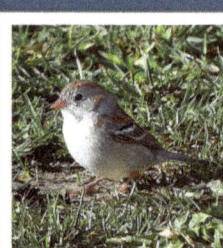
Field Sparrow
February 15, 2024
Texas

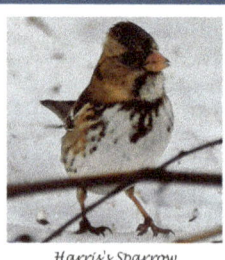
Harris's Sparrow
March 2, 2024
Texas

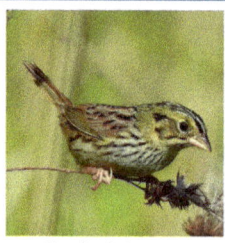
Henslow's Sparrow
April 14, 2024
Illinois

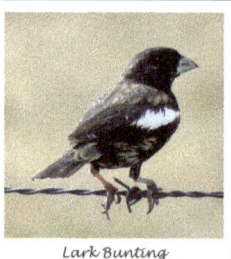
Lark Bunting
February 19, 2024
Texas

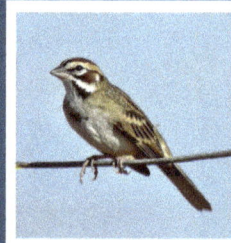
Lark Sparrow
February 25, 2024
Texas

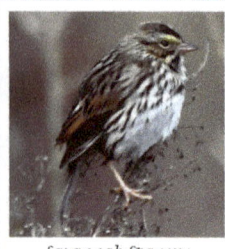
Savannah Sparrow
January 19, 2024
Maine

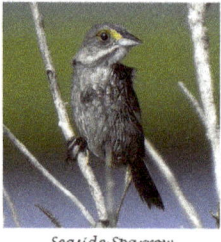
Seaside Sparrow
May 13, 2024
Masschusetts

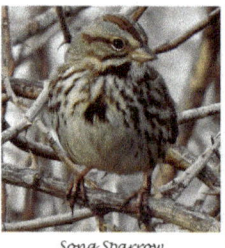
Song Sparrow
January 1, 2024
Masschusetts

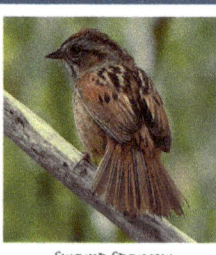
Swamp Sparrow
January 31, 2024
North Carolina

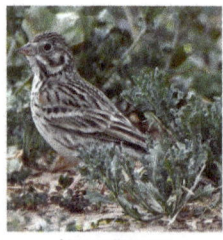
Vesper Sparrow
February 13, 2024
Florida

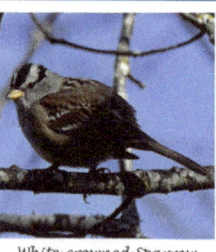
White-crowned Sparrow
February 24, 2024
Texas

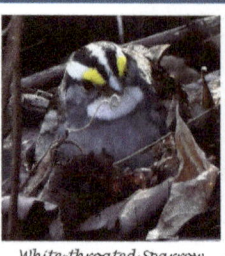
White-throated Sparrow
January 8, 2024
Maine

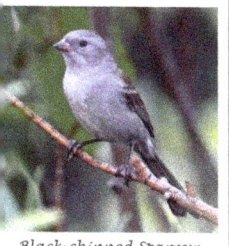
Black-chinned Sparrow
August 10, 2024
Arizona

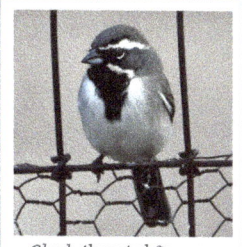
Black-throated Sparrow
February 25, 2024
Texas

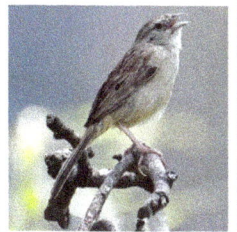
Botteri's Sparrow
August 9, 2024
Arizona

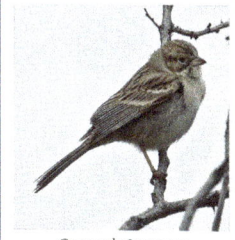
Brewer's Sparrow
Ferbruary 18, 2024
Texas

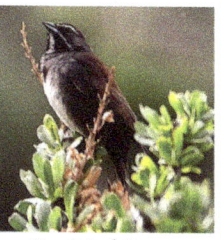
Five-striped Sparrow
August 8, 2024
Arizona

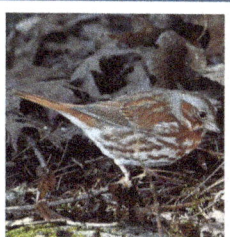
Fox Sparrow
January 9, 2024
Florida

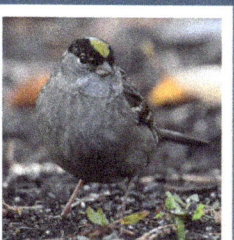
Golden-crowned Sparrow
September 13, 2024
California

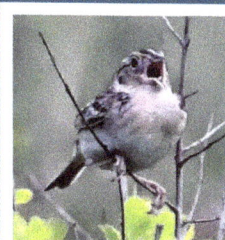
Grasshopper Sparrow
February 22, 2024
Texas

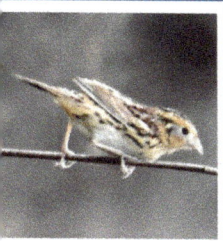
LeConte's Sparrow
February 29, 2024
Texas

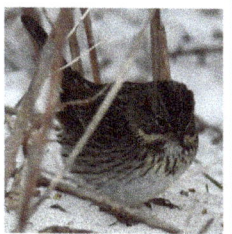
Lincoln's Sparrow
February 16, 2024
Texas

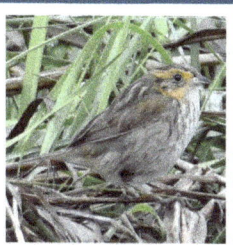
Nelson's Sparrow
May 19, 2024
New Hampshire

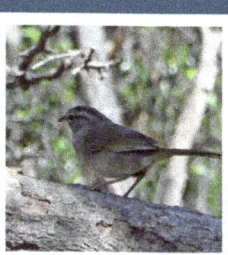
Olive Sparrow
February 17, 2024
Texas

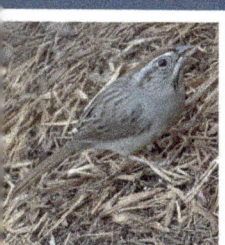
Rufous-crowned Sparrow
March 24, 2024
Texas

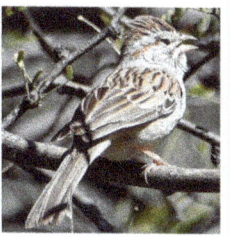
Rufous-winged Sparrow
April 3, 2024
Arizona

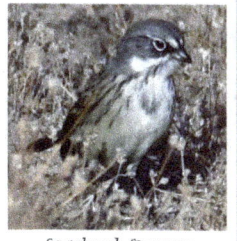
Sagebrush Sparrow
April 7, 2024
Utah

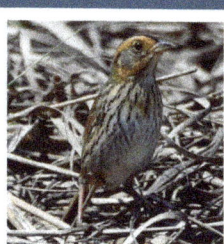
Saltmarsh Sparrow
May 13, 2024
Massachusetts

209

Wood Warblers — 1 of 2

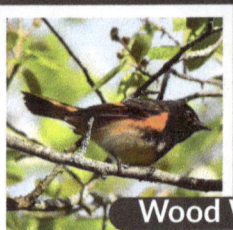
American Redstart
May 5, 2024
Florida

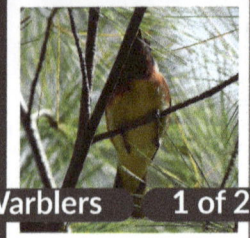
Bay-breasted Warbler
May 10, 2024
Maine

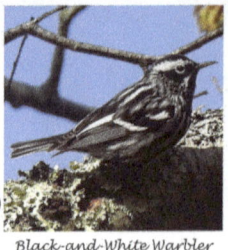
Black-and-White Warbler
February 9, 2024
Florida

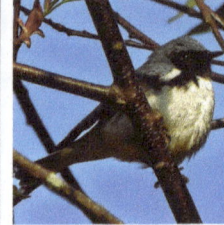
Black-throated Blue Warbler
May 2, 2024
Maine

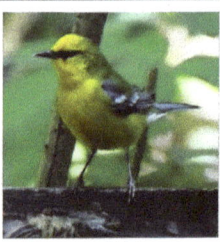
Blue-winged Warbler
April 17, 2024
Massachusetts

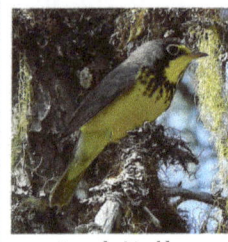
Canada Warbler
May 12, 2024
Maine

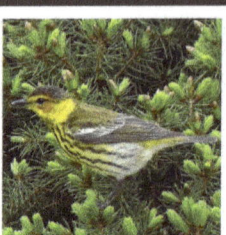
Cape May Warbler
April 2, 2024
Arizona

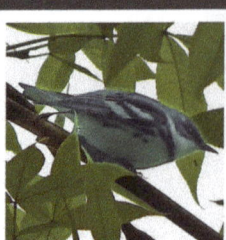
Cerulean Warbler
May 18, 2024
Maine

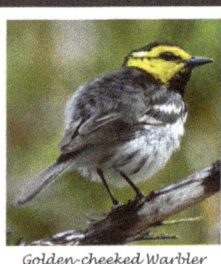
Golden-cheeked Warbler
March 24, 2024
Texas

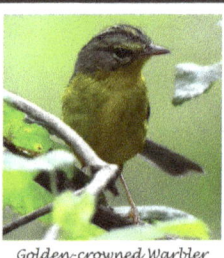
Golden-crowned Warbler
February 18, 2024
Texas

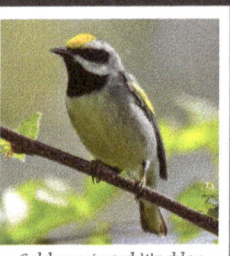
Golden-winged Warbler
June 6, 2024
Michigan

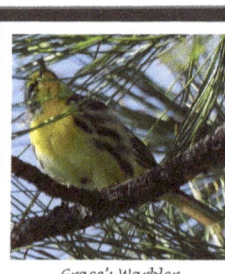
Grace's Warbler
March 30, 2024
Arizona

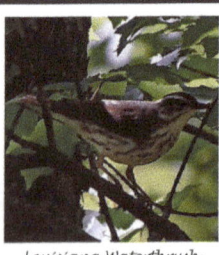
Louisiana Waterthrush
April 21, 2024
New Hampshire

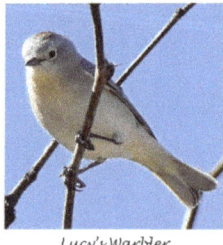
Lucy's Warbler
March 28, 2024
Arizona

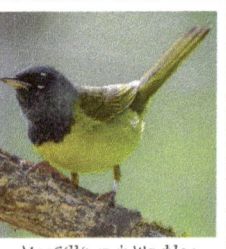
MacGillivray's Warbler
June 24, 2024
Washington

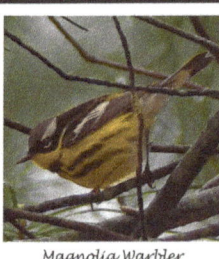
Magnolia Warbler
May 2, 2024
Maine

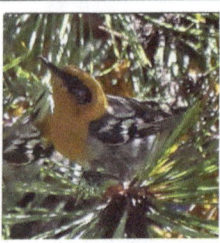
Olive Warbler
August 10, 2024
Arizona

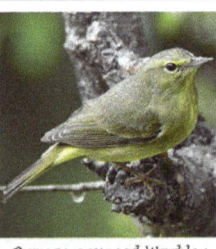
Orange-crowned Warbler
February 13, 2024
Florida

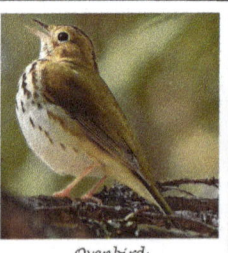
Ovenbird
April 29, 2024
Massachusetts

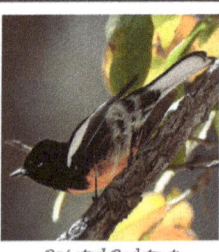
Painted Redstart
March 29, 2024
Arizona

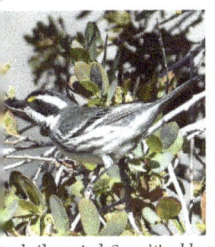
Black-throated Gray Warbler
February 26, 2024
Texas

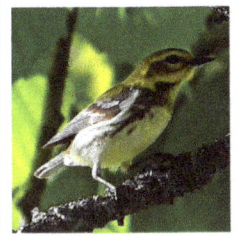
Black-throated Green Warbler
February 18, 2024
Texas

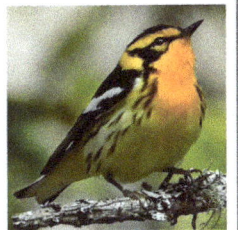
Blackburnian Warbler
May 11, 2024
Maine

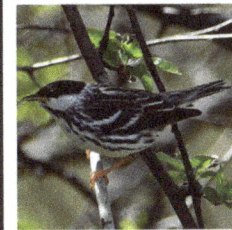
Blackpoll Warbler
May 6, 2024
Florida

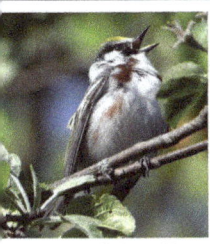
Chestnut-sided Warbler
May 11, 2024
Maine

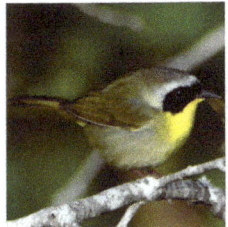
Common Yellowthroat
February 3, 2024
Florida

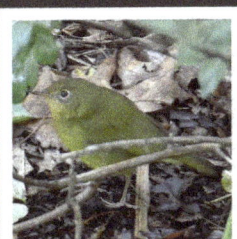
Connecticut Warbler
September 22, 2024
Massachusetts

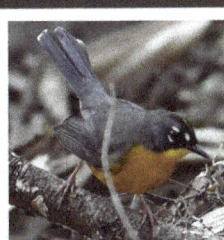
Fan-tailed Warbler
February 10, 2024
Texas

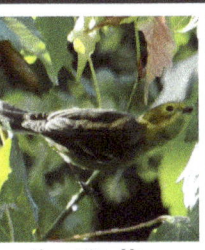
Hermit Warbler
February 18, 2024
Texas

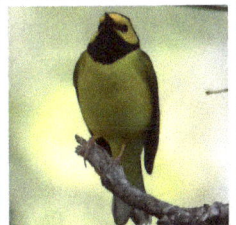
Hooded Warbler
May 31, 2024
Virginia

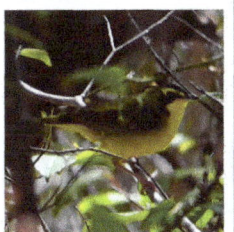
Kentucky Warbler
May 13, 2024
Massachusetts

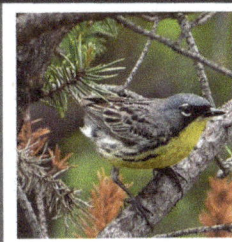
Kirtland's Warbler
June 6, 2024
Michigan

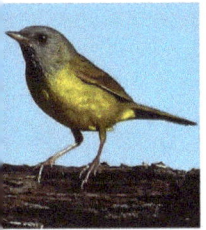
Mourning Warbler
June 9, 2024
Maine

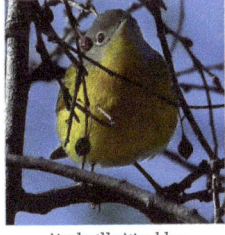
Nashville Warbler
February 24, 2024
Texas

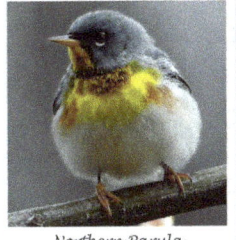
Northern Parula
February 9, 2024
Florida

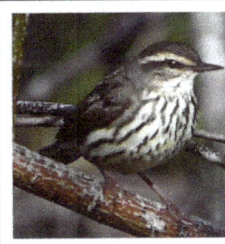
Northern Waterthrush
April 29, 2024
Massachusetts

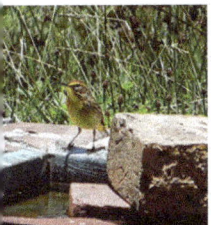
Palm Warbler
January 31, 2024
North Carolina

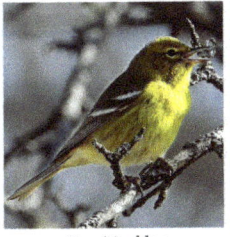
Pine Warbler
January 12, 2024
Maine

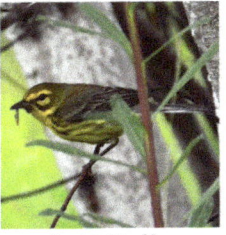
Prairie Warbler
Feebruary 11, 2024
Florida

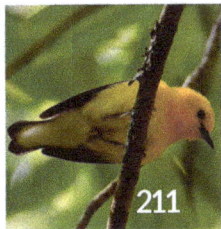
Prothonotary Warbler
May 18, 2024
Massachusetts

Wood Warblers 2 of 2

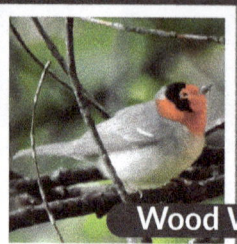
Red-faced Warbler
August 10, 2024
Arizona

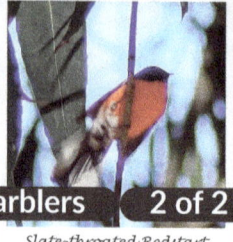
Slate-throated Redstart
September 12, 2024
California

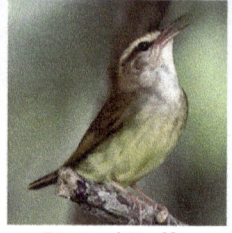
Swainson's Warbler
May 31, 2024
Virginia

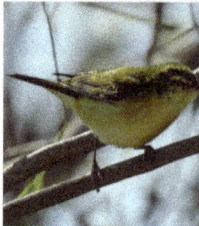
Tennessee Warbler
February 17, 2024
Texas

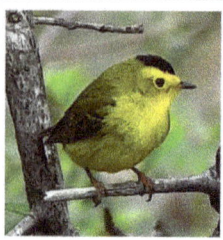
Wilson's Warbler
January 20, 2024
Maine

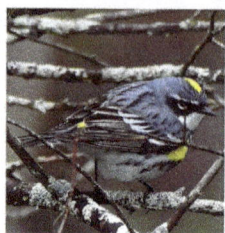
Yellow-rumped Warbler
January 30, 2024
Maryland

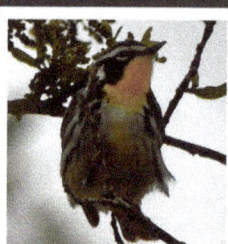
Yellow-throated Warbler
Feruary 8, 2024
Florida

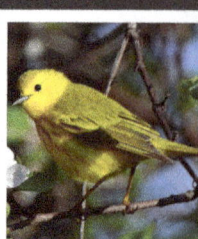
Yellow Warbler
February 6, 2024
Florida

Orioles

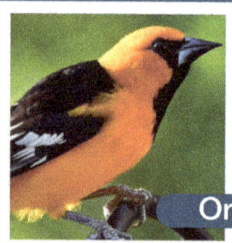
Altamira Oriole
February 17, 2024
Texas

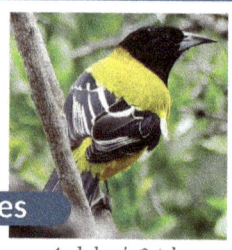
Audubon's Oriole
February 25, 2024
Texas

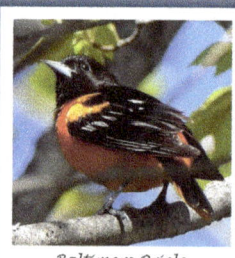
Baltimore Oriole
April 17, 2024
Masshusetts

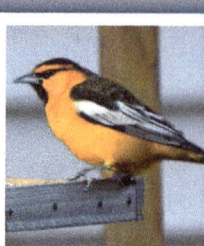
Bullock's Oriole
June 25, 2024
Washington State

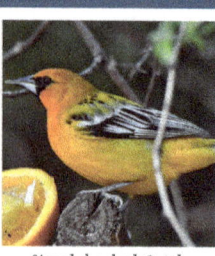
Streak-backed Oriole
April 5, 2024
Arizona

Blackbirds

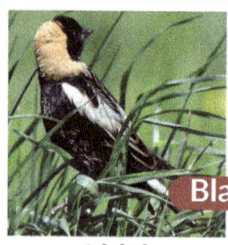
Bobolink
May 6, 2024
Florida

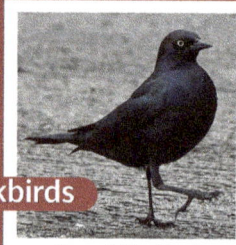
Brewer's Blackbird
February 18, 2024
Texas

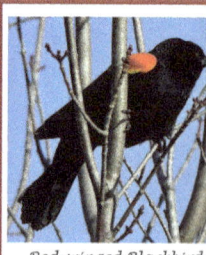
Red-winged Blackbird
January 31, 2024
North Carolina

Cowbirds

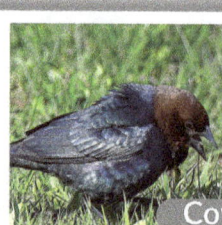
Brown-headed Cowbird
February 6, 2024
Florida

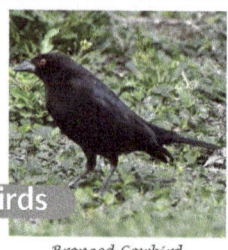
Bronzed Cowbird
February 19, 2024
Texas

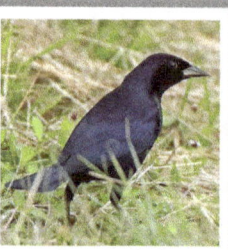
Shiny Cowbird
May 6, 2024
Florida

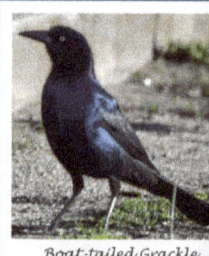
Boat-tailed Grackle
January 30, 2024
North Carolina

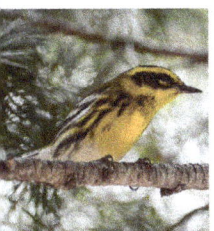
Townsend's Warbler
June 23, 2024
Washington State

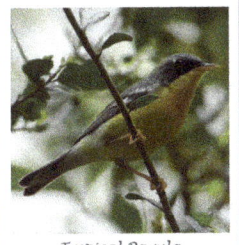
Tropical Parula
February 18, 2024
Texas

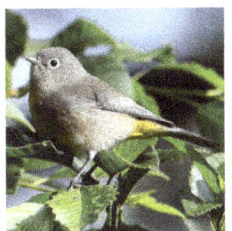
Virginia Warbler
February 5, 2024
Arizona

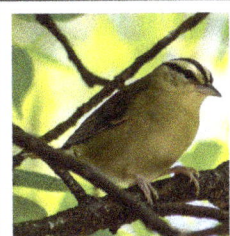
Worm-eating Warbler
May 8, 2024
Florida

Swifts

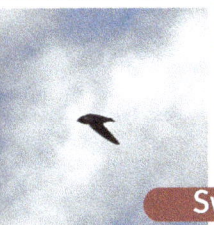
Black Swift
June 22, 2024
Washington State

Chimney Swift
March 23, 2024
Texas

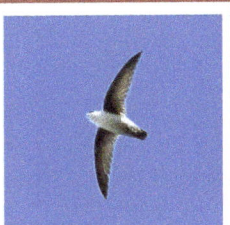
Vaux's Swift
June 22, 2024
Washington State

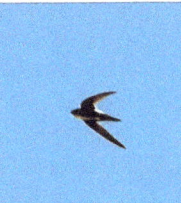
White-throated Swift
March 28, 2024
New Mexico

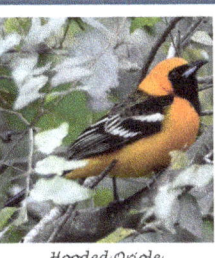
Hooded Oriole
March 29, 2024
Arizona

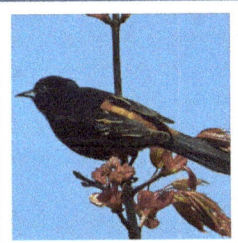
Orchard Oriole
April 30, 2024
Massachusetts

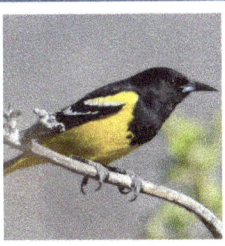
Scott's Oriole
March 29, 2024
Arizona

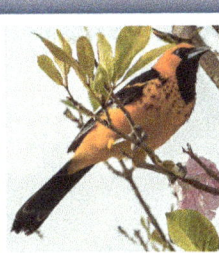
Spot-breasted Oriole
February 11, 2024
Florida

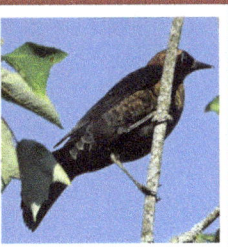
Rusty Blackbird
March 17, 2024
Maine

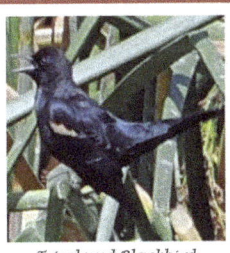
Tricolored Blackbird
September 8, 2024
California

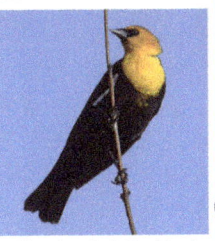
Yellow-headed Blackbird
February 19, 2024
Texas

Chachalacas

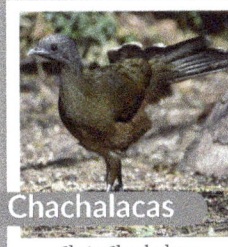
Plain Chachalaca
February 16, 2024
Texas

Grackles

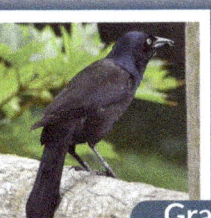
Common Grackle
February 1, 2024
South Carolina

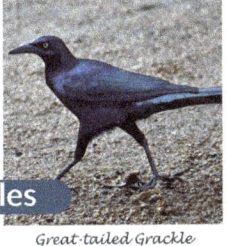
Great-tailed Grackle
February 15, 2024
Louisiana

Wagtails

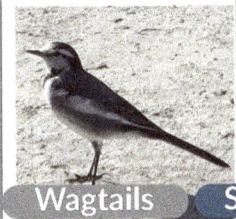
White Wagtail
September 17, 2024
California

Skimmers / 213

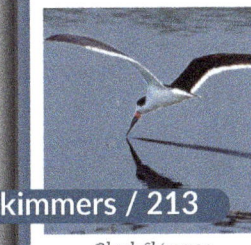
Black Skimmer
February 3, 2024
Florida

Index

A

ABA 1, 13, 14, 138
ABA Area 1
ABA Continental 138
Abert's Towhee 56
Abraham Lincoln 69
Acadian Flycatcher 93
Acorn Woodpecker 121
Africa 44, 110, 144, 167
AirBnB 53
Alabama 27, 31, 37
Alaska 1, 76, 77, 92, 118, 134, 138, 140, 144, 146, 157
Albatross 137, 191
    Black-footed Albatross 137
Albuquerque 50, 52
Alex Lamoreaux 83, 124, 161
Allen's Pond 86
Alligator Alley 113
Altamira Oriole 41, 42
Amazons 107, 145, 161, 168, 198
    Lilac-crowned Parrots 45
    Orange-winged Amazons 78
    Yellow-headed Amazons 138
American Barn Owl 107
American Birding Association 1
American Bittern 30
American Dipper 67, 102, 103, 105
American Flamingo 3
American Herring Gull 30, 107
American Ornithological Society 107
American Redstarts 84
American Three-toed Woodpecker 117, 152
American Woodcock 49
Andy Baker 69
Anhingas 191
Anis 183
    Groove-billed Ani 162, 163
Anna 8, 56, 91, 150, 152
Anna Hodgkins 91
Anna's Hummingbirds 150
Antarctica 116
Antelope Squirrel 130
Antillean Nighthawk 81
April 38, 54, 58, 60, 62, 71, 83, 102, 108, 125, 146, 155, 172
Arches National Park 65
Arctic 17, 89, 91, 92, 114, 144, 146
Arctic Terns 89
Arizona 12, 18, 27, 42, 47, 52, 53, 54, 58, 59, 60, 64, 65, 74, 77, 108, 120, 121, 122, 123, 124, 125, 127, 128, 136, 139, 143, 146, 149, 150, 151, 154, 170, 172, 173
Arthur Fiedler 85
Ash-Canyon Bird Sanctuary 121
asparagus 85
Atlantic Puffins 87, 89, 101
Audubon 51, 52, 71, 74, 82, 87, 91, 97, 107, 121, 158, 165
Audubon's Oriole 165
Audubon's Shearwater 82, 107
August 74, 81, 82, 120, 121, 144, 172
Auklets 101, 108, 187
    Cassin's Auklet 134
    Rhinoceros Auklet 101
Auks 186
    Atlantic Puffins 87, 89, 101
    Common Murre 101
    Dovekie 17, 20, 21, 133, 167
    Razorbills 20
    Thick-billed Murre 17, 21
Austin 46

B

Bainbridge Island 100
Baltimore Oriole 71
Band-rumped Storm-Petrel 97
Bare-throated Tiger Heron 45
Bar Harbor 116
Barnacle Goose 28, 29
Barn Owl 107
Bath 85
Becards 195
    Gray-Collared Becard 40
Belgrade 87
Bendire's Thrasher 123
Berylline Hummingbird 59
Bicknell's Thrush 88, 89, 90, 92, 93

Biddeford Pool 21, 127
Big Year 1, 5, 7, 12, 13, 14, 15, 17, 18, 23, 26, 27, 28, 31, 35, 37, 40, 42, 44, 45, 50, 66, 67, 69, 71, 74, 78, 87, 92, 96, 99, 100, 106, 107, 109, 110, 115, 116, 117, 122, 123, 124, 125, 127, 138, 142, 144, 145, 146, 148, 150, 151, 152, 159, 162, 164, 167, 168, 169, 170, 172
Big Year Assistant 67
Big Years 1, 17, 18, 57, 138, 145
Bill Baggs Cape Florida State Park 112
Birders 1, 17, 18, 141
Birding 1, 5, 7, 39, 42, 72, 74, 80, 116, 123, 128, 145
Bitterns 191
  American Bittern 30
Black-backed Woodpeckers 100
Black Bear 122
Black-billed Magpie 24
Blackbirds 212
  Bobolink 89
  Red-winged Blackbird 137
  Tricolored Blackbird 137
Blackburnian Warblers 100
Black-capped Chickadee 76
Black-capped Petrel 82, 97
Black-chinned Hummingbirds 126
Black-chinned Sparrow 125
Black-crowned Night-Heron 37, 107
Black-footed Albatross 137
Black-headed Gull 18
Black-legged Kittiwakes 20
Black Noddies 82
Black Phoebe 44
Black Rail 160
Black Rosy-Finches 51
Black Skimmer 36
Black Squirrel 130
Black Storm-Petrel 136
Black Terns 87
Black-throated Blue Warbler 75
Black-throated Gray Warblers 125
Black-Throated Sparrow 54
Black-vented Shearwater 134
Black-whiskered Vireos 80
Blue-and-Yellow Macaw 38

Bluebirds 66, 140, 204
Blue Grosbeak 68
Blue Mesa Reservoir 66
Blue-throated Mountain-Gem 10
Blue-winged Warbler 71, 73
Boat Trips 16, 34, 47, 58, 78, 95, 110, 120, 132, 143, 156, 166, 172
Bobolink 89
Bob Ross 69
Bohemian Waxwings 27
Bonaparte's Gulls 115
Boobies 82, 188
  Brown Boobies 82
  Brown Booby 107
  Cocos Booby 3, 107, 137, 152
  Masked Boobies 82
  Red-footed Booby 83
Booby 82, 188
  Cocos Booby 3, 107, 137, 152
Boreal 22, 24, 76, 99, 148
Boreal Chickadee 24, 76
Boreal Owl 148
Bosque del Apache 52
Boston 23, 36, 71, 72, 85, 98, 100, 133, 140, 142, 146
Botteri's Sparrow 124
Box Canyon 60, 125
Boyce Thompson Arboretum 149
Brad 47
Bradley 8, 161
Brandon Sullivan 66
Brewer Park 78
Brian Patterson 96
Bridled Terns 83
Broad-billed Hummingbirds 126, 150
Brown Boobies 82
Brown Booby 107
Brown-capped Rosy-Finches 51
Brown-crested Flycatcher 123
Brown Jay 43, 165, 168
Brown Noddies 82, 83
Brownsville 39, 40, 44
Brownsville Landfill 40
Buff-breasted Flycatcher 121
Buff-breasted Sandpiper 133, 135
Bulbuls 160, 195
  Red-vented Bulbul 160
  Red-whiskered Bulbul 44
Buller's Shearwater 140

Bullock's Oriole 103
Buntings 48, 49, 205
   Snow Buntings 48, 49
   Varied Bunting 124, 125
Burrage Pond 74
Burrowing Owl 37
Burrowing Parakeets 134
Butler Head 85

C

Cackling Goose 151
California 12, 32, 33, 62, 63, 65, 77, 100, 103, 110, 118, 130, 132, 133, 134, 135, 136, 137, 138, 139, 140, 141, 150, 153, 154, 170, 172, 173
California Condors 62, 65
California Gnatcatchers 134
California Gull 100
California Quail 103, 153
California Scrub-Jay 32, 103, 139
California Thrasher 134, 135
California Towhee 133
Calliope Hummingbird 105, 106, 173
Cambridge 92
Canada 1, 17, 22, 28, 44, 48, 50, 99, 113, 118, 138, 151
Canada Goose 151
Canada Jays 99
Canoa Ranch 60
Canyon Towhee 52, 55
Cape Canaveral 31, 34
Cape Cod 127, 167, 168
Cape Elizabeth 20, 30
Cape Henlopen 146
Cape May Warbler 84
Capisic Pond 75, 85
Caracaras 195
   Yellow-headed Caracara 80, 112, 113, 114, 115, 173
Cardinals 206
   Dickcissel 98
Carolina Chickadee 76
Carolina Wren 22
Cascades 103, 106
Casco Bay 91
Cassin's Auklet 134
Cassin's Vireo 102

Cattle Tyrant 38, 39
Cave Creek Ranch 54
Cave Swallows 159
Cedar Waxwings 27
Celtics 100
Central America 39, 42, 50, 112, 118
Cerulean Warbler 71, 85, 86
Chachalacas 213
Charles River 85
Chats 203
   Yellow-breasted Chat 98
Chestnut-collared Longspur 43, 46
Chicago 22, 23, 69, 70
Chickadees 22, 51, 56, 76, 77, 173, 202
   Black-capped Chickadee 76
   Boreal Chickadee 24, 76
   Carolina Chickadee 76
   Mexican Chickadee 55, 56, 77
   Mountain Chickadees 51
Chihuahuan Meadowlark 52
Chihuahuan Ravens 40
Chuck-will's-widow 85, 86
Chukars 146, 148
Civil War 82, 93
Clark's Grebes 53
Cliff Island 90, 91
Coal Canyon 148
Coalville 65
Cocoa Beach 112
Cocos Booby 3, 107, 137, 152
Cohasset 158
Colima Warbler 117
Colorado 27, 58, 65, 66, 67, 69, 102, 143, 146, 150, 152, 172
Colorado River 65
Colorado Springs 67
Columbia Ridge Winery 108
Columbia River Valley 108
Common Gull 18, 157, 158, 159
Common Murre 101
Common Mynas 35
Common Nighthawk 78, 80
Common Paruque 81
Common Ringed Plover 140, 142
Common Shelduck 141, 144
Common Tern 128
Connecticut 16, 18, 141, 142, 145,

157, 172
Connecticut Warbler 141, 142
Continental Divide 67, 146
Cormorants 190
Cornell 56, 67
Corpus Christi 39
Cory's Shearwater 97
Costa's Hummingbirds 150
County Big Year 1
Cowbirds 212
   Shiny Cowbird 80
Crandon Park 78
Cranes 38, 39, 42, 182
   Whooping Cranes 38, 39, 42
Crazy Chicken Tour 66
Creepers 201
Crossbills 17, 23, 50, 206
   White-winged Crossbill 48, 50
   White-winged Crossbills 17, 50
Crows 198
   Tamaulipas Crow 40
Cuckoos 87, 182
   Mangrove Cuckoo 35
   Yellow-billed Cuckoos 87
Curlews 185

D

Dartmouth 86
David McQuade 145
David Simpson 37
D-Day Invasion 146
December 18, 40, 110, 166, 167, 168, 172
Delaware 16, 28, 95, 98, 172
Denver 146
Deschutes National Forest 106
Dickcissel 98
Dippers 102, 203
   American Dipper 67, 102, 103, 105
Dominican Republic 90
Doug Hitchcox 158, 161
Douglas Fir 103
Dovekie 17, 20, 21, 133, 167
Doves 182
Dowitchers 184
Dry Tortugas 78, 80, 81, 82, 173
Duck Boat 100
Ducks (Dabbling) 178

Common Shelduck 141, 144
Garganey 72
Tufted Duck 18
Ducks (Diving) 178
Dusky Flycatcher 106
Dusky Grouse 153

E

Eagles 193
   Steller's Sea Eagle 114
Eastern Egg Rock 87, 89
Eastern Meadowlark 52
Eastern Screech-Owl 17
Eastern Whippoorwills 81, 86
Eastern Whippoorwills, 81
Eaton Farm 48, 49
eBird 1, 15, 22, 47, 56, 57, 67, 107, 128, 145, 151, 158
Eddy Edwards 39
Edinburg 45
Edward Abbey 53
Egrets 12, 192
   Snowy Egrets 12
Egyptian Goose 35
Eiders 179
Elegant Tern 133
Elegant Trogon 54, 122, 173
Elephant Butte 53
Elephant Seals 137
Elf Owl 56
Ell Pond 142
El Niño 40, 42
Esplanade 85
Ethan 7, 12, 13, 14, 15, 21, 22, 26, 37, 40, 42, 51, 52, 54, 64, 67, 69, 71, 72, 74, 80, 83, 88, 90, 92, 100, 102, 103, 108, 113, 114, 116, 122, 128, 140, 142, 144, 146, 149, 151, 153, 157, 158, 164, 167, 168, 169, 173
Eurasia 144
Eurasian Escapees 193
Eurasian Tree Sparrow 70
European Goldfinch 3, 68
European Goldfinches 70
Evening Grosbeak 24
Everglades 35
Every Bird in Maine 13

Exotics 37, 198
  Common Mynas 35
  Northern Red Bishop 134
  Pin-tailed Whydah 133
Ezekiel Dobson 145, 161, 168

F

Falcons 194
Fan-tailed Warbler 39, 41
February 12, 34, 35, 37, 44, 78, 80, 112, 138, 164, 172
Fenway Park 42
Ferruginous Hawk 47, 67
Ferruginous-Pygmy Owl 161, 162
Ferry 144, 145, 146, 167
Finches 48, 51, 56, 205, 206
  Pine Siskins 140
  Purple Finch 48, 49
Five-striped Sparrow 124
Flagstaff 62
Flame-colored Tanager 121
Flamingos 29, 31, 32, 36, 37, 183
  American Flamingo 3
Flammulated Owl 106
Flesh-Footed Shearwaters 140
Florida 18, 27, 31, 32, 33, 34, 35, 37, 44, 67, 72, 73, 74, 78, 81, 90, 110, 112, 113, 128, 139, 145, 155, 169, 172, 173
Florida Keys 81, 173
Florida Scrub-Jay 32, 33, 139
Flycatcher
  Scissor-tailed Flycatcher 3, 159
Flycatchers 100, 121, 197, 200
  Acadian Flycatcher 93
  Brown-crested Flycatcher 123
  Buff-breasted Flycatcher 121
  Dusky Flycatcher 106
  Gray Flycatcher 62
  Great Crested Flycatcher 74
  Olive-sided Flycatchers 100
  Scissor-tailed Flycatcher 3, 159
  Sulphur-bellied Flycatcher 121, 123
Fort Jefferson 82
Fort Myers 35, 36, 110
Fowl 14, 80, 181
  Indian Peafowl 6, 78
  Red Junglefowl 80, 81
Frigatebirds 4, 189
  Magnificent Frigatebirds 4
Fulmars 114, 190
  Northern Fulmars 114

G

Galveston 160
Galveston Island 160
Gambel's Quail 54, 55
Gannets 189
  Northern Gannet 20, 21, 30
Garden Key 82, 84
Geese 28, 37, 42, 178
  Barnacle Goose 28, 29
  Cackling Goose 151
  Canada Goose 151
  Egyptian Goose 35
  Pink-footed Goose 27, 28, 29
  Ross's Goose 42, 67
  Snow Geese 42
Geology Vista 125
George Walker House 123, 126
Gila Woodpecker 56

Glaucous Gull 18, 19
Glaucous-winged Gull 100
Glenn Hodgkins 91
Gnatcatchers 134, 205
  California Gnatcatchers 134
Godwits 185
Golden-cheeked Warbler 50
Golden-Crowned Kinglets 21
Golden-crowned Sparrow 140
Golden-crowned Warbler 40
Goldeneyes 178
Golden-fronted Woodpeckers 161
Golden Road 117
Golden-winged Warblers 98
Goldfinch
  European Goldfinch 3, 68
Goldfinches 70, 206
  European Goldfinch 3, 68
  European Goldfinches 70
Gordon Payne 113
Grace's Warbler 125
Grackles 213
Grand Canyon 13, 62, 64
Grand Junction 66, 146
Gray-Cheeked Thrush 92
Gray-Collared Becard 40
Gray-crowned
  Rosy-Finches 51
Gray Flycatcher 62
Gray Fox 60
Gray-headed
  Swamphens 35
Grayling 99
Gray Partridge 153
Gray Vireo 125, 126
Gray Whale 130
Great Black-backed Gulls 18, 157

Great Crested Flycatcher 74
Great Dismal Swamp 93
Greater Prairie-Chickens 69
Greater Roadrunner 40, 41
Greater Sage-Grouse 3, 63, 65
Greater Yellowlegs 72
Great Gray Owl 22, 23, 24, 26, 173
Great-Horned Owl 60
Great Northern Paper 117
Great Plains 49, 121
Great Shearwater 97
Grebes 53, 180
  Clark's Grebes 53
  Western Grebes 53
Green Jay 41, 42
Greenland 28, 144
Green Mountains 72
Green Parakeet 43
Greg Miller 90, 91
Grondin Pond 30
Groove-billed Ani 162, 163
Grosbeaks 71, 206
  Blue Grosbeak 68
  Evening Grosbeak 24
  Pine Grosbeak 24
  Yellow Grosbeak 147, 149, 150, 173
Ground Squirrel 130
GroupMe 21, 91, 92
Grouse 3, 26, 63, 64, 65, 66, 69, 98, 99, 100, 101, 153, 181
  Dusky Grouse 153
  Gray Partridge 153
  Ruffed Grouse 26
  Sharp-tailed Grouse 99, 153
  Sooty Grouse 101
  Spruce Grouse 98, 99, 100
Guillemots 108, 187
  Pigeon Guillemots 108

Gulf of Maine 116
Gulls 18, 30, 40, 100, 107, 115, 157, 158, 188
  American Herring Gull 30, 107
  Black-headed Gull 18
  Black-legged Kittiwakes 20
  Bonaparte's Gulls 115
  California Gull 100
  Common Gull 18, 157, 158, 159
  Glaucous Gull 18, 19
  Glaucous-winged Gull 100
  Great Black-backed Gulls 18, 157
  Heerman's Gull 100
  Herring Gulls 18, 30, 157
  Iceland Gull 18
  Little Gull 114, 115, 116
  Mew Gull 157
  Ring-billed Gulls 18, 158
  Short-billed Gull 157
  Western Gull 100
  Yellow-footed Gull 138
Gunnison Sage-Grouse 66

H

Hadley 85
Hamilton 74
Hampton Beach 49
Hanyang Ye 145
Hardy Boat 87
Harlingen 40
Harriers 195
Harrisburg 71
Hatteras Pelagic 96
Hawks (Accipiters) 193
Hawks (Buteos) 192
  Ferruginous Hawk 47, 67
  Red-tailed Hawk 47, 48
  Swainson's Hawk 44
Hays 67, 69, 83
Heerman's Gull 100
Henefer 65
Hepatic Tanager 18
Hermit Warblers 125

Herons 191, 193
Herring Cove 128
Herring Gull 30, 107
Herring Gulls 18, 30, 157
Hidden Valley Nature Center 85
Himalayan Snowcock 117
Hinckley Park 85
Homestead 35
Hometown Bakery 69
Hooded Oriole 154
Hooded Warbler 74, 87, 93
Hook-billed Kites 163
Horned Lark 18, 48
Horned Puffin 105, 107, 108
Hospital Key 82
Houghton Lake 99
House Wren 107
Houston 160, 167
Houston Reservoir 160
Hudsonian Godwit 126, 127
Hummingbird
  Rivoli's Hummingbird 3, 59, 61, 121, 173
Hummingbirds 56, 59, 60, 126, 150, 182
  Anna's Hummingbirds 150
  Berylline Hummingbird 59
  Black-chinned Hummingbirds 126
  Black-chinned Hummingbirds, 126, 150
  Blue-throated Mountain-Gem 10
  Broad-billed Hummingbirds 126, 150
  Broad-tailed Hummingbirds 126
  Calliope Hummingbird 105, 106, 173
  Costa's Hummingbirds 150
  Lucifer's Hummingbird

122, 123
Magnificent Hummingbird 59
Plain-capped Starthroat 149, 150, 152
Rivoli's Hummingbird 3, 59, 61, 121, 173
Rufous Hummingbirds 126, 150
White-eared Hummingbird 122, 123, 125, 127
Humpback Whale 116, 130
Hyannis Ferry 167

I

Ibises 193
Iceland Gull 18
Illinois 16, 58, 69, 172
Indiana 71, 99
Indian Peafowl 6, 78
Ingrid 7, 12, 13, 22, 24, 27, 28, 35, 38, 50, 51, 54, 60, 71, 72, 74, 83, 85, 88, 90, 92, 100, 102, 116, 122, 125, 127, 133, 139, 140, 144, 153, 157, 164, 167, 168, 173
Ipswich 71
Island Fox 139
Island Scrub-Jay 32, 33, 139

J

Jack Black's 92
Jaegers 97, 128, 187
  Long-tailed Jaeger 127, 128
  Parasitic Jaeger 97
Jake Molhmann 124
Jake Thompson 59
Janice Travis 161
January 13, 16, 17, 18, 22, 27, 30, 31, 71, 139, 144, 157,
172, 173
Javelinas 60
Jays 32, 33, 99, 106, 198, 201
  Brown Jay 43, 165, 168
  Canada Jays 99
  Green Jay 41, 42
  Pinyon Jays 106
  Steller's Jay 62
Jefferson 82, 85
John Yerger 125
Jourdanton 163
Judd Brink 23, 24
July 110, 113, 119, 121, 140, 151, 172
Juncos 205
June 89, 95, 103, 141, 152, 172
Juniper 50

K

Kadynn Hatfield 150
Kanab 65
Kansas 27, 31, 58, 67, 69, 83, 172
Kathie Brown 56
Keith Lockhart 85
Kentucky Warbler 86
Keurig 70
Key West 80, 81, 82, 84
Killdeer 134
Kill Devil Hills 28
Killian Sullivan, 66
Kingbirds 73, 125, 196
  Thick-billed Kingbird 125
Kingfishers 183
Kinglets 22, 203
  Golden-Crowned Kinglets 21
King Rail 74, 75
King Ranch 161
Kirtland's Warbler 98
Kiskadees 197
Kites 74, 163, 164, 192
  Hook-billed Kites 163
  Swallow-tailed Kites 74
  White-tailed Kite 39
krummholz 89, 90

Krummholz 124

L

Lake Huron 99
Lake Michigan 99
Lake Superior 99
Land of Lincoln 70
Lapland Longspur 48, 49, 50
Lapwings 184
  Northern Lapwing 144, 167, 168
Large-billed Tern 110, 112
Larks 49, 201
  Horned Lark 18, 48
Las Cienegas Grasslands 124
Laudholm Farm 74
Least Storm-Petrel 136
Legacy Whale Watch 134
Lesser Scaup 30
Lesser Yellowlegs 72
Lewis's Woodpecker 105
Lewis' Woodpeckers 103
Lifer Pie 26
Lilac-crowned Parrots 45
Limpkin 181
  Limpkins 44
Limpkins 44
Lindo Lake 137
Lisa Bonato 113
Little Gull 114, 115, 116
LL Bean 59, 114
Logan Airport 100, 133
Long Beach 133, 134
Long-eared Owl 17, 19
Long Island 144, 145, 146
Longmire 103
Longspurs 204
  Chestnut-collared Longspur 43, 46
  Lapland Longspur 48, 49,

220   EVERY BIRD FROM SEA TO SHINING SEA

50
Long-tailed Jaeger 127, 128
Long-tailed Tits 199
Loons 189
   Yellow-Billed Loon 146
Los Angeles River 134, 140
Louis Bevier 161
Louisiana 27, 31, 34, 37, 38, 172
Lovebirds 9, 61, 62, 197
   Rosy-faced Lovebirds 9, 61
   Rosy-face Lovebirds 9
Loveland Pass 146
Lower 48 State Big Year 1, 23, 27, 138, 144, 145
Lower 48 States 22, 67, 151
Lucifer's Hummingbird 122, 123
Lucy's Warbler 54
Luxembourg 161

M

Macaws 37, 199
   Blue-and-Yellow Macaw 38
MacGillivray's Warbler 102
Madera Canyon 59, 121, 125
Magill Weber 158
Magill Weber, 158
Magnificent Frigatebirds 4
Magnificent Hummingbird 59
Magnolia Warbler 75
Magpies 67, 139, 199
   Black-billed Magpie 24
   Yellow-billed Magpie 139
Maine 7, 12, 13, 16, 17, 18, 19, 20, 21, 22, 23, 27, 30, 40, 47, 48, 49, 50, 53, 58, 62, 69, 71, 72, 73, 74, 75, 78, 82, 83, 85, 86, 87, 89, 90, 91, 95, 99, 101, 110, 113, 114, 115, 116, 117, 120, 127, 128, 133, 136, 139, 141, 144, 146, 148, 152, 157, 158, 159, 163, 167, 169, 172 173
Maine Audubon 91, 158
Maine Big Year 13
Maine Coon Cats 27
Maine North Woods 117
Mangrove Cuckoo 35
Marblehead 71, 74, 87
March 47, 48, 49, 50, 53, 54, 172
Marita 8, 65
Mary Jo Ballator 122
Maryland 16, 28, 172
Masked Boobies 82
Massachusetts 16, 19, 27, 30, 58, 71, 72, 73, 74, 78, 85, 86, 92, 120, 127, 132, 140, 142, 156, 158, 159, 166, 172
May 73, 75, 78, 80, 81, 82, 83, 84, 85, 86, 87, 88, 89, 90, 91, 93, 141, 172
Mayo Clinic 127
McAllen 45
McDonald's 80, 173
Meadowlarks 207
   Chihuahuan Meadowlark 52
   Eastern Meadowlark 52
Medicine Bow Curve, 148
Melrose 142
Mennonite 99
Mergansers 180
Messalonskee Lake 87
Mew Gull 157
Mexican Chickadee 55, 56, 77
Mexican Whip-poor-will 121
Mexico 27, 32, 39, 42, 45, 47, 50, 51, 52, 53, 59, 77, 117, 118, 120, 121, 123, 140, 149, 150, 164, 172
Miami 35, 44, 78, 80, 112, 113, 114
Michigan 31, 95, 98, 99, 159, 172
Millinocket 117
Mimics 202
   Bendire's Thrasher 123
   California Thrasher 134, 135
   Sage Thrashers 66
Minnesota 16, 23, 26, 141, 169, 172
Minor Islands 108
Mississippi 27, 37
Missouri 58, 69, 172
Monterey Bay 140
Montezuma Quail 125, 127
Montosa Canyon 124, 125
Moose 128
mosquitoes 110, 141, 160
Mottled Owl 42, 45, 173
Mountain Bluebird 62, 64
Mountain Chickadee 76
Mountain Chickadees 51
Mountain Picas 146
Mountain Plover 45, 67
Mountain Quail 153
Mount Auburn Cemetery 92
Mount Rainier 103
Mourning Warbler 74
Mt. Lemmon 124, 126

INDEX   221

Mt. Washington 88, 89, 92
Murrelets 101, 187
  Scripp's Murrelet 133, 135
Murres 101, 108, 186

N

Nantucket 167, 168
Nantucket Island 167
Naples 110, 113
Naples Zoo 110
National Audubon Society 87
National City 134
Navajo Bridge 65
Newburyport 17, 86
New England 18, 27, 47, 71, 72, 78, 80, 89, 142, 144, 159, 167
New England Patriots 144
New Hampshire 16, 47, 49, 58, 73, 78, 132, 133, 144, 159, 172
New Harbor 87
New Jersey 16, 17, 18, 19, 28, 78, 144, 172
New London 145
New Mexico 27, 47, 50, 51, 52, 53, 77, 117, 120, 154, 172
Newport 106, 107
Newton 27
New World Quail 181
  California Quail 103, 153
  Gambel's Quail 54, 55
  Montezuma Quail 125, 127
  Mountain Quail 153
New York 27, 89, 143, 144, 145, 172
Night-Herons 191
  Black-crowned Night-Heron 37, 107
  Yellow-crowned Night-Heron 37, 107
Nightjars 184
  Antillean Nighthawk 81
  Chuck-will's-widow 85, 86
  Common Nighthawk 78, 80
  Common Paruque 81
  Eastern Whippoorwills 81, 86
  Mexican Whip-poor-will 121
Nights Away 16, 34, 47, 58, 78, 95, 110, 120, 132, 143, 156, 166, 172
Nobleboro 89
Noddies 82, 83, 189
  Black Noddies 82
  Brown Noddies 82, 83
North Carolina 16, 28, 30, 31, 92, 93, 95, 96, 128, 172
Northern Fulmars 114
Northern Gannet 20, 21, 30
Northern Hawk Owl 18, 22, 23, 24
Northern House Wren 107
Northern Lapwing 144, 167, 168
Northern Pygmy-Owl 60
Northern-Pygmy Owls 60
Northern Red Bishop 134
Northern Saw-whet Owl 48, 49
Northern Waterthrush 74
Northern Wheatear 144, 145
November 39, 156, 157, 158, 159, 160, 172
Nutcrackers 199
Nuthatches 202

O

Oak 50, 161
Ocotillo cactus 60
October 30, 143, 144, 146, 150, 151, 160, 172
Ohio 31, 66, 159
Old Baldy Trail 59
Old World Sparrows 207
  Eurasian Tree Sparrow 70
Oliveira Park 40
Olive-sided Flycatchers 100
Olive Warbler 125
Olympia 102
Olympic National Park 101
Olympus's OM 1- Mark II 128
Ontario 113
Orange County 134
Orange-winged Amazons 78
Orchard Oriole 155
Oregon 32, 95, 106, 152, 169, 172
Oregon Trail 106
Orioles 62, 212
  Altamira Oriole 41, 42
  Audubon's Oriole 165
  Baltimore Oriole 71
  Bullock's Oriole 103
  Hooded Oriole 154
  Orchard Oriole 155
  Scott's Oriole 154
  Spot-breasted Oriole 155
  Steak-backed Oriole 155
Ospreys 193
Outer Banks 30
Ovenbird 74
Owen Wilson 12, 14
Owls (Barn) 194
  American Barn Owl 107
  Barn Owl 107
Owls (Typical) 194
  Boreal Owl 148
  Burrowing Owl 37
  Eastern Screech-Owl 17
  Elf Owl 56

Ferruginous-Pygmy Owl 161, 162
Flammulated Owl 106
Great Gray Owl 22, 23, 24, 26, 173
Great-Horned Owl 60
Long-eared Owl 17, 19
Mottled Owl 42, 45, 173
Northern Hawk Owl 18, 22, 23, 24
Northern Pygmy-Owl 60
Northern-Pygmy Owls 60
Northern Saw-whet Owl 48, 49
Short-eared Owls 21
Snowy Owl 67, 144, 145, 159, 160
Snowy Owl's 67
Spotted Owl 60, 149, 150, 151, 152
Spotted Owls 60
Western Screech Owl 149, 152
Western Screech-Owl 56, 150
Whiskered Screech-Owl 60
Oystercatchers 183

P

Pacific Flyway 137
Pacific-Golden Plover 138
Pacific Wren 101
Packing 27, 70
Painted Desert 65
Painted Redstarts 125
Palm Warblers 84
Parakeets 36, 37, 45, 78, 134, 198
Burrowing Parakeets 134
Green Parakeet 43
Rose-ringed Parakeet 110, 112
White-eyed Parakeets 78
Yellow-chevroned Parakeets 78
Parasitic Jaeger 97
Parker River National Wildlife Refuge 86

Parrotbills 199
Wrentit 105, 106
Parrots 40, 41, 45, 78, 80, 107, 138, 198
Patagonia 42, 56, 59, 60
Paton Center 56, 60
Paula Aschim 70
Pease Air Force Base 73
Pelicans 37, 191
Pennsylvania 71
Petrels 97, 136, 188
Black-capped Petrel 82, 97
Pewees 196
Phainopepla 54
Phalaropes 75, 114, 116, 187
Red Phalaropes 114
Wilson's Phalarope 52, 75
Pheasants 180
Chukars 146, 148
Phoebes 197
Black Phoebe 44
Phoenix 60, 62, 149
Pigeon Guillemots 108
Pigeons 80, 180
White-crowned Pigeons 80
Pine Grosbeak 24
Pine Lake Park 139
Pine Siskins 140
Pine Warbler 22
Pink-footed Goose 27, 28, 29
Pink-footed Shearwaters 136
Pin-tailed Whydah 133
Pintails 80, 178
White-cheeked Pintails 80
Pinyon Jays 106
Pipits 204
Plain-capped Starthroat 149, 150, 152
Plane Flights 16, 34, 47, 58, 78, 95, 110, 120, 132, 143, 156, 166, 172
Plovers 69, 141, 184

Common Ringed Plover 140, 142
Mountain Plover 45, 67
Pacific-Golden Plover 138
Semipalmated Plovers 141
Wilson's Plover 36
Plymouth 74
Ponderosa Pines 62
Portal 52, 53, 54, 56, 127
Port Aransas 42
Portland 20, 75, 78, 85, 91, 127, 160
Portland Jetport 78
Port Reyes 140
Port Townsend 100, 108
Prairie-Chickens 180
Greater Prairie-Chickens 69
Lesser Prairie-Chickens 69
Prineville 106
Prisoner's Harbor 139
Prothonotary Warbler 71, 85
Ptarmigans 91, 146, 149, 181
Willow Ptarmigan 90, 91, 92
Publix 80
Puffins 87, 89, 100, 101, 108, 186
Horned Puffin 105, 107, 108
Tufted Puffin 101
Puget Sound 101
Purple Finch 48, 49
Purple Sandpiper 17

Q

Quebec 89
Queen Mary 133

R

Race Point Beach 127, 128
Rails 99, 184

Black Rail 160
Gray-headed Swamphens 35
King Rail 74, 75
Yellow Rail 99, 173
Randall Davey Audubon Center 52
Ravens 40, 198
Chihuahuan Ravens 40
Razorbills 20
Red-Billed Tropicbird 136
Red-breasted Sapsucker 118
Red-Breasted Sapsucker 100
Red-cockaded Woodpecker 31
Red-faced Warbler 124, 125
Red-flanked Bluetail 17, 19
Red-footed Booby 83
Red Junglefowl 80, 81
Red-naped Sapsucker 106, 118
Red Phalaropes 114
Red Sox 36, 42
Red-tailed Hawk 47, 48
Red-vented Bulbul 160
Red-whiskered Bulbul 44
Red-winged Blackbird 137
Rehoboth 74
Rental Cars 16, 34, 47, 58, 78, 95, 110, 120, 132, 143, 156, 166, 172
Rhinoceros Auklet 101
Rhode Island 86, 161
Richard Garrigus 75
Ring-billed Gulls 18, 158
Rio Grande 27, 39, 42, 44, 45, 122, 162, 163, 164
Rio Grande River 39, 42, 44, 45

Rivoli's Hummingbird 3, 59, 61, 121, 173
Roadrunners 182
Greater Roadrunner 40, 41
Rosencrantz Avenue 134
Rose-ringed Parakeet 110, 112
Ross's Goose 42, 67
Rosy-faced Lovebirds 9, 61
Rosy-face Lovebirds 9
Rosy-Finches 51, 56, 205
Black Rosy-Finches 51
Brown-capped Rosy-Finches 51
Gray-crowned Rosy-Finches 51
Ruff 72, 73
Ruffed Grouse 26
Rufous-backed Robin 150, 173
Rufous Hummingbirds 126, 150
Ryan Dibala 146

S

Saddleback Ski Resort 50
Sage-Grouse 3, 63, 181
Greater Sage-Grouse 3, 63, 65
Gunnison Sage-Grouse 66
Sage Thrashers 66
Saguaro cactus 60, 124
Salineño 163
Salineño Wildlife Preserve 163
Salt Bay Farm 89
Saltmarsh Sparrow 86
Salton Sea 137, 138, 173
Samoset Resort 157
San Andreas Fault 137
San Antonio 47, 50, 52, 163
Sandia Crest 50, 51, 52
Sandia-Manzano Mountains 51
San Diego 134, 138, 140
San Diego Pelagic 134, 140
Sandpipers 19, 73, 186
Buff-breasted Sandpiper 133, 135
Killdeer 134
Purple Sandpiper 17
Ruff 72, 73
Surfbird 134
Upland Sandpipers 73
Wandering Tattler 133, 135
Sandy Komito 14
San Francisco 139
San Juan Wetlands Park 162
San Pedro Fishing Pier 133, 134
Santa Cruz Island 33, 139
Santa Fe 52
Santa Margarita Ranch 42, 43, 44, 163, 164
Santa Rita Mountains 59, 125
Sapsuckers 118, 119, 194
Red-breasted Sapsucker 118
Red-Breasted Sapsucker 100
Red-naped Sapsucker 106, 118
Williamson's Sapsucker 106, 119
Yellow-bellied Sapsucker 118
Sargasso Shearwater 107
Sax-Zim Bog 22, 23, 24, 173
Scapoli's Shearwater 107
Scarlet Tanager 71

Scaups 179
  Lesser Scaup 30
Scissor-tailed Flycatcher 3, 159
Scoters 181
Scott's Oriole 154
Scripp's Murrelet 133, 135
Scrub-Jays 32, 33, 201
  California Scrub-Jay 32, 103, 139
  Florida Scrub-Jay 32, 33, 139
  Island Scrub-Jay 32, 33, 139
  Woodhouse's Scrub-Jay 32, 139
Seaside Sparrow 86
Seattle 100, 103, 107, 108
Semipalmated Plovers 141
September 132, 133, 134, 139, 140, 142, 152, 172, 173
Sharon Goldwasser 124
Sharp-tailed Grouse 99, 153
Shearwaters 97, 116, 136, 140, 190
  Audubon's Shearwater 82
  Black-vented Shearwater 134
  Buller's Shearwater 140
  Cory's Shearwater 97
  Flesh-Footed Shearwaters 140
  Great Shearwater 97
  Pink-footed Shearwaters 136
  Sargasso Shearwater 107
  Scapoli's Shearwater 107
  Sooty Shearwaters 140
Shiny Cowbird 80
Short-beaked Dolphin 137
Short-billed Gull 157
Short-eared Owls 21
Shrikes 194
Sierra Vista 56

Silky Flycatchers 197
  Phainopepla 54
Skimmers 213
  Black Skimmer 36
Skuas 116, 187
  South Polar Skua 116
Slate-throated Redstart 139
Small Point 91, 92
Smith Island 101, 108
Snow Buntings 48, 49
Snow Geese 42
Snowy Egrets 12
Snowy Owl 67, 144, 145, 159, 160
Snowy Owl's 67
Song Sparrows 140
Sooty Grouse 101
Sooty Shearwaters 140
Sooty Terns 83
South Bend 71
South Carolina 31, 34, 74, 172
Southeast Arizona Birding Festival 74, 123, 128
Southeastern Arizona Bird Observatory 122
South Padre Island 163
South Polar Skua 116
South Portland 85
Sparrows 70, 140, 207, 208
  Black-chinned Sparrow 125
  Black-Throated Sparrow 54
  Botteri's Sparrow 124
  Five-striped Sparrow 124
  Golden-crowned Sparrow 140
  Saltmarsh Sparrow 86
  Seaside Sparrow 86
  Song Sparrows 140
Spotted Owl 60, 149, 150, 151, 152
Spotted Owls 60
Springfield 69

Spruce 22, 98, 99, 100
Spruce Grouse 98, 99, 100
State Big Year 1, 23, 27, 138, 144, 145
Steller's Jay 62
Steller's Sea Eagle 114
Stephen Kress 87
Stilts 183
Storks 182
Storm-Petrels (Northern) 188
  Band-rumped Storm-Petrel 97
  Least Storm-Petrel 136
Storm-Petrels (Southern) 188
  Black Storm-Petrel 136
  Townsend's Storm-Petrels 136
  Wilson's Storm-Petrel 89, 97
Streaked-backed Oriole 61
styrofoam 39, 40
Subaru 17, 26, 27, 29, 35, 51, 56, 70
Subaru Outback 17, 26, 27, 29, 35, 70
Sulphur-bellied Flycatcher 121, 123
Surfbird 134
Swainson's Hawk 44
Swainson's Warbler 93
Swallows 159, 204
  Cave Swallows 159
Swallow-tailed Kites 74
Swans 18, 28, 30, 178
  Trumpeter Swans 18
  Tundra Swan 18
  Tundra Swans 28, 30
Swifts 213

T

Tamaulipas Crow 40
Tammy McQuade 145
Tanagers 206
  Flame-colored Tanager 121

Hepatic Tanager 18
Scarlet Tanager 71
Tanner 47, 161
Teal 180
Telos Road 117
Terns 83, 87, 89, 110, 115, 190
Arctic Terns 89
Black Terns 87
Bridled Terns 83
Common Tern 128
Elegant Tern 133
Large-billed Tern 110, 112
Sooty Terns 83
Texas 12, 18, 27, 31, 32, 34, 39, 40, 42, 44, 46, 47, 48, 50, 51, 52, 67, 70, 110, 117, 138, 139, 154, 156, 157, 160, 162, 163, 164, 166, 167, 170, 172
Thanksgiving 163
The Big Year 12, 14, 67, 92
Thick-billed Kingbird 125
Thick-billed Murre 17, 21
Thrushes 71, 92, 204
American Robin 144
Bicknell's Thrush 88, 89, 90, 92, 93
Gray-Cheeked Thrush 92
Northern Wheatear 144, 145
Red-flanked Bluetail 17, 19
Rufous-backed Robin 150, 173
Townsend's Solitaire 67
Varied Thrush 103
Western Bluebirds 140
Titmice 202
Tova Mellen 75, 116
Towhees 196
Abert's Towhee 56
California Towhee 133

Canyon Towhee 52, 55
Townsend's Solitaire 67
Townsend's Storm-Petrels 136
Townsend's Warbler 101
Tricolored Blackbird 137
Trogons 54, 122, 207
Elegant Trogon 54, 122, 173
Tropicbirds 136, 190
Red-Billed Tropicbird 136
Trumpeter Swans 18
Tucson 59, 60, 121, 122, 123, 124, 125, 127, 150
Tucson Audubon 121
Tufted Duck 18
Tufted Puffin 101
Tundra Swan 18
Tundra Swans 28, 30
Turkeys 180
Turnstones 185
Tyrants 196
Cattle Tyrant 38, 39

U

Umbazookus Road 117
United States 1, 31, 33, 51, 70, 76, 110, 113, 114, 118, 119, 138, 141, 144, 148, 159, 161
Upland Sandpipers 73
Utah 32, 58, 65, 66, 69, 172, 173

V

Vancouver 108
Varied Bunting 124, 125
Varied Thrush 103
Verdins 201
Vermont 58, 72, 172
Victoria 39
Vireos 73, 80, 200
Black-whiskered Vireos 80
Cassin's Vireo 102

Gray Vireo 125, 126
Yellow-Green Vireo 112
Yellow-throated Vireo 85
Virginia 31, 78, 93, 95, 98, 172
Vultures 40, 192
California Condors 62, 65

W

Wagtails 213
White Wagtail 134, 140
Waldoboro 91
Wandering Tattler 133, 135
Washington 88, 89, 92, 93, 95, 102, 103, 106, 108, 117, 150, 152, 170, 172, 173
Waxwings 27, 199
Bohemian Waxwings 27
Cedar Waxwings 27
Wells 74, 75
Wescalo 45
Western Bluebirds 140
Western Bluebirds, 140
Western Grebes 53
Western Gull 100
Western Screech Owl 149, 152
Western Screech-Owl 56, 150
Westport 86
Whale Watch 116, 134
Wheatears 144, 200
Whiskered Screech-Owl 60
Whistling-Ducks 179
White-cheeked Pintails 80
White-crowned Pigeons 80
White-eared Hummingbird 122, 123, 125, 127
White-eyed Parakeets 78
White-headed Wood-

pecker 106
White-tailed Deer 128, 131
White-tailed Kite 39
White Wagtail 134, 140
White-winged Crossbill 48, 50
White-winged Crossbills 17, 50
Whooping Cranes 38, 39, 42
Wigeons 179
Wiley E. Coyote 40
Williamson's Sapsucker 106, 119
Willow Ptarmigan 90, 91, 92
Wilson's Phalarope 52, 75
Wilson's Plover 36
Wilson's Storm-Petrel 89, 97
Wiscasset 7, 85
Wisconsin 31, 70, 159
Woodcocks 185
   American Woodcock 49
Woodhouse's Scrub-Jay 32, 139
Woodpeckers 100, 103, 161, 196
   Acorn Woodpecker 121
   American Three-toed Woodpecker 117, 152
   Gila Woodpecker 56
   Golden-fronted Woodpeckers 161
   Lewis's Woodpecker 105
   Lewis' Woodpeckers 103
   Red-cockaded Woodpecker 31
   White-headed Woodpecker 106
Wood Warblers 210, 212
   American Redstarts 84
   Black-backed Woodpeckers 100
   Blackburnian Warblers 100
   Black-throated Blue Warbler 75
   Black-throated Gray Warblers 125
   Blue-winged Warbler 71, 73
   Cape May Warbler 84
   Cerulean Warbler 71, 85, 86
   Colima Warbler 117
   Connecticut Warbler 141, 142
   Golden-cheeked Warbler 50
   Golden-crowned Warbler 40
   Golden-winged Warblers 98
   Grace's Warbler 125
   Hermit Warblers 125
   Hooded Warbler 74, 87, 93
   Kentucky Warbler 86
   Kirtland's Warbler 98
   Lucy's Warbler 54
   MacGillivray's Warbler 102
   Magnolia Warbler 75
   Mourning Warbler 74
   Northern Waterthrush 74
   Olive Warbler 125
   Ovenbird 74
   Painted Redstarts 125
   Palm Warblers 84
   Pine Warbler 22
   Prothonotary Warbler 71, 85
   Red-faced Warbler 124, 125
   Slate-throated Redstart 139
   Swainson's Warbler 93
   Townsend's Warbler 101
   Worm-eating Warbler 84
Worm-eating Warbler 84
Wrens 202
   Carolina Wren 22
   House Wren 107
   Northern House Wren 107
   Pacific Wren 101
Wrentit 105, 106
Wright Brothers 28
Wyoming 143, 146, 172

Y

Yakima 103
Yellow-bellied Sapsucker 118
Yellow-billed Cuckoos 87
Yellow-Billed Loon 146
Yellow-billed Magpie 139
Yellow-breasted Chat 98
Yellow-chevroned Parakeets 78
Yellow-crowned Night-Heron 37, 107
Yellow-footed Gull 138
Yellow-Green Vireo 112
Yellow Grosbeak 147, 149, 150, 173
Yellow-headed Amazons 138
Yellow-headed Caracara 80, 112, 113, 114, 115, 173
Yellowlegs 72, 186
   Greater Yellowlegs 72
   Lesser Yellowlegs 72
Yellow Rail 99, 173
Yellow-throated Vireo 85

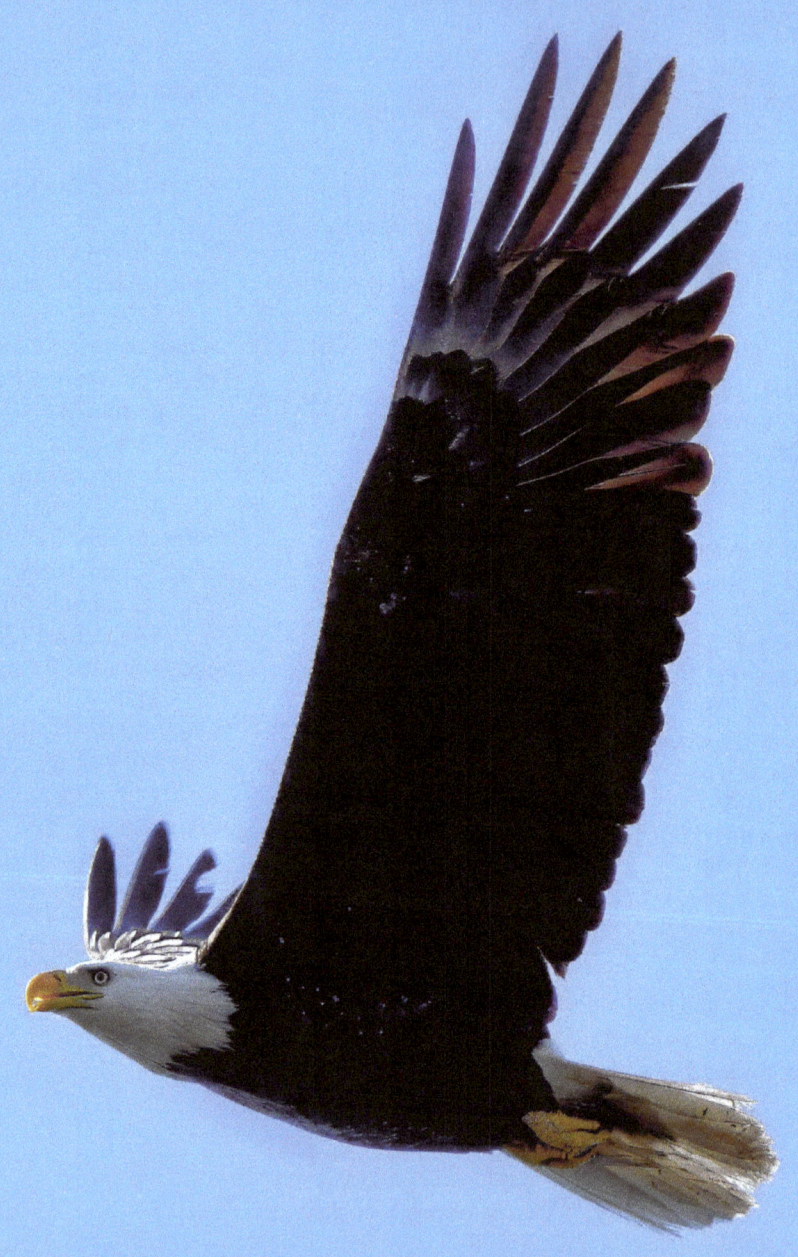
Bald Eagle

www.ingramcontent.com/pod-product-compliance
Lightning Source LLC
Chambersburg PA
CBHW052029030426
42337CB00027B/4919